YO-EIB-551

HISTOLOGY

Fourth Edition

MEDICAL OUTLINE SERIES

PETER S. AMENTA, PhD
Professor and Chairman
Department of Anatomy
Hahnemann University School of Medicine
Philadelphia

Howard T. Chang, Ph.D.
The University of Tennessee, Memphis
The Health Science Center
Department of Anatomy & Neurobiology
875 Monroe Avenue, Memphis, Tennessee 38163

MEDICAL EXAMINATION PUBLISHING COMPANY

No responsibility is assumed by the publisher for any injury and/or damage to persons or property as a matter of products liability, negligence or otherwise, or from any use or operation of any methods, products, instructions, or ideas contained in the material herein. No suggested test or procedure should be carried out unless, in the reader's judgment, its risk is justified. Because of rapid advances in the medical sciences, we recommend that independent verification of diagnoses and drug dosages should be made. Discussions, views, and recommendations as to medical procedures, choice of drugs, and drug dosages are the responsibility of the authors.

Medical Examination Publishing Company
A Division of Elsevier Science Publishing Co., Inc.
655 Avenue of the Americas, New York, New York 10010

© 1990 by Elsevier Science Publishing Co., Inc.

This book has been registered with the Copyright Clearance Center, Inc. For further information please contact the Copyright Clearance Center, Inc., Salem, Massachusetts.

This book is printed on acid-free paper.

Library of Congress Cataloging-in-Publication Data

Amenta, Peter S. (Peter Sebastian), 1927–
    Histology / Peter S. Amenta. — 4th ed.
    p.   cm. — (Medical outline series)
    Bibliography: p.
    Includes index.
    ISBN 0-444-01493-4 (alk. paper)
    1. Histology—Outlines, syllabi, etc.   I. Title.   II. Series.
    [DNLM: 1. Histology.   QS504 A511h]
QM553.A46 1990
611'.018'0202—dc20
DNLM/DLC
for Library of Congress   89-12412
                                                                                   CIP

Current printing (last digit):
10 9 8 7 6 5 4 3 2 1

Manufactured in the United States of America

This fourth edition is dedicated to
Rose, Rosemarie, Mary Vin,
Larry, and Sam

Howard T. Chang, Ph.D.
The University of Tennessee, Memphis
The Health Science Center
Department of Anatomy & Neurobiology
875 Monroe Avenue, Memphis, Tennessee 38163

Contents

ORGANS AND SYSTEMS OF THE BODY

Preface

Today's structural biologists are contributing vast amounts of new knowledge, some resolving old problems, and some posing new questions. Today's student accesses numerous information sources, especially via computer, to complement and broaden lecture and textbook information. Histology teachers should encourage students to (1) read and research the literature, (2) acquire a disciplined approach to self-learning, (3) explore the subject matter, (4) develop problem-solving skills, and (5) integrate information with other disciplines. A sixth goal must not be overlooked: prepare for Part I National Board Examinations (NBME). To this end, a new feature has been added to this fourth edition: 300 NBME-type questions distributed at the end of each chapter for pretesting and reviewing.

The text has three major objectives: (1) introduce the latest histological nomenclature (*Nomina Anatomica* 1983, fifth edition, Williams & Wilkins, Baltimore); (2) build a firm base for subsequent courses; and (3) stimulate students to read in their never-ending quest for knowledge. In the text, the nomenclature recommended by the International Nomenclature Committee (*Nomina Histologica* of the *Nomina Anatomica*) is set in bold print. Older names and eponyms and translations are enclosed in parentheses. (A sixth edition of *Nomina Anatomica* has just been published by Churchill Livingstone.)

Electron and light micrographs are minimal because there are many excellent large texts and atlases that serve as important reference sources. This text uses a minimal number of figures and diagrams, anticipating that the outline presentation is easy to read and facilitates learning. A selected list of reference texts and atlases has been included to direct the student to those resources.

Literature citations at the end of the text are referred to in each chapter by senior author name rather than by number to acquaint students with those who have made significant contributions to the literature. Students are encouraged to read some of the pertinent literature, which is enlightening and exciting. Literature citations are invaluable sources for attracting perceptive students to research and academic careers.

The term *structural biology* reflects the dynamic role of anatomy in providing answers to fundamental questions in human biology. The research laboratory of the modern anatomist is equipped with instrumentation at the cutting edge of science, and thus it is natural that academic histology reflects this research influence. The author recognizes that it is impossible to teach every bit of information flowing in from the research laboratory, nor should it be taught. Thus the text emphasizes important concepts and information that will benefit other courses (particularly pathology) and includes research information as a starting point to a lifetime of self-study.

Acknowledgments

The author gratefully acknowledges the support and encouragement of Harry Wollman, MD, Vice President for Academic Affairs and Dean of the School of Medicine. Special gratitude is offered to Mr. Iqbal Paroo, President of Hahnemann University, for his efforts in providing an environment conducive to academic pursuits.

The author is grateful for the significant contributions of the following members of the Department of Anatomy: Ms. Thelma Ward, Ms. Marsha Brown, Ms. Valine Irons, Mr. Renaldo Williams, and Mr. Albert E. Geiser.

Editorial assistance was provided by Judy Churchill, PhD; D.M. DePace, PhD; A.J. Ladman, PhD; R.P. Meyer, PhD; S.J. Wieland, PhD; and S.C. Zarro, MD.

The author is indebted to Lynn Reynolds, who illustrated the text.

Chapter 4 was contributed by Peter S. Amenta, MD, PhD, of the Department of Pathology, Robert Wood Johnson Medical School.

Most importantly, the author is grateful to his wife Rose and daughter Rosemarie for their love, understanding, graciousness, and support at home, where most of the reading, writing, and editing was conducted.

Tissues of the Body

1 Introduction to Histology

Histology investigates the normal microscopic and submicroscopic structural biology of cells, tissues, and organs as a basis for understanding biochemical, physiological, and pathological processes.

Older proven, plus newer methods and techniques are available to investigate nucleocytoplasmic relationships and the association of cells with each other and with their environment. Early investigators, limited by the resolution of optical microscopy, concerned themselves with the structure of cells and tissues. Today's technological advances are helping us to understand how the molecular structure of cells influences functional and morphological characteristics of tissues and organs. While current research methods make distinctions between disciplines difficult, teaching histology in the medical curriculum emphasizes structural biology in the light of cell, tissue, and organ histogenesis.

Some of the instruments, techniques, and methods employed by histologists are described briefly.

I. *Microscopy* (the optical microscopes)

A. The bright-field or light microscope (LM) (Fig. 1-1) (Abramowitz, 1985), which employs the visible portion of the spectrum, permits a theoretical resolution of about 0.2 μm or 20 nm. The *resolving power* of a microscope is the ability of an objective lens to distinguish clearly two points lying close together in a specimen. Useful magnifications of about 1000 diameters can be achieved with the following basic components: (1) a condenser that focuses visible light through a prepared tissue, (2) an objective lens that collects heterochromatic wavelengths of light, and (3) an eyepiece that projects a magnified image of tissues to the eye. Total magnification for a lens system is obtained by multiplying the magnification numbers of the objective and eyepiece. Study the comparison diagrams of the bright-field microscope and the transmission electron microscope (Fig. 1-2).

3

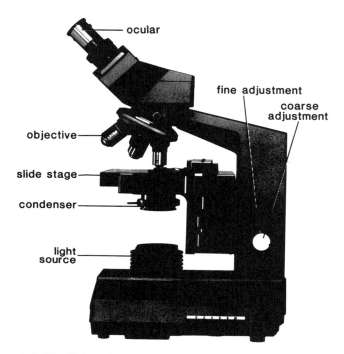

Figure 1-1 The light microscope. (Courtesy Olympus Corporation of America.)

B. The phase-contrast microscope (Abramowitz, 1987) permits visualization of living unstained cells in tissue culture and unstained tissue sections prepared for light or electron microscopy. As visible light waves are transmitted through a cell, their phase is altered. Differences in the phase of visible light waves cannot be detected by our eyes. If, however, phase differences are converted to amplitude differences, then our eyes can distinguish one cell component from the other. Thus, the dark medium phase-contrast microscope causes chromosomes to appear darker than the surrounding cytoplasm.

C. The interference microscope (Abramowitz, 1987), a variation of the phase-contrast microscope, is available in two types:

1. The Nomarski type (differential interference contrast) causes the surface of single cells in tissue culture to present a three-dimensional shadowed appearance.

2. The Baker type (Davies, 1958) utilizes optics that "shear" an

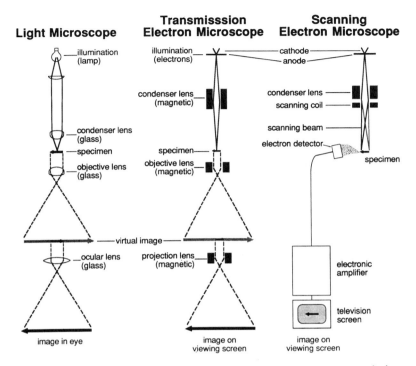

Figure 1-2 Diagram comparing the light microscope vs transmission electron microscope vs scanning electron microscope. (After Cormack, Ham's Histology, 9th Edition.)

image, so that from two resulting images quantitative measurements can be made, ie, recorded optical densities can be inserted into a formula to calculate the dry mass (relative weights) of cell parts (Blumenstein and Amenta, 1981).

D. The polarizing microscope (Barer, 1955) detects linearly oriented structures of living cells in tissue cultures or in fixed stained tissue preparations, ie, the birefringent spindle fibers of dividing cells or the banding patterns of striated muscle.

E. The fluorescence microscope (Hamashima, 1982) requires specific wavelengths of ultraviolet light, which excite cell structures or substances to emit visible light. Vitamin A, a naturally occurring substance, is autofluorescent, ie, on absorption of ultraviolet light it emits detectable visible light. Binding fluorescent dyes to antibodies in cells now is performed routinely.

F. The electron microscope (EM) is indispensable in studying biological structure. To achieve its potential magnifications, electron beams are "focused" by electromagnetic coils rather than glass lenses. Two types of instruments are used routinely:

1. The transmission electron microscope (TEM) (Wischnitzer, 1970) channels streams of negatively charged electrons through apertures in electromagnetic coils ("lenses") located relative to where optical microscopes have condensers, objectives, and eyepieces. The eyepiece is represented by a coil that projects the diverging electron beam onto a fluorescent screen. The column housing the coils must be devoid of air, thus a vacuum pump is an integral part of the instrument. Specimens must be sectioned to about 0.025 μm or 2.5 nm thick in contrast to specimens for light microscopy, which could be 2.5 μm or thicker. Magnifications are feasible to 500,000 diameters, with resolutions down to 0.2 nm. Electrons will fail to penetrate denser cell parts (coated with heavy metallic molecules of lead, uranium, osmium, or vanadium). The image appearing on the fluorescent screen may be recorded on film. Lighter areas on negatives represent areas where electrons impinged on the film plate, while the positive print demonstrates the reverse (Fig. 1-3).

2. The scanning electron microscope (SEM) (Hearle et al, 1972) permits examination of whole cells, tissues, and organs (coated with conductors such as gold or platinum) in a seemingly three-dimensional appearance (Fig. 1-4). Like the TEM, the subject to be studied must be in a vacuum, thereby negating the possibility of studying living cells. Electrons strike the coated surface of a specimen, which in turn emits secondary electrons. These are collected by an electron detector, which relays a signal to an electronic amplifier for projection onto a video screen. A black-and-white micrograph can be recorded. While most scanning electron micrographs are of lower resolution (2 to 10 nm) than the TEM, the depth of focus is generally ~500 times that of the light microscope at relatively equal magnifications. Newer developments in SEM technology permit the localization of cytochemical characteristics of cells. There is a new SEM (the ESEM) on the market (Science, Oct. 21, 1988, *242*:453), which "allows the direct observation of unprepared specimens. Wet specimens can be examined in their natural state, without drying, freezing, fracturing, or coating. The microscope's vacuum system permits continuous observation of wet samples, including liquids, under fully saturated water

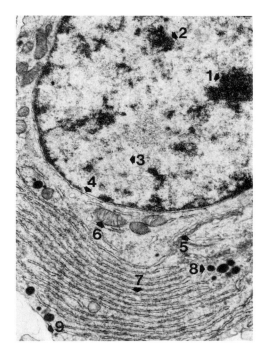

Figure 1-3 Transmission electron micrograph, ×8000. 1 = nucleolus, 2 = heterochromatin, 3 = euchromatin, 4 = nuclear membrane, 5 = golgi complex, 6 = mitochondrion, 7 = granular (rough) endoplasmic reticulum, 8 = secretory granules, 9 = plasmalemma.

vapor conditions. Dynamic processes can be observed and recorded as they happen." It will be interesting to see the variety of applications, particularly in tissue culture.

II. *Histological techniques* (Sheehan and Hrapchak, 1973): Preparation of a tissue for the bright field microscope entails:

A. *Fixation:* Excised tissues are fixed (killed) to stabilize intercellular and intracellular substances in a state as close to the living as possible. The most common fixative is an aqueous, neutral buffered 4% solution of formaldehyde. Many fixatives take advantage of the fixative properties of several chemicals and combine these (eg, Zenker-formol). Fixatives crosslink, denature, or precipitate proteins by replacing associated water, resulting in tissue hardening. Enzymes

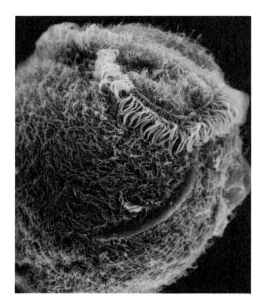

Figure 1-4 Scanning electron micrograph of *Stentor coeruleus,* a single-celled, ciliated protozoan. (Courtesy P.S. Amenta, MD, PhD, Department of Pathology, Robert Wood Johnson Medical School.)

are inactivated by some fixatives, thus localizing sites of enzymatic activity requires judicious selection of a fixative.

B. *Embedding:* Fixed tissues are so brittle that they cannot be sliced thin enough to be useful. The histologist takes advantage of the properties of melted paraffin and paraffin-like substances, which can penetrate the recesses of fixed, dehydrated tissue. Dehydration is imperative because paraffin does not mix with the water in fixatives.

C. *Sectioning:* The hardened block of embedded tissue is shaped to facilitate slicing on a microtome. Most tissues are "sliced" or sectioned at about 5 μm along a desired plane (horizontal, longitudinal, or tangential). The section is placed on a clean glass slide, to which it adheres, and is deparaffinized and rehydrated.

D. *Staining:* aqueous stains are selected to reveal specific cell or tissue components. Several stains may be combined to reveal a number of entities. The most common combination of stains is hematoxylin and eosin (H&E). Special stains distinguish the **stroma** (tissue framework) from the **parenchyma** (the functional cells of the tissue). Before mounting, the stained tissue is rehydrated.

E. *Mounting:* The dehydrated, fixed, and stained tissue is covered with a medium of appropriate refractive index (similar to glass). The medium (eg, balsam) does not mix with water, thus the reason for dehydration. Balsam protects the tissue from drying and facilitates viewing when sealed.

F. *Sealing:* The mounted preparation is covered with a thin glass coverslip to protect the tissue and the mounting medium from the external environment and from rough handling. The exposed peripheral edge of the mounting medium dries and hardens, while the interior remains gel-like. When cleaning the coverslip of a completed slide, care must be exercised not to crack the coverslip or the dried peripheral seal. Carelessness will cause the coverslip to slide off and perhaps destroy the tissue.

III. *Electron microscopic techniques* (Hayat, 1972)

A. Preparing tissues for TEM

1. *Fixation:* Tissues are fixed for the same reasons that are valid for light microscopy, to avoid postmortem changes that occur very rapidly and influence the appearance of cells at the EM level. The widely used fixative, glutaraldehyde (usually followed by postfixation in osmium tetroxide), initiates precipitation of proteins with minimal distortion of cellular structure. When choosing a fixative one must consider the pH, tonicity, temperature, and length of fixation. The tonicity of most fixatives (Palade, 1952) is usually strongly hypertonic to red blood cells but good results are obtained.

2. *Dehydration:* To facilitate the infiltration of plastic embedding medium, the small piece of fixed tissue must have all water removed from it, by sequential immersion in ascending concentrations of ethyl alcohol to 100%. Later the alcohol is replaced by another solution (eg, propylene oxide) that is soluble in the epoxy resin. Commercially available water-soluble resins are available to perform cytochemical analyses.

3. *Embedding:* Unpolymerized epoxy resins or acrylics are used routinely as the embedding medium. While these substances shrink less than the old methacrylates and preserve fine structure better, they do not penetrate as well. Subsequent polymerization (with low heat or ultraviolet light) hardens the resin so that ultrathin sections may be obtained.

4. *Sectioning:* An ultramicrotome equipped with glass or diamond knives cuts 60-nm-thick sections. The specimen must be ultrathin and be able to withstand both the high vacuum of the TEM and the effects of the electron beam. The microtome introduced by Porter and Blum in 1953 was the instrument that overcame all the problems inherent in previous mechanisms to produce routine serial sections of uniform thickness for both the TEM and the LM.

5. *Mounting:* Sections floating in the water trough attached to the knife are picked up on small copper grids that have small enough apertures to support an entire cell. Though grids may be coated with a thin layer of formvar or carbon, some microscopists prefer the uncoated grid. Care must be exercised in the latter case to prevent excessive damage by the electron beam. Without support, sections have a tendency to drift in the electron beam, making photography impossible. Carbon-coated copper grids overcome this difficulty of section stability.

6. *Staining:* The term "staining" is not appropriate in electron microscopy, for instead of chemical dyes, salts of heavy metals such as uranium, lead, or vanadium (singly or in combinations) are deposited onto cellular components to render them electron dense in varying degrees. Salts such as uranyl acetate (useful to increase contrast of nucleic acids; Huxley and Zubray, 1961) and lead citrate (Reynolds, 1963) are applied to the sections mounted on the small copper grids.

7. *Studying:* Grids (on a special holder) are inserted into the stage vacuum chamber of the electron microscope. Electrons penetrating cell areas with minimal deposition of heavy metals strike a fluorescent screen where an image appears. A permanent image may be recorded on a very-fine-grained photographic film plate.

B. Preparing tissues for SEM (Hayat, 1978)

1. *Fixation:* Whereas TEM uses hypertonic fixatives, SEM requires isotonic solutions to avoid osmotic shock to the superficial cell layers of the tissue block.

2. *Drying* (dehydration): The specimen must be thoroughly dried before inserting into the SEM vacuum chamber.

a. *Air:* Though the most rapid method, it is also the most uncontrollable. Distortion and shrinkage of soft tissues are inherent disadvantages.

b. *Critical point:* The critical-point method uses a simple pressure container surrounded by a water jacket for either heating or cooling. The apparatus facilitates dehydration of tissues as they pass through intermediate and transition fluids to a gas (eg, carbon dioxide). At certain temperatures and pressures a fluid may exist as a vapor in equilibrium with the liquid. Between these two phases exists a sharp interface. Heating the two phases in the critical point apparatus causes thermal expansion until a "critical point" is reached when the liquid phase is indistinguishable from the vapor phase. Following removal of the liquid surface interface, drying proceeds. This method has the advantage of controllability and minimal artifactual shrinkage.

     c. *Freeze-dry-cleave:* This process eliminates most problems encountered with chemical fixatives or dehydration solvents. Tissues are immersed in liquid nitrogen and dried in a vacuum apparatus. The frozen tissue (without ice crystals) is cleaved with a blade to initiate a fracture plane, which travels between membranes. Exposed membrane surfaces are coated by evaporating a heavy metal over them. This technique produces not only high fidelity replicas of cell surface membranes, but also the intermediate faces of the fractured or cleaved membranes (Fig. 2-2).

IV. *Special methods*

    A. *Autoradiography:* Intracellular localization of radioactivity in sectioned tissues results from in vivo introduction of radioactive isotopes. If the isotope (tritiated thymidine) is introduced into an animal, it binds to deoxyribonucleic acid (DNA) which is undergoing synthesis. The procedure is applicable to LM and TEM. A tissue sectioned from this animal is

    1. coated with a very fine layer of silver halide crystals embedded in a gel and

    2. kept in a dark room for a rather long period of time. Beta (β) particles emitted from the isotope strike the silver halide crystals, which are converted to metallic silver granules. The latter are easily visualized under the microscope, thus localizing rather precisely the sites of DNA synthesis. This technique can be used to determine whether specific cells can assimilate specific amino acids to incorporate them into proteins.

    B. *Histochemistry:* Special biochemical techniques are adapted to localize biological activity of enzymes and other substances in tissue sections. Color reactions in the tissue reveal sites of specific activity, ie, glucose-6-phosphatase activity, intracellular localization of individual antigens, nucleic acid sequencing, and many more (Troyer, 1980).

    C. *Immunocytochemistry:* Specific sites of macromolecular activity are revealed by this technique. In earlier applications, only the immune response was studied. Today a vast area has been opened with the localization of endogenous proteins.

D. *Microdissection:* Cell biologists "forge" their own microscopic instruments to perform cell surgery under the microscope. Parts of cells may be removed (eg, the nucleus) and transferred to other cells or a variety of substances can be injected directly through the cell membrane.

E. *Tissue culture:* This technique permits observation of excised cells from the body in vitro (in glass containers) where they are maintained in a synthetic medium simulating the tissue fluids of liquid component of the blood.

V. *How to study histology:* In histology laboratories, students are issued boxes containing glass slides with tissue sections stained for study with the bright-field microscope. Students today also must have access to EM atlases emphasizing the submicroscopic biological structure of cells and tissues. Please see atlases listed at the end of this chapter.

A. *Understand the microscope.* Students should consult the manuals that accompany new microscopes or the sections on microscopy found in some of the listed texts.

B. *Understand tissue sections.* A tissue section is but one slice from a three-dimensional block of tissue.

1. A tissue section is analogous to a single page from a book. Obviously, one page cannot provide sufficient information. However, it may provide clues to the type of book or its identity. If one previously read the book, then one page might be useful. It is clear then that understanding histology requires some basic biology and perhaps even gross anatomy.

2. Recognize several tissue characteristics. If only one characteristic is learned, that one is invariably absent in an unknown. In a pathological tissue, that characteristic may be destroyed.

C. *Learn the proper approach.*

1. Examine each slide with the naked eye to
   a. avoid placing the coverslipped surface down,
   b. count the number of sections on the slide, and
   c. determine the size, stain, and type of tissue.

2. Examine each slide with a hand lens (or with an inverted eyepiece) to obtain an overall view.

3. Examine first with low-power objectives. Gradually work up to higher powers.

4. Conceive a 3-D image of the tissue, to relate the tissue section to the organ as a whole.

D. *Compare similar tissues and cells.* Students should develop the habit of examining look-alike tissues under the LM. Compare micrographs from TEMs, SEMs, and freeze-fracture preparations and relate to the LM.

E. *Determine the type of section.* Examples include transverse (cross), longitudinal, or oblique. Constructing a three-dimensional model with colored clay to represent organ layers and slicing it in planes similar to the tissue section will prove useful.

VI. *Measurements in microscopy*

A. The microscopic and submicroscopic structure of cells and tissues requires comprehension of comparative units of measurement.

B. The accepted system of measurement is the SI System, or Systeme Internationale d'Unities, emphasizing the following units: millimeter [mm], micrometer [μm], and nanometer [nm]. The terms micron [μ] and angstrom [A] are obsolete (cf Table 1-1).

Table 1-1 International System of Units

Units of measurement			Comparative structures	
mm	= μm	= nm	Size	Identity
1	1000 (10^3)	10^6	1 mm	intestinal villus
0.1 (10^{-1})	100 (10^2)	10^5	150 μm	human ovum
10^{-2}	10 (10^1)	10^4	7.5 μm	erythrocyte
10^{-3}	1	1000	1 μm	mitochondrion (x-s)
10^{-4}	10^{-1}	100	100 nm	microvilli (x-s)
10^{-5}	10^{-2}	10	10 nm	cell membrane

Questions

DIRECTIONS: Each of the questions or incomplete statements below is followed by four suggested answers or completions. Select the single best answer for each question.

---

1. The resolving power of a microscope is defined as the
   A. magnification of the objective times the magnification of the eyepiece
   B. ability to distinguish two points lying close together in a specimen
   C. conversion of phase differences to amplitude differences
   D. detection of linearly oriented structures in cells

2. Ultraviolet light excitation of cell structures causing them to emit visible light is a function of which microscope?
   A. Polarizing
   B. Dark-field
   C. Interference
   D. Fluorescence

3. Specimens for study with the transmission electron microscope are sectioned to a thickness of
   A. 0.025 μm
   B. 2.5 μm
   C. 5.0 μm
   D. 20.5 μm

4. Scanning electron microscopy facilitates the following *except*
   A. viewing living cells in tissue culture
   B. a depth of focus far greater than the optical microscopes
   C. localization of cytochemical characteristics of cells
   D. a seemingly three-dimensional appearance

5. Fixation accomplishes all of the following *except*
   A. hardening the tissue
   B. denaturing proteins
   C. stabilizing intracellular substances
   D. keeping cells alive in suspended animation

6. Staining
   A. reveals specific tissue or cell components
   B. protects the tissue from the environment
   C. dehydrates tissues
   D. is not carried out in aqueous solutions

7. Tissues for transmission electron microscopy are embedded in
   A. formvar
   B. epoxy resins
   C. uranyl acetate
   D. glutaraldehyde

8. Revealing cellular structures for TEM requires the use of
   A. salts of heavy metals
   B. aqueous chemical dyes
   C. formaldehyde
   D. isotonic solutions

9. Specimens prepared for SEM must be
   A. thoroughly dried
   B. stained with hematoxylin and eosin
   C. thin enough to permit electrons to penetrate
   D. hypertonic solutions

10. Which of the following units is considered obsolete?
   A. mm
   B. μm
   C. μ
   D. nm

Explanatory Answers

1. B. Resolving power also can be defined as the number of parallel lines individually visible in 1 mm. Answer A defines total magnification. Answer C describes the phase-contrast microscope. Answer D describes the polarizing microscope.

2. D. Ultraviolet light is in the invisible portion of the spectrum, and uniquely it excites either naturally occurring substances or the bound fluorescent dyes to emit visible light that can be detected.

3. A. Answers B and C are section thicknesses for use in light microscopy. Answer D is a section thickness not usually used.

4. A. Because of the necessity to dry a tissue and place it in a vacuum, it is not possible to study living cells in the common SEM.

5. D. Fixation kills the cells in a tissue accomplishing the statements in Answers A, B, and C.

6. A. A variety of stains used singly or in combinations are selected to bring out the variety of cells and components in the connective tissue.

7. B. Answer A (formvar) is used to coat copper grids to support tissue sections. Answer C (uranyl acetate) is the salt of the heavy metal uranium, used to "stain" cellular structures. Answer D (glutaraldehyde) is a tissue fixative used in TEM.

8. A. Heavy salts coat cells and tissues where structural components reside. Electrons do not penetrate these now "electron dense" structures and hence will appear as light areas on a negative. Answer B (aqueous dyes) are used to stain tissues for LM. Answer C (formaldehyde) is the primary component of most fixatives prepared for LM. Answer D (isotonic solutions) are required in SEM fixatives to prevent osmotic shock to superficial cell layers of a tissue block.

9. A. Tissues must be thoroughly dehydrated by processes that do not cause excessive shrinkage or distortion to the tissue. Answer B refers to the H&E stain used most routinely. Answer C is incorrect because in SEM electrons do not penetrate but are reflected from the prepared tissue. Answer D refers to the hypertonicity of solutions used for TEM. See question 8, where SEM uses isotonic solutions.

10. C. The μ is superseded by μm and the numbers remain the same: the old 5 μ is now 5 μm. Additionally, the angstrom unit is obsolete. However, what was 10 angstroms is now 1 nm (nanometer), and what was 100 angstroms is now 10 nm, and so forth. Use of the nm unit permits using smaller numbers in the literature, as structural biology delves into increasingly smaller domains.

2 The Cell

Knowledge of the living cell and its nucleocytoplasmic relationships, intercellular mechanisms of communication, and responses to stimuli is a major objective of histology. A dynamic concept of the cell is difficult to achieve from studying only fixed stained tissues. Students usually concentrate on tissues prepared for light microscopy, which reveal specific cell types situated in the intercellular (interstitial) substances. These static images are reinforced by complex electron micrographs. Histology courses must emphasize the dynamism and inherent vitality of cells via:

I. Studying living cells:

    A. viewing ameba cultures.

    B. studying simple tissue cultures, eg, respiratory epithelium to demonstrate ciliary activity.

    C. demonstrations of living cells undergoing mitosis, in tissue culture.

    D. examining blood circulating in capillaries in the web of frog's foot.

II. Viewing films of a variety of cells in tissue culture.

    A. A catalogue containing film descriptions may be obtained by writing to: TCA Business Office, 19110 Montgomery Village Avenue, Suite 300, Gaithersburg, MD 20879.

    B. Viewing films speeded up by time-lapse microcinematography will aid immensely in developing a sense of cellular dynamism. A few of the many functional activities recorded in a variety of cells are:

        1. *Locomotion:* the ability of a cell to move from one point to another (Amenta, 1967; DeBruyn, 1944).

2. *Phagocytosis:* the mechanism by which cells ingest particles larger than 0.2 µm in diameter (Dean and Jessup, 1985).

3. *Pinocytosis:* the process by which macromolecules in solution are drawn into a cell and processed (Dean and Jessup, 1985).

4. Mitosis, cell division in somatic cells, and **meiosis,** a form of cell division peculiar to reproductive germ cells (Schlegel et al, 1987).

5. *Pyknosis:* a phenomenon heralding cell death, in which the nuclear contents detach from the nuclear membrane and concentrate in a tight ball (Amenta, 1962).

6. *Chemotaxis:* the attraction of one cell to another, induced by chemicals released by one of the cells (Amenta, 1967).

7. *Response to irradiation:* effects of microirradiation on specific parts of cells (McNeil and Berns, 1981).

The *cell* is the basic unit of structure and function. Two compartments compose the cell (Fig. 2-1): the *nucleus* and *cytoplasm.* Enclosing both is the *cell membrane* or **plasmalemma,** which selectively regulates the entrance or exit of substances. Upon cessation of cellular functions (death), the plasmalemma loses this specialized regulatory facility and substances freely enter or leave the cell.

III. The **plasmalemma** (Finian, 1977) (cell membrane, unit membrane) pertains to the outer 6- to 10-nm-thick "trilaminar appearing membrane" enclosing the cell contents. Other membranes within the cell (eg, endoplasmic reticulum, golgi complex, nuclear membrane, and mitochondria) are modifications of the plasmalemma. In addition to its regulatory facility (termed permeability), it provides a wall of protection from the external milieu.

A. The "Fluid Mosaic Model" (Fig. 2-2) proposed by Singer and Nicholson (1972), explaining the molecular organization of the plasmalemma, emphasizes three points:

1. The plasmalemma is composed of a bilayer of ionic and polar head groups (phospholipid molecules attached to fatty acid chains). Integral proteins and lipids embedded in a "mosaic" configuration move freely within the plasmalemma.

2. Extrinsic protein molecules arranged on the outer (external) and inner (cytoplasmic) surfaces of the plasmalemma impart an asymmetry to the molecular structure.

3. Oligosaccharide chains protruding from the external surface of the plasmalemma increase the asymmetry.

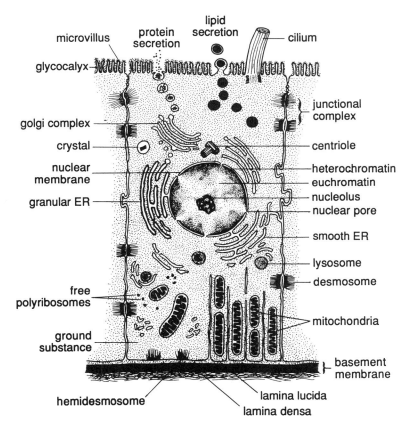

Figure 2-1 Diagram of a highly idealized cell. Processes of lipid and protein secretion appear at lumenal surface. Arrangement of mitochondria in columns (as in striated duct cells of salivary glands) between plasmalemmal invaginations is depicted at the basal surface.

B. Appearance of the plasmalemma via TEM

    1. "Fluidity" can be reasoned but not demonstrated.

    2. The trilaminar appearance is attributed to osmium deposition (from fixation) in the protein and hydrophilic polar heads of the phospholipid molecules.

    3. The hydrophobic ends of the molecules, situated between the

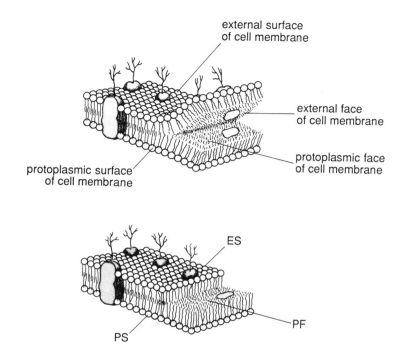

Figure 2-2 The *fluid mosaic model* of the **plasmalemma**. The recommended nomenclature for surfaces and faces is incorporated. The glycocalyx attaches to the protein globules at the external surface.

blackened layers, are devoid of osmium and hence are "electron lucent."

C. Freeze-fracture or freeze-etch preparations cause the plasmalemma to appear as if it were pulled apart (Fig. 2-2). The fractured plasmalemma exposes two surfaces and two faces, which are named as follows (Branton et al, 1975):

1. *external or extracellular surface* (ES) viewing the external hydrophilic surface.

2. *internal* or *protoplasmic surface* (PS) viewing the internal hydrophilic surface.

3. *external or extracellular face* (EF) viewing the external hydrophobic ends.

4. *internal* or *protoplasmic face* (PF) viewing the internal hydrophobic ends.

D. The **glycocalyx** (sweet husk) (Rambourg, 1966), coating the external apical surface of most eucaryotic cells, is a carbohydrate-rich zone consisting of 9 of the more than 100 monosaccharides occurring naturally (Roseman, 1975). Its thickness measures from 10 to 20 nm according to specialized functions of the cell. The glycocalyx provides

1. *protection.* Intestinal cells possess a thicker glycocalyx to protect them from the variety of ingested substances that come in contact with their surfaces.

2. an effective *filtration* barrier.

3. a suitable *environment* for materials to enter and exit.

4. a means for *cell–cell interactions* by virtue of the complexity of some of its oligosaccharides. Some cells possess surface proteins that bind and thus "recognize" only certain oligosaccharides. While increasing experimental evidence supports this phenomenon in plants, demonstration in animal cells has proved difficult. *Cell–cell recognition* may play an important role in tissue grafts and organ transplant histocompatibility.

5. a special identity to each cell, imparted by the following membrane glycoproteins and glycolipids: fucose, glucose, glucosamine, galactose, galactosamine, mannose, and sialic acid.

IV. The *cytoplasm* (Watson, 1982)

A. The cytoplasmic matrix or ground substance (Porter and Tucker, 1981), termed the *hyaloplasm,* is subdivided into:

1. *endoplasm,* usually in the sol phase, is characterized by active cytoplasmic streaming. Cellular components are carried along by rapid, seemingly directed movements.

2. *exoplasm,* usually in the gel phase, is relatively free of cellular components and occupies the cell periphery of the cell where it is limited by the plasmalemma.

B. *Organelles* and *inclusions:* Previously defined as living and nonliving, these are now classified together, because the rapid flow of information provided by newer techniques defies classification.

1. Cytocentrum or cell center: a relatively organelle-free zone of the cytoplasm adjacent to the nucleus is important to the process of cell division because in it are embedded the *centrioles,* which give rise to the mitotic apparatus. The cytocentrum is usually found nestled in an indentation of the nucleus.

2. *Centrioles* (Sorokin, 1968), via light microscopy, are resolved as two dots called the *diplosome* (Fig. 2-3). Via electron microscopy they appear as two "rigatoni-like" bodies set at right angles to one another. Each cylinder measures about 200 to 500 nm long and 150

Figure 2-3 *A.* 3-D diagram of *centrioles* at right angles to each other. *B.* Cross section of one centriole depicting tubulomicrotubules, forming the centriole wall.

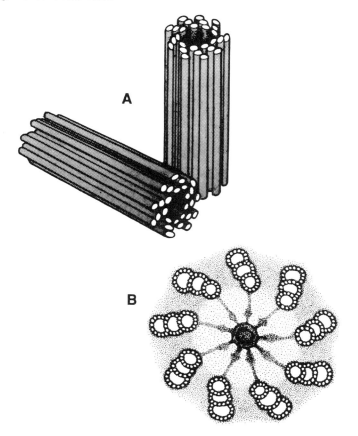

nm wide with nine circumferentially arranged microtubular units embedded in a dense homogeneous substance. Greater resolution reveals that each microtubular unit is composed of three tubular subunits, the *triplomicrotubules*. During cell division the *centrioles* replicate, not by horizontal or longitudinal division as once speculated, but de novo. A new centriole develops in close proximity to a preexisting centriole in an end-to-end relationship. Following replication, each pair of centrioles migrates to opposite poles of the cell where peripheral microtubules radiate from the *diplosome* to form the structural components of the **fusus mitoticus,** freely translated as the *mitotic spindle*. The microtubules form a star-like configuration, the **aster,** surrounding the diplosome. The term "astral rays" refers to the radiating microtubules. Evidence supports the concept that spindle microtubules originate from the diplosome microtubules.

3. Mitochondria (Fig. 2-4) (Lehninger, 1964) studied via TEM are the most recognizable cytoplasmic bodies, averaging about 5 μm in length and 100 nm in width. In tissue cultures of fibroblasts, one can study (via time-lapse microcinematography) the fragmentation of long, filamentous mitochondria into smaller rod-like or granular forms or vice versa, reflecting their pleomorphic dynamic nature. The size and shape of the mitochondria and their internal membranes reflects the function of the "host" cell.

a. A double *membrane* encloses the *mitochondrial matrix* or ground substance (Palmer and Hall, 1972). Within the matrix are small electron-dense *mitochondrial granules* composed of calcium and magnesium, which are required for some enzymes to function. The *internal mitochondrial membrane,* in contact with the mitochondrial matrix, is folded into a series of **cristae,** which may be lamelliform (leaf-like) or tubular, according to the cell type. For example, steroid-secreting cells have tubular cristae, while pancreatic protein-secreting acinar cells are characterized by lamelliform cristae. This membrane and the *external mitochondrial membrane* surrounding the entire mitochondrial complex are 7 nm thick each. Confined between the internal and external mitochondrial membranes is the *intermembranous space,* which continues into the cristae (Munn, 1975).

b. *Elementary particles* (small spherules) (Fernandez-Moran et al, 1964), attached by short rods to the internal mitochondrial membrane, protrude into the mitochondrial matrix. As revealed by "negative staining" in the TEM, they measure approximately 9 nm $\times$ 3 nm. The particles contain the enzyme necessary for phosphorylation of adenosine diphosphate (ADP) to adenosine triphosphate (ATP).

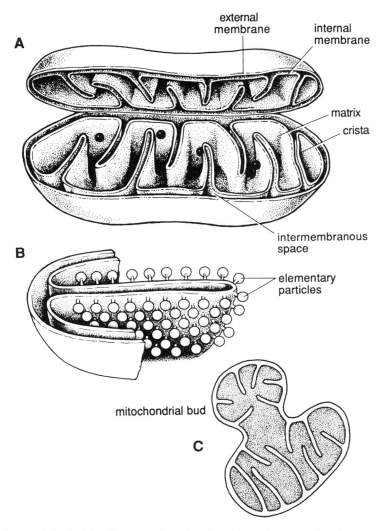

Figure 2-4 *A*. 3-D diagram of a **mitochondrion** sliced longitudinally to reveal internal structure. *B*. A segment of a **crista** depicting attachment of elementary particles. *C*. Mitochondrial replication by "budding."

c. Mitochondrial deoxyribonucleic acid (DNA), ribonucleic acid (RNA), and ribosomes bear a striking resemblance to the DNA, RNA, and ribosomes of bacteria, leading to the speculation that mitochondria have a potentiality for independent life. Like some bacteria, mitochondria are considered by some to be symbionts. Like bacteria, mitochondria replicate by budding (Fig. 2-4C).

d. References to the mitochondria as the "powerhouse" of the cell reflect their importance in the citric acid cycle (Krebs cycle). Mitochondria are capable of sequestering the energy released by oxidation of nutrients and fix that energy in the usable form of ATP.

4. In 1898, Camillo Golgi discovered a cellular structure that he named the **apparatus reticulatus internus.** Investigators since his time have used his name as an eponym for this structure. Despite international efforts to delete all eponyms, the term *golgi complex* or *golgi apparatus* remains entrenched. It is the only acceptable eponym, but it must be spelled with a lower-case *g*, as in *golgi*. The golgi complex had a long and difficult history and was considered by many to be an artifact (Farquhar and Palade, 1981). TEM confirmed not only its existence, but revealed its complex membranous structure and its participation in protein secretion.

a. Structure (Fig. 2-5): TEM reveals layers of parallel *lamelliform sacs* stacked like several hot-water bags one on top of the other, with convex and concave surfaces (Rambourg et al, 1974). The interior of each bag can be compared to the interior or **cisterna** of each golgi sac. Individual golgi sacs are embedded in the *ground substance* of the cell (the gel-like substance). The 7-nm-thick golgi membranes lack ribosomal granules, but are totally dependent on the *granular endoplasmic reticulum* (rER) for continued formation, development, and survival. The complex of lamelliform sacs (**sacculus lamelliformis**) have two faces, an *immature face* (forming or cis face) and a *mature face* (trans face). In Figure 2-5, the convex surface of the golgi sac closest to the rER is the immature or forming face. *Transfer vesicles* from the rER are received by the outer membrane of the immature face. Thus, transfer vesicles add membrane to the immature face. The *mature face* (trans face), with a concave surface, is involved in the final packaging of secretory products.

b. Functionally, the golgi complex accumulates and concentrates secretory products. *Proteins* are synthesized in the granular endoplasmic reticulum and delivered to the golgi complex in vesicles to be concentrated. The *carbohydrate* (CHO) moiety of a carbohy-

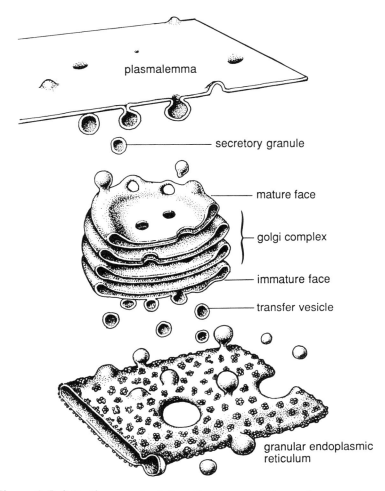

Figure 2-5 3-D diagram depicting the process of protein secretion. The granular endoplasmic reticulum produces protein, which is sequestered in small transfer vesicles devoid of polyribosomes. Transfer vesicles migrate to the convex surface of the immature surface of the golgi complex. Membrane-bound secretion granules form from the mature face and move to the plasmalemma to release the products. The golgi membranes are endowed with properties that facilitate fusion with the plasmalemma.

drate-protein complex is synthesized in the golgi complex, where the membranes have been shown to possess the required enzymes. *Polysaccharides* plus *protein* are conjugated in the golgi complex. In nonsecretory cells, CHO components of the plasmalemma are synthesized in the golgi complex.

    c. Mechanism of secretion is unique to cells. A portion of the mature face membrane containing the secretory product pinches off to form a "secretory granule." This granule migrates to the surface of the cell where its membrane fuses with the cell membrane followed by discharge of the contents. Thus while membrane is continually lost on the mature face, additional membrane forms at the immature (forming) face. This dynamic process conserves and replenishes precious membranous material. It should be recalled that the plasmalemma thickness is about 10 nm thick, in contrast to the 7-nm-thick intracellular membranes.

    d. Summary of golgi complex involvement:

    (1) conservation and replenishing of membranes.

    (2) concentration of secretory products.

    (3) transport of secretory products.

    (4) release of secretory products.

    (5) synthesis of some products (mucopolysaccharides, glycoproteins).

    5. The *endoplasmic reticulum* (ER) (Palade and Porter, 1954) is a cytoplasmic structure composed of a complex network of tubules or flattened membranes (7 nm thick) enclosing a space, the **cisterna**. This cisterna is similar to that enclosed by the golgi complex membranes. The myriad connections of ER membranes to the plasmalemma and nuclear membrane leads to the reasoning that the ER is derived from invaginations of the plasmalemma. The organizational complexity and intricacy of the ER may be as varied as the number of cell types. Although two distinct forms are described, *granular* (rough) and *nongranular* (smooth), there are transitional forms between the two. Indeed it is accepted that granular (rough) ER gives rise to nongranular (smooth) ER (Fig. 2-6).

    a. *Granular* (rough) *ER,* abbreviated *rER,* appears "rough" via TEM because its membrane surfaces are studded by evenly spaced, small ribonucleoprotein granules termed *ribosomes.* The ribosomes, measuring 13.5 nm to 15 nm in diameter, are sites of synthesis of protein, which is ultimately packaged by the golgi for extramural secretion (see above). The ribosomes are responsible for the basophilia observed in the light microscope. In subsequent chapters, reference

cisternal lumen

tubules of smooth
endoplasmic reticulum

ribosomes

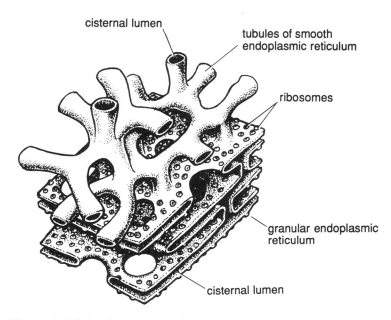

granular endoplasmic
reticulum

cisternal lumen

Figure 2-6 3-D diagram showing the relationship between smooth and granular endoplasmic reticulum. In the liver, smooth endoplasmic reticulum arises from granular endoplasmic reticulum when drugs are detoxified.

will be made to the cytoplasmic basophilia of fibroblasts, osteoblasts, plasma cells, pancreatic acinar cells, stomach gland principal cells, and many others. The basophilia is due to the prominent rER, indicating cellular activity in protein synthesis.

   b. *Nongranular* (*smooth*) *ER,* or *sER,* membranes lack attached ribosomal granules, hence the name *smooth.* The membranes are arranged in an anastomosing network of tubules that develop from rER. Smooth ER is abundant in *striated muscle cells* for liberation and reuptake of ionic calcium required for muscle contraction and relaxation, in *endocrine gland cells* involved in the synthesis of steroid hormones (eg, suprarenal cortex, testes, ovary), in *hepatocytes* (liver cells) involved in cholesterol and lipid metabolism and possibly in glycogen metabolism, in *parietal* cells of the stomach involved in producing free hydrochloric acid, and in *columnar absorptive cells* of the intestine where sER occurs during synthesis and transport of lipids. Barbiturates and other drugs stimulate the proliferation of sER tubules directly from rER, resulting in detoxification. Failure of sER to develop increases detoxification time, resulting in drug sensitivity. Detoxification is the process by which a toxic substance is broken down and rendered inactive.

6. *Ribosomes* (Porter, 1953; Palade, 1955) are small, electron-dense cytoplasmic particles measuring about 15 nm wide and 25 nm in height. Each ribosome unit consists of two portions, a larger subunit capped by a smaller subunit. The *large subunit* is composed of at least two RNA molecules and some 40 associated proteins. The *small subunit* consists of one RNA molecule plus up to 30 associated small proteins.

a. *Free ribosomes,* which exist singly in the cytoplasmic ground substance, cannot function effectively. To be functional, they must aggregate.

b. *Polyribosomes* (*polysomes*) are linked aggregates of 10 to 20 free ribosomes associated with one strand of *messenger RNA* (mRNA), the carrier of genetic information (codons) which determines sequencing of amino acids into polypeptides. Polyribosomes first link linearly, then spiral into a rosette configuration. *Free polyribosomes* synthesize proteins destined for intracellular use. *Polyribosomes* attached to the flat lamellar membranes of the ER (to form *rER*) synthesize proteins within the rER cisterna. Newly manufactured protein is transported to the golgi complex in membranous vesicles where it is packaged for transfer to the plasmalemma to be discharged for extracellular use.

c. Cytoplasmic *basophilia* (the attraction of basic dyes by acidic substances) is attributed to the high content of ribosomes containing both RNA and protein.

7. *Lysosomes* (DeDuve, 1963) are characterized by TEM as cytoplasmic organelles containing important hydrolytic enzymes (acid hydrolases) packaged in membrane units. These dense bodies may assume spherical, ovoid, or irregular shapes and vary in size from 0.25 μm to 0.5 μm.

a. Functionally, these organelles serve

(1) a *defense* role for the organism. Bacteria and foreign bodies engulfed by cells are destroyed by some 50 hydrolytic enzymes.

(2) a *self-destruct* role at death. If a tissue biopsy is not "fixed" immediately, the cells undergo *autolysis* (self-dissolution) following release of the packaged lysosomal enzymes. Lowering temperature will help delay autolysis.

(3) as an intracellular *digestive system.*

b. Lysosomes developed from membrane-bound ribosomal granules and packaged by the golgi complex are referred to as *nascent granules.* As they enlarge into *primary lysosomes* they appear (via TEM) to have an electron-dense, uniform-appearing material enclosed by membranes. Fusion of phagocytized material with a primary lysosome forms a *secondary lysosome.* Lysosomal activity occasionally forms a *residual body,* which may remain within the cell.

c. Lysosomes probably arise by the same mechanism as secretory vesicles, with enzymes synthesized from the rER membranes and packaged by the golgi complex. Evidence exists that implicates a special region associated with the ER close to the golgi complex mature face. This area is considered to be a specific organelle, the "*g*olgi-*a*ssociated *e*ndoplasmic *r*eticulum from which *l*ysosomes form," better known by the acronym *GERL* (Novikoff et al, 1971).

d. In healthy cells, lysosomal activity is responsible for breaking down ingested proteins by proteases, lipids by lipases, and phosphates by phosphatases. Other important enzymes found in lysosomes are the nucleases, glycosidases, phospholipases, and certain sulfatases.

e. *Tay-Sachs disease* is one of a group of several important genetic diseases involving lysosomal activity. If particular lysosomal enzymes are deficient or fail to function, then substances that should have been degraded accumulate in the cytoplasm to such a degree that proper cell activity is impaired. Since the enzyme hexosaminidase A (Devlin, 1986) is deficient, the principal storage substance ganglioside GM12 accumulates in nerve cells of the cerebral cortex. Diagnostic TEMs reveal the accumulation of lamellated electron-dense bodies. The patient presents with mental retardation, blindness, a macular red spot, and death between the second and third years.

8. *Phagolysosomes, phagosomes, autophagosomes,* and *heterophagosomes*

a. The *phagolysome* is the generalized structure that performs *endocytosis* (Silverstein et al, 1977), the process by which extracellular substances are wrapped in a plasmalemma-derived vesicle and internalized.

(1) The process by which extracellular fluids, with or without suspended substances, are internalized is *pinocytosis.*

(2) *Phagocytosis* (Hirsch, 1965) is the process by which extracellular particles or bacteria are engulfed and internalized to form *phagosomes.* Lysomes fuse with the phagosome and destroy the bacteria. Subclassifications of this process are *autophagy* and *heterophagy.* *Autophagy* is the process of controlled digestion of aging intracellular structures to form an *autophagosome*. Lysosomes fuse with the auto-phagosome. Structures that fail to be completely digested accumulate in the cytoplasm as wear and tear pigment or lipofuscin. *Hetero-phagosomes* digest extracellular material by the process of *heterophagy*.

    b. *Exocytosis* (Allison and Davies, 1974), the opposite of en-docytosis, expels secretory products extracellularly. Membranes of the golgi complex or ER form vesicles that fuse with the plasmalemma. This seemingly extra membranous material will be recovered by endocytosis.

    9. *Peroxisomes* (microbodies) (Novikoff and Allen, 1973) are membrane-bound organelles, larger than lysosomes, which may be continuous with sER. They function primarily in peroxide metabo-lism where the enzyme catalase converts generated hydrogen peroxide into water. They are numerous in macrophages, hepatocytes, and kidney tubules. Evidence implicates the peroxisomes in α-keto acid formation.

    10. *Multivesicular bodies* containing multiple smaller vesicles are presumed to be a form of lysome. The presence of acid phospha-tase can be detected histochemically, but a specific function in cellular defense has yet to be confirmed.

    11. *Multitubular bodies* resemble multivesicular bodies, except that elongate tubular vesicles predominate. This structure found in endothelial cells once was called by the eponym "Weibel-Palade body."

    12. *Microfilaments* are structural proteins existing as two distin-guishable types, *contractile microfilaments* and *intermediate filaments* (Pollard, 1981).

    a. *Contractile microfilaments* (the major one, *actin* [5 to 6 nm in diameter], comprises at least 10% to 15% of all cells) are responsible for (1) *undulations* of the plasmalemma of cells completing the mi-totic phase (this phenomenon is best studied in time-lapse movies of cells in tissue culture), (2) *locomotion* (ameboid motion) of cells, (3) *contraction* of cells and microvilli, (4) *constriction* of mitotic cells, by a sphincter of actin microfilaments (Schroeder, 1975), (5) *vesicle forma-tion* during pinocytosis and phagocytosis, (6) *expulsion* of secretory products, (7) *cytoplasmic streaming* seen during locomotion.

    b. *Intermediate filaments* (Lazarides, 1980; Steinert et al, 1985) (9 to 12 nm in diameter) participate in strengthening, support-ing, and forming the *cytoskeleton* or cell framework. Several important classes exist: (1) *keratin tonofilaments* provide support and strength to stratified squamous epithelial cells, (2) *desmin filaments* are wrapped around muscle fibrils to hold them in place, (3) *vimentin* (a structural protein) forms a meshwork around the nucleus and probably contributes to the maintenance of nucleocytoplasmic communications, (4) *neurofilaments* (Shelanski and Liem, 1979) provide the structural support to nerve cells.

13. *Microtubules* (Olmstead and Borisy, 1973; Burnside, 1975): The heterodimer *tubulin,* a proteinaceous substance, is organized into elongated tubular structures, with a *size* of 24 nm in diameter, 14 nm lumen, therefore a 5-nm-thick wall. They originate from a specific terminal of a preexisting microtubule called the *nucleation site.* Microtubules form the walls of centrioles, cilia, and flagellae, and help maintain characteristic cellular shapes and facilitate *intracellular transport.*

14. *Transitory substances* are those that have a limited period of time within the cell. Such substances are *lipid droplets, glycogen deposits* (eg, liver and muscle), *protein deposits* (in the form of secretory granules), and *pigment granules* (lipofuscin, an aging pigment, and melanin pigment present in the epidermal melanocytes).

V. The *nucleus*

A. The nucleus contains the major portion of the genetic material deoxyribonucleic acid (DNA), which not only governs the visible features of our bodies, but also the specific morphological and chemical profiles of all cell types and their metabolic activities. For example, DNA "directs" the pancreatic beta (β) cells to produce and release insulin (1) in set amounts, (2) under set circumstances, and (3) at set times. DNA combines with small basic proteins called histones (and others) to form the visible structural component the *chromatin* (Kornberg, 1977). The DNA content of chromatin causes it to be *basophilic* (love = philia for basic [baso-] dyes). During the *interphase* period of **mitosis** (cell division), chromatin can exist in two phases:

1. *Heterochromatin* (the condensed form): In this "clumped" basophilic form, it is relatively *inactive.*

2. *Euchromatin* (the extended form) (Fig. 2-1): This is the *active* form, which directs and provides instructions for important cellular activities (ie, protein secretion). In the extended form, via LM, it appears very lightly basophilic. Via TEM it is electron lucent or minimally electron dense, depending on the degree to which it is extended. Nuclei with a maximum quantity of euchromatin are named *vesicular nuclei.*

B. The nucleus assumes various shapes: *annular, bacilliform* (rod-shaped), *fusiform* (spindle shaped), *ovoid, planus* (flat), *polymorphus* (many shapes or segments), *reniformis* (kidney shaped), *segmental,* and *spherical.*

C. During mitosis, chromatin condenses into visible "stripes" (Amenta et al, 1973) associated with the nuclear membrane. In prophase and metaphase of the mitotic cycle, the stripes increase in thickness and shorten to become recognizable as *chromosomes.*

D. The **nucleolemma** or *nuclear membrane* (Gerace, 1986) consists of two thin membranes, each about 7 nm thick, separated by a 15- to 25-nm electron-lucent space, the *nuclear cisterna.* In some pathological cases, the cisterna may increase in width as a result of accumulated fluid as occurs in normal antibody-producing cells (ie, plasma cells). The *external nuclear membrane* is continuous with the rER and is similarly roughened with ribosomes. The *internal nuclear membrane* (somewhat thinner and smooth) forms an attachment surface for heterochromatin.

E. Complexus pori or the *pore complex* of the nuclear membrane are spaced between 100 nm and 200 nm apart around the entire nucleus. These are very complex structures consisting of three basic parts: (1) the *nuclear pore* ranging in size from 30 to 100 nm, (2) the **annulus pori** (ring) with eight granules at each of nuclear membranes (internal and external), and (3) the **diaphragma pori** (pore diaphragm), with a central granule connected attached to the granules of the annulus. The internal nuclear membrane is joined to the external nuclear membrane, and the diaphragm is a separate membrane associated by the rays from the granules to cover the pore. Pores appear to control which materials can enter or exit the nucleus to facilitate nucleocytoplasmic exchange.

F. Nucleolus (nucleolus principalis) (Brinkley, 1965; Ghosh, 1976), the nuclear organelle containing large quantities of ribonucleic acid (RNA), are sites where ribosomal RNA is synthesized. In living cells, viewed by dark medium phase-contrast microscopy, and in sections prepared for LM and TEM, nucleoli generally appear darker than adjacent chromatin. Cells may have more than one nucleolus and may vary in size. Frequently, protein-secreting cells may exhibit enlarged nucleoli. The fewer the nucleoli, the longer the interphase period.

1. *Nucleolar fusion* (Amenta, 1961): Time-lapse microcinematographic recordings clearly demonstrate the ability of nucleoli to fuse and separate. This phenomenon results in a variable nucleolar number, an important consideration when classifying normal or pathological cells via nucleolar number. It appears that fusion occurs in interphase soon after *telophase* (in mitosis) and that separation occurs prior to a new interphase. The mass of fused nucleoli is not necessarily the sum of two component nucleoli, indicating that this occurrence is not per chance, but rather an active functionally important process.

2. **Nucleolonema:** Electron microscopic studies do not reveal a membrane around the nucleolus, which is composed of a **pars filamentosa** (a filamentous part), a **pars granulosa** (a granular part), and an amorphous medium in which the filamentous and granular portions are embedded.

3. The nucleoli are important as sites for nucleic acid synthesis and as dynamic organelles through which materials are continuously flowing (Perry, 1964).

VI. *Cell division:* Cells may divide either by *direct cell division (amitosis)* or *indirect cell division (mitosis).*

A. *Direct cell division,* studied best in the unicellular organisms such as the ameba, occurs by **nucleokinesis** (nuclear constriction) followed by **cytokinesis** (cytoplasmic constriction). In humans, direct cell division, to form two cells, occurs most frequently in liver cells and rarely in other cells. Nucleokinesis without cytokinesis results in increasing the *ploidy* (chromosome number) of a cell.

1. A *haploid* cell has one half the chromosome number or "n" (eg, in spermatocytes or ovocytes of the human, there are 23 chromosomes). In spermatozoa, one of these 23 chromosomes is called the sex or *Y chromosome*, while in the ovum it is the *X chromosome*.

2. A *diploid* cell resulting from the union of sperm and ovum has a 2n number or 46 chromosomes. Two of these 46 are sex chromosomes. In the male one chromosome is a *Y* and the other is an *X (XY).* In the female, both sex chromosomes are *X (XX).*

3. Repeated nucleokinesis of diploid cells results in *triploid* or 3n, *tetraploid* or 4n, etc. In abnormal cells the condition with more than two sets of chromosomes is called *polyploidy.* Normal *ploidy* in bone marrow *megacaryocytes* may reach a 64n number of chromosomes. Departures from the normal diploid number that do not involve entire *"n"* sets of chromosomes are designated as *aneuploid.*

B. *Indirect cell division* or the *mitotic cycle* (Fig. 2-7): In the total life span of a cell, the time devoted to mitosis is extremely short. The life cycle of a cell is divided for convenience into a period of *mitosis* (M) of up to 1 hour and an *intermitotic (interphase) period* lasting up to 30 hours depending on cell type. The *intermitotic period* is divided into three phases:

1. The *first gap phase* (G_1) may take 8 to 10 hours following mitosis. Most of the reconstruction of the nucleus occurs during this phase.

2. The *synthesis phase* (S) will take 7 to 8 hours to complete, during which time duplication of DNA molecules occurs in preparation for distribution in the upcoming mitotic period. All cellular energy is directed to synthesizing new DNA.

3. The *second gap phase* (G_2), prior to mitosis proper, lasts 4 or more hours. Protein secretion and other specialized cellular functions are confined primarily to G_2 and some to G_1.

Figure 2-7 Diagram of the cell cycle.

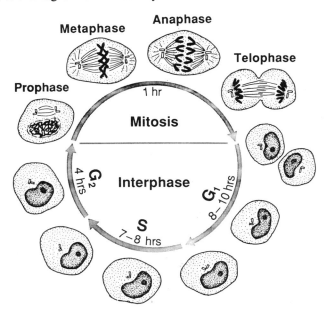

4. The entire cell cycle (including mitosis) continues to occur unabated in embryonic cells, until cellular *differentiation* transforms the cell into a *determined* or *specialized* cell. If further division is not required, the cell in G_1 may exit the cycle permanently (as in central nervous system neurons). In the adult, intestinal epithelial cells are produced daily via this mechanism.

5. Cells may remain in the G_1 phase for extended periods of time (beyond the 8–10 hours). In this condition they may be called upon to perform their specialized tasks or be stimulated to reenter the cell cycle and continue into the S phase.

C. Mitosis (Mazia, 1964)

1. The fertilized ovum divides into two cells (daughter cells) and thereby initiates prenatal development through a series of changes from an embryo into a fetus. Postnatal development continues with the following stages: neonatal, childhood, adolescence, adulthood, and the aged adult. Intensive study, clinical practice, and research have produced specialists concerned with various phases of human development: the embryologist, fetologist, geneticist, pediatrician, internist, and geriatric physician. In development, countless billions of new cells are "born" in the body's ceaseless program of self-renewal, at the rate of some three billion cells per minute by the process of **mitosis**. Mitosis is responsible for distributing to the new "daughter" cells an equal heritage of DNA, RNA, and organelles and inclusions. This process is remarkable indeed, if one considers that a mature human being possesses some 50 trillion cells. In the natural process of day to day living, cellular death from wear and tear is expected and normal, but these cells must be replaced.

2. Mitosis also occurs by nucleokinesis and cytokinesis, but with very special differences. For convenience, mitotic phases are delineated, but one should understand that the process is continuous and not fragmented. Two daughter cells like the mother cell are produced. One may remain in the cycle to generate more cells, while the second may differentiate into a determined cell with a specific function(s) to perform. The following stages are defined:

a. *Prophase* is characterized by retardation of cytoplasmic streaming as the cell mobilizes for division. The chromatin threads contract and thicken into conspicuous chromosomal strands. The pars filamentosa of the nucleolonema is distributed and wrapped around the chromosomes, thus rendering the nucleoli invisible. The nucleolemma disappears to mark the end of prophase.

b. *Prometaphase* is the interval between prophase and *meta-*

phase. The centrioles replicate and migrate to opposite poles of the nucleus. The region surrounding each pair of centrioles is termed the **cytocentrum** or the cell center (centrosome). Microtubular filaments extending from one cytocentrum to the other form a fusiform structure, the *spindle* (Inoue, 1981). Additional microtubular filaments attach to the chromosomes at the *primary constriction* known as the *centromere* (kinetochore). Although experimental evidence implicates the microtubules as factors in pulling the chromosomes apart into *chromatids*, no completely satisfactory explanation of the precise mechanism has been forthcoming.

   c. *Metaphase* is characterized by an arrangement of the chromosomes around the equator of the spindle, or *equatorial plane*, equidistant from the ends of the spindle. The centromeres (at the apex of V- or J-shaped chromosomes) attach to the microtubules. Phase-contrast, time-lapse microcinematographic studies reveal a display that tissue culturists call "the dance of the chromosomes" in which metaphase chromosomes are jostled to and fro at the centromere while the dragging arms dangle freely in the cytoplasm.

   d. *Anaphase* commences with the simultaneous snapping apart of all chromosomes at the centromere and gradual separation through the chromosome arms to the ends. Newly separated chromosomes, now termed *chromatids*, are aimed centromere first toward each cytocentrum located at opposite ends of the spindle. The centromeres seem to be pulled as the ends drag behind. Equal numbers of chromatids (2n) move rapidly toward each cytocentrum, appearing as two bunches of bananas moving apart.

   e. *Telophase* is the finale of chromatid movement. The chromatids are bunched closely together with all the centromeres focused toward the cytocentrum. Thereafter, **cytokinesis** begins at the equator of the cell, perpendicular to the axis of the mitotic spindle, and continues until separation is complete. Normal completion distributes an equal number of chromosomes and an equal amount of cytoplasm to each daughter cell.

   f. *Reconstruction* of the interphase nucleus occurs when the shortened telophase chromosomes revert to their filamentous interphase condition and attach to the reappearing nuclear membrane. The nucleolonema reorganizes into visible interphase nucleoli. Chromosomes possessing *secondary constrictions* are designated *nucleolus-organizing chromosomes* because they participate in reorganization of *nucleoli*. Following completion of cytokinesis, the daughter cells reenter interphase and the mitotic cycle starts again. A single, newly formed cytocentrum nestles close to the nucleus.

VII. *Tissue culture observations:* In the tissue culture, it is interesting to observe the periphery of the cell membrane of a new daughter cell as it attempts to flatten and attach to the coverglass surface. Wildly undulating movements subside once the plasmalemma attaches to the coverslip. When approaching prophase, a cell rounds up, but retains attachment to the coverslip at a few points (perhaps by the secreted glycocalyx). Then at metaphase, a peculiar bubbling phenomenon occurs in which the cell membrane is distorted by the cytoplasm extruding into the peripheral bubbles. Bubbling intensifies severely if the cytoplasm is irradiated with microbeams of ultraviolet light, to the extent that even the *mitotic apparatus* (centrosomes, spindle, and chromosomes) is extruded en masse into a large bubble and returned to the cell proper.

VIII. *The four basic tissues:* Similar cells functioning in harmony are classified into four basic tissues, to be discussed in subsequent chapters:

A. Epithelial tissue

B. Connective tissue

C. Muscle tissue

D. Nerve

Questions

DIRECTIONS: For each of the items in this section, one or more of the numbered options is correct. Select

A if only *1, 2, and 3* are correct
B if only *1 and 3* are correct
C if only *2 and 4* are correct
D if only *4* is correct
E if *all* are correct

1. The "Fluid Mosaic Model" emphasizes that
   1. the plasmalemma is composed of a bilayer of phospholipid molecules attached to fatty acid chains
   2. extrinsic protein molecules arranged on the inner and outer surfaces of the plasmalemma impart an asymmetry to the molecular structure
   3. oligosaccharide chains protrude from the external surface
   4. the cytoplasmic surface is studded with polyribosomes

2. The glycocalyx
   1. participates in protection of the plasmalemma
   2. is arranged on the matrix surface of mitochondrial cristae
   3. provides a means for cell – cell communication
   4. forms the electron-lucent hydrophobic molecule ends of the plasmalemma

3. The cytocentrum (centrosome)
   1. exists at the primary constriction of a chromosome
   2. contains the centrioles
   3. forms the nucleolar organizer region of a chromosome
   4. resides in the cytoplasm, close to the nucleus or in a nuclear indentation

4. Mitochondria possess which of the following structural features?
   1. An internal membrane modified by a series of folds or tubules which extend into the matrix
   2. Mitochondrial matrix granules composed of calcium and magnesium
   3. Elementary particles
   4. A relatively smooth external membrane

5. The golgi complex
   1. is covered by ribosomes on the protoplasmic surface
   2. is composed of membranes arranged in a tubular complex
   3. possesses an immature face involved in packaging secretory products
   4. is dependent on granular endoplasmic reticulum for its continued formation

6. Nongranular (smooth) endoplasmic reticulum characterizes which of the following cell types?
   1. Striated muscle cells
   2. Steroid-secreting endocrine cells
   3. Hepatocytes (liver cells)
   4. Parietal cells of the stomach

7. Free ribosomes
   1. exist singly in the cytoplasm
   2. synthesize proteins destined for intracellular use
   3. are functionally inactive
   4. transport new proteins to the golgi complex

		Directions Summarized		
A	**B**	**C**	**D**	**E**
1,2,3	1,3	2,4	4	All are
only	only	only	only	correct

8. Cellular lysosomes
   1. function primarily in peroxide metabolism
   2. contain important enzymes
   3. are transitory substances
   4. may develop into residual bodies

9. Nucleoli are nuclear structures
   1. where ribosomal RNA is synthesized
   2. surrounded by the nucleolemma
   3. composed of a nucleolonema
   4. that possess complex pores

10. During mitosis
    1. microtubular filaments extend from one cytocentrum to the other
    2. chromosomes move from the equatorial plane toward the spindle poles, trailing their arms
    3. the nucleoli and the nuclear membrane disappear during prophase
    4. nucleokinesis occurs without cytokinesis

Explanatory Answers

1. A. 1, 2 and 3 are correct. Answer 4 is false for the plasmalemma, but true for the nucleolemma (nuclear membrane).

2. B. 1 and 3 are correct. A thick glycocalyx is found on cell surfaces (eg, intestinal epithelial cells) that require protection from harsh substances. Communication is facilitated by the complexity of oligosaccharides in the glycocalyx. Answer 2 is incorrect. Mitochondrial cristae are coated with elementary particles. Answer 4 is incorrect. The glycocalyx, which is hydrophilic, resides on the exterior of cell surfaces.

3. C. 2 and 4 are correct. In histological preparations the cytocentrum is devoid of cytoplasmic organelles except for the centrioles. Answer 1 relates to the centromere of the chromosome. Centromere should not be confused with cytocentrum. Microtubules originating from the cytocentrum do attach to the centromeres in mitosis. Answer 3 is a chromosome secondary constriction usually associated with nucleolar ogranization following telophase.

4. E. All are correct. The folded cristae are characteristic of cells involved in protein synthesis for external export, while tubular cristae (as well as tubular smooth ER) exist in steroid-secreting cells. The calcium and magnesium mitochondrial granules are required for some enzymes to function. Elementary particles contain the enzyme required for phosphorylation of ADP to ATP. The external mitochondrial membrane confines the intermembranous space between itself and the inner mitochondrial membrane.

5. D. Only 4 is correct. Answer 1 granular (rough) endoplasmic reticulum and the nucleolemma are the only cellular structures covered with ribosomes. Answer 2, a complex of tubular membranes is characteristic of the agranular (smooth) endoplasmic reticulum of steroid-secreting cells and their mitochondria. Answer 3 is incorrect because the mature face is involved in the final packaging of secretory granules.

6. E. All are correct. Answer 1, sER occurs in striated muscle for the liberation and reuptake of ionic calcium required for muscle contraction and relaxation. Answer 2, the steroid-secreting endocrine cells are those of the suprarenal cortex, the testes, and the ovaries. Answer 3, hepatocytes with sER are involved in cholesterol and lipid metabolism. Answer 4, the sER in parietal cells participates in producing free hydrochloric acid.

7. B. 1 and 3 are correct. Ribosomes that exist singly associate linearly with a molecule of messenger RNA to form a polyribosome. In this form they can be functionally effective in producing protein for intracellular use. Individual ribosomes are ineffective. New proteins are transported from rER to the golgi complex in rER-derived membranes.

8. D. 2 and 4 are correct. *Answer 1*, peroxisomes are responsible for peroxide metabolism. *Answer 2*, the hydrolytic enzymes are usually the acid hydrolases. *Answer 3*, transitory substances have a limited period of existence in the cell. Examples are lipid droplets, glycogen droplets, and lipofuchsin pigment. *Answer 4*, a primary lysosome which fuses with the membranous sac containing a phagocytized material (eg, bacteria) can become a residual body following enzymatic activity.

9. D. 1 and 3 are correct. *Answer 1* is true. *Answer 2*, the nucleolus has no surrounding membrane, the nucleolemma is the membrane surrounding the nucleus. *Answer 3* is correct, and the nucleolonema is subdivided into a pars filamentosa and a pars granulosa embedded in an amorphus medium. *Answer 4* is false. The nuclear membrane, or nucleolemma, has complex pores.

10. A. 1, 2, and 3 are correct. Answers 1, 2, and 3 are straightforward. Answer 4 is incorrect because in mitosis nucleokinesis (division of the nuclear material) is always followed by cytokinesis.

3 Epithelium

I. During early *embryogenesis* (development of the embryo), three differentiated primary germ cell layers are distinguishable (Moore, 1988):

A. *ectoderm*, the external monolayer of closely related cells, destined to develop into skin, its appendages, and the nervous system. The ectoderm covers an underlying germ layer, the *mesoderm*.

B. *mesoderm*, a middle layer of diffuse stellate-shaped cells, embedded in a gelatinous extracellular matrix (ground substance) (Hay, 1981). The mesoderm develops into the major supporting tissues (bone, cartilage, and connective tissues), the vascular system, and the serosal linings of the body cavities.

C. *endoderm* (entoderm), the inner monolayer of closely related cells, which will differentiate into the digestive tube and associated glands, and the respiratory tree and its glands. The prefix *ent-* is found in the word *enteron* (signifying primitive gut), and *enteritis* (inflammation of the intestines).

II. A practical understanding of epithelium should emphasize

A. functionally related parenchymal cells with little or no extracellular matrix are held together by intercellular junctions,

B. provision of a modulating influence between underlying tissues and materials exposed to the *luminal* surface, hence cells are polarized to facilitate transportation of materials in and out of the cells (Sabatini et al, 1983),

C. derivation from one of the primary germ layers with retention of some embryonic powers for renewal and repair,

D. avascularity, ie, epithelia receive nourishment from underlying capillary beds since there are no blood vessels in the epithelium proper.

III. Classification: Epithelia are classified structurally according to cell shapes, height, and the degree of complexity. Structural integrity of cells is maintained by intracellular intermediate filaments. Cells in a monolayer form a *simple epithelium* and multiple layers of cells form a *stratified epithelium*. (Two other forms are discussed below.) The *basal surface* of epithelial cells attaches to a substrate called the *basement membrane*. The opposite surface is the *free* or *luminal surface* (facing a *space*). The *lateral surfaces* adhere to adjacent cells by cellular junctions and extracellular matrix. The exposed luminal surface subjects epithelia to a variety of mechanical, thermal, and toxic stresses and hence they must be adequately developed for repair and renewal.

A. *Simple epithelium* is arranged in a monolayer of similar cells (Fig. 3-1) closely attached by intercellular junctions plus minimal extracellular matrix.

1. Simple squamous epithelium is a monolayer of flattened cells resembling fried eggs. The yolk represents the cell nucleus and the egg white, the cytoplasm. Simple epithelium is composed of numerous interdigitating cells anchored to a basement membrane.

a. One form, the **mesothelium**, lines the pleural, pericardial, and peritoneal cavities. It is proper to refer to this variety of simple squamous epithelium as a *serosal lining*.

b. Another form, the **endothelium**, lines the *lumena* of blood vessels, the heart, and lymphatic channels. The *lumen* is the open portion of any tube. Holding a tube up to a light source allows light to enter, hence the name lumen. The free surface of epithelial cells lining any tube faces the lumen.

c. Endothelium and mesothelium are derived from mesoderm.

2. *Simple cuboidal epithelium* appears as a monolayer of cubes when viewed in cross-sectional profile. However, viewed from the luminal surface, it presents the profile of tightly fitting hexagonal polygons. This epithelium forms the secretory portions of many glands (eg, liver, thyroid), the lining of exocrine gland ducts, pigmented epithelium of the retina, inner surface of the lens capsule and some ducts and tubules of the kidney, and the covering epithelium of the ovary.

3. *Simple columnar epithelium* is a monolayer of elongated cells. Functionally, cells may change shape, height, and width. For example, the epithelium enclosing the thyroid colloid may at one time appear cuboidal and at another, columnar, reflecting the physiological activity and plasticity of cells.

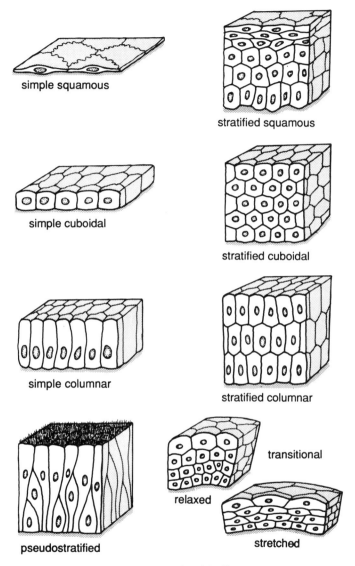

Figure 3-1 The known varieties of epithelium.

a. The luminal surface of columnar cells presents hexagonal profiles. Nuclei may be polarized closer to the basal surface (as in the digestive tract) or closer to the luminal surface (as in the oviduct).

b. Simple columnar epithelium is encountered in the lining of the uterus, smaller bronchi of the lung, paranasal sinuses, and central canal of the spinal cord.

B. *Stratified epithelium* is multilayered (Fig. 3-1), reflecting response to the degree and type of stress. One obvious functional characteristic of stratified epithelium is protection to underlying tissues.

1. The basal layers of cells are anchored to a *basement membrane*, to laterally located cells, and to the cells above. The superficial layer of cells is generally exposed to the external environment (skin) or to a lumen (esophagus).

2. The thicker the stratification, the more distant the upper cell layers will be from nutrient capillaries lying beneath the basement membrane. Malnutrition may be accompanied by dehydration and death of the more superficial cell layers.

3. Aged or dead cells are replaced by cells residing in the deeper layers undergoing disciplined mitoses. Rampant mitoses may lead to carcinomas.

4. *Classification* is similar to that used for simple epithelia, except that the word *stratified* is substituted for simple.

a. *Stratified squamous epithelium* possesses cell layers that vary in shape. Only the *superficial layers* (toward the lumen) are characterized as squamous, with nuclei flattened in a plane parallel to the basement membrane. Cells of the *basal layer* (resting on the basement membrane) are usually columnar with oval nuclei oriented perpendicular to the base. The cells, with a remarkable regenerative capacity, serve as the last reserve for replenishing more superficial cells. The *middle layers*, the normal reserve cells frequently undergoing mitoses, are populated by polygonal "cuboidal-appearing" cells with more spherical nuclei.

(1) *noncornified stratified squamous epithelium* possesses superficial squames that remain alive and functional until they age and are loosened by friction or abrasion. Loss of cells stimulates deeper layers to produce new cells. Local glandular secretions provide a lubrication that prevents dehydration of the superficial cells. This epithelium lines the oral cavity, esophagus, anus, and vagina.

(2) *cornified stratified squamous epithelium* is characterized by superficial squames lacking nuclei, resulting from dehydration from exposure to air. The excessive distance from the capillary bed beneath the basement membrane leads to their death from lack of nutrition. Because superficial cell layers usually become cornified (hardened), they serve admirably as a major protective layer. The skin is an example where *keratin* in the superficial layers prevents dehydration of underlying cells. The keratin also prevents cells in deeper layers from taking in too much water.

b. *Stratified cuboidal epithelium* is a rarity. In man only the ducts of sweat glands possess this form of epithelium. The minimal cell layers have superficial cells that appear cuboidal with spherical nuclei in each layer. One could argue that the seminiferous tubules are lined with stratified cuboidal cells.

c. *Stratified columnar epithelium* is rare in standard student collections. It exists at confined junctions where stratified squamous epithelium changes abruptly to pseudostratified columnar epithelium as in the nasopharynx, oropharynx, and larynx. Sometimes it is encountered as small patches in the male cavernous urethra and in short portions of the excretory ducts of the lacrimal and salivary glands. Nuclei appear at every level of columnar cells.

C. *Pseudostratified columnar epithelium* resembles stratified columnar epithelium because nuclei appear at different levels in at least one half to two thirds of the epithelial thickness.

1. In other stratified epithelia only the basal cells anchor into the basement membrane, but in pseudostratified epithelium (almost) every cell is anchored.

2. Small basal cells are pushed aside by taller cells that are narrow at the base and wider at the apex. The more bulbous superficial cells may be anchored to the basement membrane only by thin processes.

3. This type of epithelium is located in the large excretory ducts of glands and in the urethra. Surface modifications, such as cilia, distinguish this epithelium in the respiratory system and in the uterine tube.

D. *Transitional epithelium* appears to be a "transition" between stratified squamous and stratified columnar epithelium, because it seems to assume both configurations in the urinary system.

1. If the urinary bladder is filled, only three or four cell layers are seen via the light microscope, and if empty, additional layers of cuboidal and/or columnar cells appear with domed surface cells. Electron microscopy reveals a unique mechanism to account for the different numbers of cell layers one sees with the light microscope. Cells may flatten in response to distension and "store" portions of their cell membranes within the cells, while the luminal cells present a scalloped boarder.

2. The basement membrane of transitional epithelium is so minimal when viewed with the light microscope that countless generations of students were taught that transitional epithelium had no basement membrane. Electron microscopy resolved a basement membrane, albeit very thin, associated with a layer of collagen fibrils.

3. Nuclei in the relaxed cells are almost all spherical, while in the stretched condition they flatten in a plane horizontal to the basement membrane.

IV. The *basement membrane* (Hay, 1981; Martinez-Hernandez and Amenta, 1983; Timpl and Dzlamek, 1986) is an extracellular matrix specialized to protect, support and provide attachment binding sites for epithelial cells and serve in an ultrafiltration capacity (especially in the kidney).

A. Two united continuous lamellae, produced by contributions from related epithelial cells (Hay, 1981), are resolved by the transmission electron microscope:

1. the **lamina lucida** [rara], an electron-lucent layer (40 to 60 nm thick), intimately follows the contours of the epithelial cells.

2. the **lamina densa** [basalis], an electron-dense layer of similar thickness, is separated from the epithelial cells by the lamina lucida.

B. Another layer, the **lamina fibroreticularis**, is produced by underlying connective tissue fibroblasts as a fibrous network of reticular fibers embedded in a protein polysaccharide *extracellular matrix* or *ground substance* (Fig. 2-1). Though not considered part of the basement membrane today, it was the basement membrane of the light microscopists.

C. Two major classes of glyoproteins contribute to the integrity and strength of basement membranes:

1. The collagenous glycoprotein *type IV collagen*, which confers great tensile strength and flexibility to accommodate stretching of tissues and

2. The noncollagenous glycoproteins:

a. *Laminin* (an adhesive bound to type IV collagen), a high-molecular-weight glycoprotein with several heterologous binding sites

(Charonis et al, 1985). It exists predominantly in the lamina lucida and to some extent in the lamina densa.

    b. *Heparan sulfate proteoglycan* has chemical binding sites not only for the other basement membrane components, but also for a number of proteases. Its importance is established by virtue of the role it plays in assisting the epithelial cells in responding to injury, cell attachment, and selective filtration (Kanwar and Farquhar, 1979).

    c. *Fibronectin, entactin,* and *nidogen* may also be found in basement membranes. Some 50 other adhesive proteins in the basement membrane are under investigation.

    D. Basement membranes, composed of the lamina lucida and lamina densa, occur where the following epithelia require attachment to underlying supportive connective tissues:

    1. the epidermis,

    2. the epithelium of the digestive, respiratory, urinary, and reproductive systems,

    3. endothelium and mesothelium,

    4. exocrine cells.

    E. Fused basement membranes (lamina lucida : lamina densa/lamina densa : lamina lucida) lacking intervening connective tissue exist between

    1. *glomerular visceral epithelium* (*podocytes* of the kidney) and capillary endothelium,

    2. *alveolar epithelium* (lung) and capillary endothelium,

    3. *endocrine cells* and capillary endothelium.

    F. A variation of the basement membrane, the *external lamina,* invests (ensheathes)

    1. *neurolemmacytes,* which form the myelin sheath of axons,

    2. *myocytes* (smooth, cardiac, and skeletal),

    3. *adipocytes.*

    G. Other variations (around vascular sinuses) will be presented with their specific tissues.

    H. Functionally, the basement membrane

    1. facilitates transfer of metabolites and oxygen from capillaries in the connective tissue bed to the avascular epithelium and removal of cellular waste products.

2. maintains a critical thickness for functional efficacy. Hyperactivity of epithelial cells may produce a thicker lamina lucida plus lamina densa. Likewise, hyperactivity of connective tissue cells produces a thicker lamina fibroreticularis. Either or both situations decreases the transfer of substances in two directions.

3. must be present and maintained in a highly efficient state. A breakdown in its integrity leads to regression of epithelial cell structures. Its absence frequently heralds the beginning of metastasis of cancer cells. In fact, some malignant tumors are distinguished from benign tumors by the absence of a basement membrane.

4. allows epithelial cells to develop an inherent morphology (polarity, cytoskeleton, etc), to perform their specialized functions and to prevent their migration and proliferation.

A. Mechanisms that hold epithelial cells together

1. Adhesive cementing substances (Fig. 3-2)

a. The *glycocalyx* (Fig. 3-2A) covers the luminal and lateral surfaces of epithelial cells and serves as the major cementing substance to hold cells together.

b. The *basement membrane* (Figs. 3-2A, 3-2D, 3-2E), at the base of the cell, attaches cells to the connective tissue.

2. Plasmalemma modifications

a. *Interdigitations* (Fig. 3-2B): Endothelial and mesothelial cells, in addition to the intervening glycocalyx, possess peripheral processes that interdigitate with neighboring cells. Silver impregnation techniques demonstrate these to best advantage. Generally a spread mesentery stained with silver provides an excellent source to reveal these interdigitations.

b. *Overlapping* (Fig. 3-2C): Only the electron microscope resolves this mechanism in capillary endothelium. If a sheet of notebook paper (representing an endothelial cell) is taken by the upper left corner and brought around to overlap with the lower right corner, then a tube is made with a large upper portion and a narrow lower portion. Where the two corners meet approximates the endothelial cell overlapping. Individual sheets so rolled and fitted together form a tube analogous to a capillary.

c. *Lock* and *key* (Fig. 3-2D): Some adjacent cells (hepatocytes) are firmly interlocked by knobs protruding from one lateral cell surface fitting into a corresponding invagination of an adjoining cell. Each lateral cell surface possesses multiple "keys" (knobs) and "locks" (invaginations).

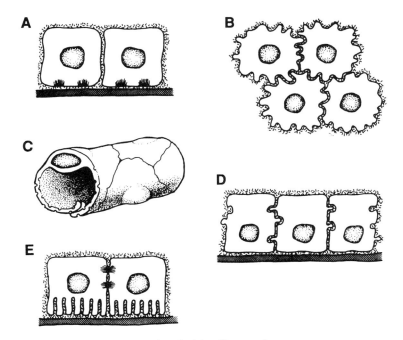

Figure 3-2 Mechanisms that hold cells together.

d. *Cell junctions*

(1) The **macula adherens** (desmosome) (Fig. 3-2E) is an electron-dense plaque of cytoplasmic condensates applied to the protoplasmic surface of the plasmalemma. Where one occurs on a lateral cell surface, another appears on the opposite cell surface. Opposing one another they resemble multiple welding spots (*macula* means spot). Although the plasmalemma retains its thickness at the macula adherens, it appears thicker due to the thickness of the plaque and the abundant extracellular matrix "adhesive" in the 20 to 30 nm space between the external surfaces of opposing plasmalemmae. A thin, electron-dense line of material in the space between the maculae distinguishes desmosomes from other junctions. Bundles of *tonofilaments* (cytoplasmic microfilaments) converge upon the macula adherens and loop back into the cytoplasm. Electron microscopic studies reveal that the hairpin-like tonofilaments anchor into the dense spot with their ends protruding into the cytoplasm. Tonofilament ends anchor into the microfilaments of the cytoskeleton.

(2) The **nexus [macula communicans]** (Fig. 3-3) (gap junction) is a specialized macular junction between cells. The minimal space between adjacent cells is narrowed to 2 nm (the "gap"). Each plasmalemmal nexus half is composed of 9 to 11 intramembranous polygonal protein particles that abut against one another (fuse?) in the intercellular space. The particles circumscribe a small hydrophilic channel that facilitates passage of certain ions from one cell to the other, hence the alternative name **macula communicans**.

(a) The nexus only provides a restricted channel that connects cell interiors. It is not open to the extracellular space. Molecules with a diameter of 1.2 nm (mw 1000) are capable of passing. Sugars and negatively charged polypeptides are able to pass through the channel. The nexus is impermeable to proteins, nucleic acids, and other macromolecules (Bennett et al, 1981).

(b) In addition to its adhesive function, the nexus provides an area of low electrical resistance that may be important in

Figure 3-3 The junctional complex.

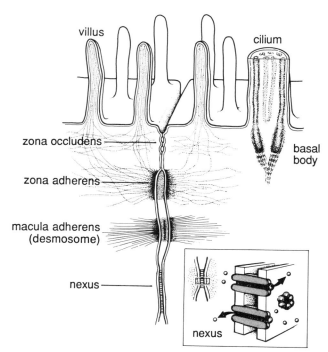

cell–cell coordination of cellular activities. In electrically excitable cells, the nexus constitutes an electrotonic synapse that transmits electrical signals (Bennett et al, 1981).

(c) The nexus also occurs between *osteocytes, smooth myocytes, cardiac myocytes*, and neuron *synapses*. The nexus can be demonstrated by TEM using special tracers (lanthanum) that fill the gap between adjacent cells. The nexus in freeze-cleave preparations appears as an array of hexagonal particles surrounding a pore.

(3) *Hemidesmosomes* (Fig. 3-2A) occur in areas where the plasmalemma contacts the noncellular material of the basement membrane. As the name implies, it is a half-desmosome, which provides additional strength to the attachment of the epithelial cell.

(4) The *junctional complex* (Fig. 3-3) is resolved by TEM and in freeze-cleave preparations at the lateral luminal border of adjacent columnar cells. Light microscopists saw a "dot" in tissue sections, which they called the "terminal bar." Via TEM three distinct morphological structures are resolved:

(a) The **zonula occludens** (*tight junction*) is formed by multiple "lines" on one cell membrane impressed into a corresponding cell membrane. This lace-like zonula, occupying 0.1 to 0.3 μm of the lateral cell membrane, encircles the cell to seal off the lumen from the intercellular space. Between the impression lines there are short regions where the opposing cell membranes are separated by a 10 to 15 nm space. This literal *tight junction* prevents large molecules leaving the lumen of an organ (intestine) via the intercellular route. The zonula occludens is revealed best in freeze-cleave preparations.

(b) The **zonula adherens**, or intermediate component of the junctional complex, resembles the desmosome structure with tonofilaments impressed into a continuous cytoplasmic band that encircles the cell. The intercellular space, measuring from 10 to 20 nm, is filled with adhesive components, but lacks the electron-dense line in the space between membranes that characterizes the macula adherens.

(c) The **macula adherens** or *desmosome* may extend to this level and become part of the junctional complex. Other desmosomes (cf above) appear as spots on all sides of cuboidal and columnar cells.

V. The *cytoskeleton* describes the cytoplasmic matrix as revealed by elegant electron microscopic studies (Porter et al, 1983). The basic architecture consists of a microtrabecular latticework (Wolosowick and Porter, 1979) of microtubules (25 nm diameter), microfilaments (6 nm diameter), and intermediate filaments (9 nm diameter). Microfilaments aggregated into bundles of *tonofilaments* not only associate with the zonulae and maculae adherens, but form an intricate *terminal web* paralleling the luminal surface of columnar cells. This web is a microfilament mesh containing myosin, a contractile protein, and several other microfilaments (cf microvilli below).

VI. *Specializations of the luminal cell surface:* To fulfill their genetically determined functions, cells must be structurally specialized. The free or luminal plasmalemmal surfaces of cells are provided with two forms of modifications: nonmotile **microvilli** and motile **cilia**.

A. Microvilli (Ito, 1965; Mooseker, 1985) are nonmotile tubular evaginations of the luminal plasmalemma that increase the absorptive surface area. A variety of enzymes involved in the absorptive process are associated with the plasmalemma covering microvilli. A core of hexagonally linked actin microfilaments, anchored in the dense cytoplasmic surface of each microvillus tip, originate from the meshwork of microfilaments in the terminal web. At the base of each microvillus exists the regulatory protein tropomyosin associated with a ring of actin microfilaments. The association of actin and terminal web horizontally arranged myosin filaments (Keller et al, 1985) may explain not only the contraction of microvilli but also their apparent stirring action.

1. *Short microvilli* (striated border), 0.5 to 1.0 μm long and 0.1 μm, occur on the luminal surface of intestinal epithelium where extensive absorption areas are required. Somewhat *longer* (2 μm) *microvilli* (brush border) characterize the absorptive epithelial cells of the kidney proximal convoluted tubules. The glycocalyx coating the microvilli expands the absorptive surface area and provides an effective barrier against larger molecules that could damage the microvilli. Small colloidal particles filter through the glycocalyx and are pumped down to the microvilli bases by their contractile activity, where they are engulfed by plasmalemma micovesicles.

2. *Long microvilli* (stereocilia), 5 to 10 μm in length, populate the epithelial surface of the ductus epididymis in the male. These differ from short microvilli by two diagnostic characteristics, branching and extreme flexibility. Flexibility is the result of fewer microfilaments in the core of these microvilli. These nonrigid branches tangle producing tufts resembling paint brushes.

B. Cilia (Fawcett, 1961; Warner and Satir, 1974) (Figs. 2-1, 3-3, 3-4) are structural modifications of the luminal cell surface capable of rapid vibratile movements. The shaft of each cilium (7 to 10 μm

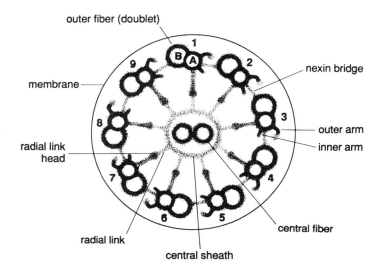

Figure 3-4 Cross section of a cilium.

long × 0.2 µm in diameter) is covered by plasmalemma. The core or *axonene* contains microtubules composed of the structural proteins *alpha* and *beta tubulin*. Nine doublets of microtubules, arranged in a ring, spiral gently around two central microtubules. While the latter resemble the microtubules of the cytoskeleton, the doublets differ. One tubule (of the doublet), designated *A*, exhibits a circular cross section, while the other, designated *B*, has a C-profile. Tubule *A* possesses two horn-like crossarms composed of *dyneins* (regulatory proteins with ATP-ase activity). The two central microtubules are surrounded by a *central sheath*, to which are attached *radial links*. Each doublet joins the other by a *nexin bridge*. Each *A* microtubule has *radial link heads* that join the radial links (of the central sheath). At the base of each cilium are *basal bodies*, structures that originated from the centrioles. Whereas the parent centrioles are two cylinders at right angles to one another, the basal body is a singular unit possessing nine triplet microtubules around the periphery (and no central microtubules). Ciliary activity may be compared with the action of a bull whip, a rapid forward movement followed by a backward slower recovery movement. Human respiratory cilia, on pseudostratified ciliated columnar epithelium, have been calculated to beat at around 1000 times per minute, creating great currents to move a mucous blanket in one direction. The uterine tube simple columnar epithelium possesses cila to move the fertilized ovum toward the uterine cavity.

VII. *Glands* differentiate from epithelial cells. Gland cells and glands may be classified on the basis of

A. *Location*

1. *intraepithelial glands*, those that reside within the epithelium.

a. *unicellular intraepithelial glands* are single cells that express their contents upon the epithelial surface. Example: the *goblet cell* in the digestive and respiratory systems.

b. *multicellular intraepithelial glands*, composed of cell groups surrounded by their own lumen, reside wholly within the thickness of the epithelium and never penetrate the basement membrane. Example: glands in the nasal epithelium.

2. *intramural glands* result from the migration of epithelial cells into the wall of a tubular organ. Examples: mucosal and submucosal glands of the esophagus and duodenal glands.

3. *extramural glands* result from migration of epithelial cells through all the layers of a tubular organ to form a gland away from the parent organ. Examples: liver and pancreas, both of which originate from the endodermal epithelium of the gut.

B. *Mode of secretion* [In the chapters that follow glands will be discussed in detail where related to a particular organ tissue.]

1. *Exocrine glands* are those that maintain structural contact with the epithelium of origin by an epithelial tubular duct. Secretions are expressed directly through the duct onto the epithelial surface.

a. They may be relatively *simple* like a test tube,

b. or *complex* with multiple branches possessing terminal cells forming acini, which are responsible for the production of secretory material.

2. *Endocrine glands* develop from epithelium but break off from the originating duct system to secrete *hormones*, which must pass into a nearby capillary.

Questions

DIRECTIONS: For each numbered item, select the one heading most closely associated with it. Each lettered heading may be selected once, more than once, or not at all.

Questions 1–4
A. Mesothelium
B. Endothelium
C. Transitional epithelium
D. Pseudostratified columnar epithelium

  1. Simple squamous epithelium
  2. Serosal lining
  3. Domed surface cells
  4. Cilia

Questions 5–8
A. Lamina lucida
B. Lamina densa
C. Lamina fibroreticularis
D. External lamina

  5. Produced by epithelial cells
  6. Produced by myocytes
  7. Found between podocytes and capillary endothelium
  8. Contain collagenous glycoproteins

Questions 9–12
A. Junctional complex
B. Terminal web
C. Cytoskeleton
D. Cilia

  9. Actin microfilaments
 10. Microtubules
 11. Tonofilaments
 12. Zonula occludens

Explanatory Answers

1. A and B. Both mesothelium and endothelium are examples of simple squamous epithelium.

2. A. The mesothelium lines the serosa of the peritoneal cavity, the pericardial cavity, and the pleural cavity.

3. C. The transitional epithelium of the relaxed (empty) bladder has surface cells that appear domed.

4. D. Pseudostratified columnar epithelium of the respiratory tract has most surface cells covered with motile cilia, which are required to move a mucous blanket.

5. A and B. The lamina lucida plus the lamina densa are produced by epithelial cells of all types, including endocrine cells.

6. C. The external lamina is a variation of the basement membrane that is produced by myocytes, adipocytes, and neurolemmacytes, none of which are considered to be epithelial cells.

7. A and B. The podocytes (like pulmonary alveolar cells) are epithelial cells that produce a layer of lamina lucida and a layer of lamina densa. Capillary endothelium (a simple squamous epithelium) also produces lamina lucida and lamina densa. In these cases the lamina densa of opposing basement membranes fuse, with no intervening connective tissue components.

8. A, B, and D. Produced by epithelial cells and the special cells invested by the external lamina, type IV collagen is found in all three layers. The collagenous glycoprotein type IV collagen has not been identified as a product of the underlying connective tissue cells that form lamina fibroreticularis.

9. B. Actin microfilaments in the core of microvilli anchor into the terminal web ring of actin. Together with the horizontal myosin filaments in the web, contraction of microvilli results.

10. C and D. Microtubules occur in the cytoskeleton and in cilia.

11. A, B, and **C.** Tonofilaments are bundles of microfilaments associated with the macula adherens and zonula adherens of the junctional complex, with the terminal web, and with the cytoskeleton.

12. A. The zonula occludens is the band surrounding the luminal lateral edges of cells, which require tight junctions to prevent luminal contents from passing between cells. The zonula occludens is the first part of the junctional complex.

4 The Connective Tissues

I. *Introduction:* The student who misses the experience of performing a dissection fails to appreciate the binding qualities of the varieties of connective tissues. Further, the opportunity is missed to feel this packing-like material that molds and permits muscles to contract, nerves to conduct impulses, and the smallest vessels of the vascular system to function.

II. *Connective tissue* describes the widely dispersed system of *cells* plus associated *extracellular matrix* that forms the *stroma* (structural framework) of muscle, nerve, vasculature, and all tissues and organs.

A. A broad range of connective tissue types are involved with the transportation of anabolic and catabolic substances through the **substantia intercellularis** to participate in tissue repair, inflammation, and blood cell development. The liberal translation *extracellular matrix* for substantia intercellularis will be used throughout because of the almost universal acceptance by investigators in connective tissue research (Hay, 1981).

B. Differentiation of closely packed, rapidly dividing cells of embryonic mesoderm forms stellate-shaped *mesenchymal cells* genetically programmed to provide structural support for rapidly developing organ systems. Packing-like material for delicate structures is derived from mesodermal and neurectodermal cells embedded in a viscid amorphous **substantia fundamentalis** (ground substance).

C. Almost all connective tissues are composed of the following, albeit in varying proportions:

1. *Extracellular matrix* (ECM), once considered an inert glue, is recognized for its role in development, differentiation, and tissue repair. It is a complex network of extracellular macromolecules that holds cells together and provides a highly organized lattice within which cells can migrate and interact. The ECM (Lennarz, 1980) is composed of four major macromolecular groups: (1) *noncollagenous structural proteins*, (2) *proteoglycans*, (3) *collagens*, and (4) *elastin* in an aqueous *tissue fluid*. The various concentrations and interactions of these components result in properties that are tissue specific. For example, both the lung and liver are endodermal derivatives, but differ dramatically in their parenchymal cell morphology and unique extracellular matrices. The following outline presents a simple approach to understanding the ECM: (a) **substantia fundamentalis**, (b) *fiber types*, (c) *cells*.

a. Substantia fundamentalis

(1) *Noncollagenous structural proteins* help create tissue cohesiveness.

(a) Represent a heterogeneous collection of macromolecules with a ubiquitous distribution. These proteins are characterized by protein chains that are attached to carbohydrate groups.

(b) Included among the defined noncollagenous glycoproteins are

[1] *Laminin*, which consists of three polypeptide chains in a cruciform structure, serves to mediate the adhesion to basement membrane collagen of certain epithelial cells that cannot utilize fibronectin for attachment to type IV collagen (Terranova et al, 1980).

[2] *Fibronectin* (Yamada et al, 1985), secreted by endothelial cells and/or fibroblasts, possesses sites that can bind to other cells, collagen fibrils, and proteoglycans.

[3] *Chondronectin* (Hewitt et al, 1980), which occurs in chondroid tissues (cartilage), mediates the attachment of cartilage cells (*chondrocytes*) to the surrounding collagens.

[4] Others identified are *entactin, vitronectin*, and *thrombospondin*.

(c) *Basement membranes* are ubiquitous extracellular matrices containing laminin, entactin, type IV collagen, and heparan sulfate proteoglycan. They

[1] surround many mesenchymal cells,

[2] underlie most epithelia, mesothelium, and endothelium.

(2) *Proteoglycans* (formerly: acid mucopolysaccharides), with a ubiquitous distribution, lubricate and interact with collagen fibrils to hold them *together* (Lindhal and Hook, 1978). Proteoglycans are essential to matrix resiliency. The *metachromasia* exhibited in the connective tissue matrix and some cells is attributed to the proteoglycans. Metachromasia is a property of basic aniline dyes whereby tissue or cell components react with a dye to change its color; in the case of toluidine blue, from blue to purple-red.

    (a) Consist of

        [1] a core protein covalently linked to

        [2] carbohydrate moieties, the glycosaminoglycans (GAG): (a) chondroitin-4-sulfate, (b) chondroitin-6-sulfate, (c) dermatan sulfate, (d) heparin, (e) heparan sulfate, (f) hyaluronic acid, (g) keratan sulfate.

    (b) The highly negatively charged proteoglycans are named according to the prominant GAG side chain, ie, heparan sulfate proteoglycan, etc.

    (3) *Tissue fluid*, resembling blood plasma in its ion content and diffusible substances, forms a small portion of the extracellular matrix. Any tissue fluid present results from hydrostatic pressure on the arterial side of the capillary network. All nutrients, oxygen, hormones, etc, plus waste products and carbon dioxide usually must pass through ECM to reach the body parenchymal cells from the blood and vice versa. Hence the amount, consistency, and nature of tissue fluid will influence the ability of these substances to pass through the ECM.

    b. *Fiber types*

    (1) *Collagen fibers:* Collagens (rod-like structures, 1.5 nm $\times$ 300 nm) are composed of three α-chains. Alpha chains are characterized by the repeating amino acid sequence of glycine $-$ X $-$ Y, where X and Y are frequently hydroxyproline and hydroxylysine. The hydroxylation of proline and lysine is critical for proper inter- and intramolecular bonds to form between various collagen molecules to form fibers and for the attachment of galactose and glucose. In routine histological preparations (H & E), the slightly refractile collagen fibers are stained pink by eosin. Collagens are sources of strength to the tissues.

    (2) *Reticular fibers* are the first fibers to appear when embryonic mesenchyme differentiates into the "loose" type of connective tissue.

    (a) In addition, these fibers are prevalent around the sinusoids of the liver, spleen, and bone marrow.

    (b) Once thought to represent type III collagen, *reticulin* is best considered a mixture of a variety of ECM components, including collagens and structural glycoproteins. These are delicate strands (0.5 nm to 2.0 nm in diameter) arranged in a "network," hence the name *reticular.*

    (c) Although difficult to stain with H & E, they are blackened by alkaline solutions of reducible silver salts. The affinity for metallic silver accounts for the former name, argyrophilic fibers.

(d) *Procollagen molecules*, precursors of collagen, are composed of three α-chains coiled in a right-handed helix. Procollagen, with amino and carboxy nonhelical ends, is secreted into the extracellular environs by *fibroblasts*. They are cleaved into collagen molecules by removal of these ends by peptidases. Collagen fibers form by the alignment of collagen molecules in staggered arrays. At least 12 genetically distinct types of collagen (Table 4-1) have been characterized and categorized into three major groups, based on size and physicochemical properties (Miller and Gay, 1987).

(3) *Elastic fibers* appear as refractile branching fibers (0.2 μm to 1 μm in diameter).

(a) Elastic fibers are composed of 10-nm bundled *fibrils* surrounding the substance *elastin*. Previously considered amorphous, elastin in now known to be composed of aggregated fibrils, each 2 nm to 4 nm thick.

(b) Elastin is rich in two amino acid derivatives: *desmosine* and *isodesmosine*. Elastin is essential to the resiliency of ECM.

Table 4-1 The Genetically Distinct Types of Collagen (Martin et al 1985)

Type	Distribution
Type I	loose and dense connective tissue, dermis, cornea, tendon, bone, dentin. Fibrils measure 20 nm to 100 nm in diameter. The predominant type of collagen.
Type II	vitreous body of embryonic and adult eyes, nucleus pulposus, embryonic notochord, hyaline cartilage of the embryo through the adult. Fibrils are 10 nm to 20 nm in diameter. Principal type of collagen in cartilage.
Type III	predominant in pliable tissues, skin, uterus, lung connective tissue, blood vessels, placenta
Type IV	predominant in all basement membranes
Type V	amnion; chorion; laminae externae of muscle, nerve, and adipocytes; minor part of interstitial tissues
Type VI	predominant in most interstitial tissues
Type VII	anchors basement membrane to underlying lamina fibroreticularis
Type VIII	produced by vascular and corneal endothelium
Type IX	occurs in cartilage
Type X	occurs in mineralizing epiphyseal cartilage
Type XI	occurs in cartilage
Type XII	cartilage

(c) Repetitive banding patterns, as seen in collagen, have not been reported in other macromolecules.

C. *Connective tissue cells:* The cell that produced ECM continues to interact with it and the ECM produced by other cells.

1. Resident cells: *fibroblasts, tissue basophils* (formerly the mast cells), *plasma cells, chondroblasts, osteoblasts.*

2. Transient cells: *macrophages, granular leucocytes,* and *lymphocytes,* which participate in tissue repair or combat infection.

III. The quality and disposition of cellular and extracellular matrix distinguishes five major categories of connective tissues:

A. *Embryonic connective tissue* (eg, umbilical cord) is composed of primitive mesenchymal cells embedded in a mucoid extracellular matrix. In the human adult, it persists in the vitreous humor of the eye as *mucous connective tissue.*

B. *Blood* consists of cells suspended in a liquid extracellular matrix. Blood is the only connective tissue variety that lacks collagen, reticular, or elastic fibers.

C. *Connective tissue proper* (CTP) possesses some pleuripotent cells and some partially differentiated cells that can produce fibers. Depending on the relative amounts of fibers in the extracellular matrix, CTP may vary from very *loose* to very *compact.*

D. *Cartilage* has all the characteristic components of CTP plus the chondroitin sulfates that impart sufficient firmness to serve as a provisional skeleton in the embryo. Cartilage persists in many places in the human adult.

E. *Bone,* a connective tissue with cells and fibers, is distinguished by an extracellular matrix with various inorganic salts, which provide remarkable strength. Bone constitutes the major portion of the adult skeleton.

IV. The classification of the connective tissues

A. The *fibrous connective tissues* differ according to the dominance and orientation of fiber types (*collagen, reticular, elastic*), the variety of cell types, and the quality and quantity of the extracellular matrix.

1. *Loose collagenous connective tissue* possesses more ground substance and cells than the fibers. Wherever loose connective tissue occurs, the component fibers (*collagen, reticular,* and *elastic*) appear to be distributed randomly. A good analogy can be made to the packing material "excelsior," representing the fibers. The space between the fibers is occupied by **substantia fundamentalis**, which permits resident cells to maneuver about to fulfill their functions. The predominant cell of loose connective tissue (and all the fibrous connective tissues) is the *fibroblast*, which has the major responsibility to produce fibers. In the embryo, the first connective tissue cell is the *primitive mesenchymal cell*, which later differentiates into the fiber-producing cell, the *fibroblast*.

      a. *Cell types* (Fig. 4-1) exist in two forms: *fixed cells* (attached to a substrate, such as a fiber) and *mobile* (free) *cells*, which move freely in the extracellular matrix.

      (1) *Fixed cell* types (*fibroblast, mesenchymal cell, reticulocytes, adipocyte,* and the *fixed macrophage* [histiocyte])

      (a) *Fibroblasts* are fusiform-shaped cells with at least three elongated processes. These processes may contact other fibroblasts to form a network of cells, as do their progenitor embryonic mesenchymal cells. The smooth-surface elliptical nucleus has a sparse dust-like euchromatin network and one or two nucleoli.

      [1] The suffix *-blast* suggests that fibroblasts possess multipotentialities, although many investigators no longer consider them to be primitive cells.

      [2] When attached or "fixed" to a substrate, the fibroblast is quiescent and does not form fibers. In this stage, it is appropriate to name it a *fibrocyte*.

      [3] TEM helps to distinguish the two functional states of this cell.

      [a] The active *fibroblast* has a large bulbous golgi complex in the vicinity of the cytocentrum that nestles against the nucleus. In tissue cultures, several elongated mitochondria are recognized hovering around the nucleus and occasionally in the long, slender cell processes. TEM confirms these observations. The presence of granular endoplasmic reticulum (rER) is responsible for a moderate cytoplasmic basophilia.

      [b] In the quiescent *fibrocyte* state, the golgi complex diminishes, while the rER becomes depleted. Some lipid droplets appear in a lightly eosinophilic cytoplasm. Eosinophilia is attributed to the decreased rER and a minimum of cytoplasmic organelles. When stimulated, the quiescent fibrocyte reverts to the active *fibroblast* by proliferating its rER content and developing the golgi complex.

      [4] Under certain pathological states, *fibroblasts* may demonstrate *osteogenic potencies* (bone forming) or *store lipids* until they resemble adipocytes (fat cells). Whether these transforming cells

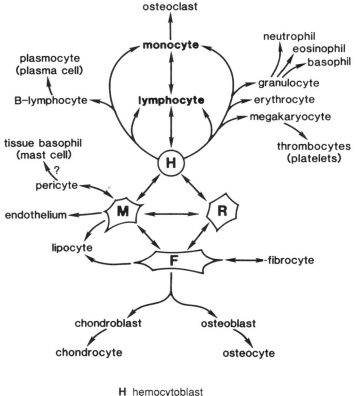

H hemocytoblast
M mesenchymal cell
R reticulated erythrocyte
F fibroblast

Figure 4-1 Interrelationships between connective tissue cells, blood cells, and primitive cells.

are actually fibroblasts or resident undifferentiated mesenchymal cells is still a subject for necessary investigation.

[5] Fibroblasts multiply extensively in vivo and in vitro. During *wound healing*, the number of fibroblasts increased by mitosis are stimulated to produce fibers and ground substance.

(b) *Mesenchymal cells* are distinguished from fibroblasts by their stellate shape, smaller size, and coarser heterochromatin. The conviction that mesenchymal cells may persist in the adult is supported by many investigators.

[1] As less-differentiated derivatives of embryonic mesenchyme, mesenchymal cells can differentiate into a variety of other cells in normal or stressed conditions.

[2] Mesenchymal cells exist in the adult by their consistent location along small blood vessels coursing through loose connective tissues.

[c] *Reticulocytes* (The name *reticulocyte*, per the *Nomina Histologica*, replaces the former name, "reticular cell." In this edition, *reticulocyte* specifies the multipotent, less-differentiated stem cell of reticular connective tissue. The immature *reticulated erythrocyte* was called the *reticulocyte*.)

[1] The reticulocyte, derived from mesenchyme, forms the reticular fiber stroma or **reticulum**, of lymphoid organs, spleen, and bone marrow. The reticulocyte attaches to the fibers produced.

[2] The reticulocyte shares many of the functional and morphological properties of mesenchymal cells and fibroblasts in many other tissues as well.

(**d**) *Adipocytes* (fat cells) store such vast quantities of lipid in the cytoplasm that the nucleus is compressed to one side as a thin film of heterochromatin, while the plasmalemma confines a thin rim of cytoplasm around the huge lipid droplet.

[1] *Formation:* Small lipid droplets accumulating in the cytoplasm coalesce to form larger droplets. With the requirement to store additional lipid, coalescence continues until all the lipid forms a single cytoplasmic droplet.

[2] *Progenitor:* Consensus points to the *mesenchymal cell* as the progenitor of the *adipocyte*. If excessive quantities of lipid must be stored, mesenchymal cells are stimulated to divide rapidly to provide the more differentiated adipocytes.

(**e**) *Fixed macrophages* (histiocytes) bear a striking resemblance to fibroblasts. A fixed macrophage attaches to neighboring structures such as fibers. When detached, it is called a *nomadic* (wandering) *macrophage*. The *fixed macrophage* (**macrophagocytus stabilis**) was formerly called the histiocyte. Because of etymology, this term (meaning "tissue cell") is considered unsatisfactory and has been deleted from the nomenclature.

[1] *Progenitor:* The *monocytes* in peripheral blood can enter the connective tissue matrix where they differentiate into *macrophages*, which can generate more macrophages as required.

[2] *Morphology:* The peripheral edges of the plasma-

lemma reflect macrophage activity. If consuming fluids, the plasmalemma is pocked by micropinocytotic vesicles. Consumption of particulate matter causes larger invaginations of the plasmalemma. There can be pleating, pseudopodia, and a variety of shapes to the plasmalemma, each reflecting the activity of the macrophage. Many lysosomes, a prominent golgi complex, and abundant rER reflect the activity of macrophages in diverse tissues.

[3] *Stimulated macrophages* exhibit increased lysosomal activity. They can secrete the enzyme collagenase to clear away collagen fibers in order to move more freely to attack unwelcomed connective tissue invaders such as cancer cells.

[4] The variety of *macrophages* throughout the body, because of similar morphology and functions, form the *macrophage system* (cf Table 4-2). The older name, "reticuloendothelial system," implies that the endothelium of lymphatic tissues have the capacity of phagocytosis. This term is unacceptable and hence only *macrophage system* or *mononuclear phagocyte system* are considered appropriate (per *Nomina Histologica*).

(2) *Mobile cells* (*Wandering macrophages, monocytes, lymphocytes, plasma cells;* blood *neutrophils, acidophils, basophils;* and the *tissue basophil granulocyte* [mast cell])

(a) The *wandering macrophages* were described above along with the *fixed macrophages*.

(b) *Monocytes* [cf Chapter 5] are the precursors of macrophages. In circulating blood their life span is limited to about 4 days. Upon entering the connective tissues they can be stimulated by inflammatory conditions to begin a new existence as tissue macrophages

Table 4-2 Cells of the Macrophage System

Cell type	Information
Monocyte	"The Macrophage"
Fixed macrophages	(histiocytes) in the connective tissues
Macrophages	in the lymph nodes and the spleen
Alveolar macrophages	of the pulmonary alveolar epithelium
Stellate macrophages	(Kupffer) in the liver
Pleural macrophages	serous cavity, lung
Peritoneal macrophages	serous cavity, abdomen
Osteoclasts	the "bone breakers"
Microglia	in the central nervous system

with voracious phagocytic appetites. Under certain conditions, monocytes may differentiate into (Vander Rhee et al, 1979)

[1] *epithelioid cells*, an aggregation of monocytes into an epithelial sheet induced by chronic inflammation or

[2] *foreign-body giant cells*, a coalescence of epithelioid cells attempting to phagocytize large indigestible particles.

(c) *Lymphocytes* [cf Chapter 5] pervade the connective tissues as *diffuse lymphatic tissue* populated by T-lymphocyte types and as *lymphatic nodules* populated by B lymphocytes.

(d) *Plasma cells*, derived from B lymphocytes, possess a rich basophilic cytoplasm, filled with rER covering a juxtanuclear area devoid of rER, the **cytocentrum**. The eccentrically located cartwheel nucleus is recognized by clumps of heterochromatin attached to the nucleolemma in spoke-like fashion. TEM reveals degrees of cisternal distention attesting to the role played by the plasma cell in storing antibodies.

[1] Although plasma cells exhibit little to no motility, they are free cells, not attached or fixed to any substrate, and live only 2 to 3 days in connective tissue.

[2] Plasma cells are not seen to any extensive degree in most loose connective tissues. They are quite numerous in the intestinal loose connective tissue immediately under the epithelium (**lamina propria mucosae**). This site is subjected to invasion by bacteria and foreign proteins.

[3] Patients with *hyperglobulinemia* have an elevated titer of antibodies and a correspondingly high population of plasma cells in the connective tissues.

[4] Patients with *agammaglobulinemia* fail to synthesize antibodies and possess few or no plasma cells.

[5] The precise mechanism for stimulating the B lymphocyte to transform into a plasma cell has not been clarified. Perhaps a macrophage that just engulfed some bacteria contacts a B lymphocyte. Apparently some chemical information released by the macrophage stimulates the B lymphocyte to become a plasma cell. In turn, the plasma cell develops specific antibodies against the specific bacterial antigens. The plasma cell, however, is not phagocytic.

(e) The *granular leucocytes* exit the blood capillaries via the process of *diapedesis*, function in the connective tissues in response to a variety of stimuli, and terminate their life span there. Leucocytes participate in *inflammation*, which occurs in vascular and connective tissues. Inflammation results from the invasion of foreign substances or bacteria. A sequelae of events occur that lower the ground substance viscosity and dilate capillaries and venules, resulting in increased blood supply and temperature in the area. Increased capillary permeability results in leakage of blood plasma into the connective tissue spaces to produce swelling or *edema*. The ensuing compression of nerve endings can produce intense pain.

(f) *Tissue basophil granulocytes* (mast cells) develop from bone marrow hemocytopoetic stem cells (Kitamura et al, 1981). The stem cells may enter the circulation, migrate into the connective tissues, and there differentiate into definitive *tissue basophils* (mast cells). The mature cells may also give rise to new tissue basophils. The *tissue basophil* appears remarkably similar to the *blood basophil granulocyte*. Distinctions between blood basophil granulocytes and tissue basophil granulocytes are presented in Table 4-3. Functionally, the *tissue basophils* act as "watchdogs" in strategic sites along blood vessels and mucosal surfaces, where they can respond to threats by foreign substances. If activated, they can rapidly release any or all of the substances stored in their granules. A slower type of deliverance of nonstored chemotactic substances attracts other cells to help ward off unwelcome invaders. Two cell types are recognized, based on their secretions. Note in Table 4-3 that the type 1 cell secretes heparin, while the type 2 cell secretes chondroitin sulfate.

[1] *Explanation of activities* of the tissue basophil granulocyte (mast cell). When stimulated, the substances listed above (plus many more) are released to promote rapid allergic reactions (within minutes). [Please consult textbooks of immunology.]

[a] Let us assume that an individual is stung by a bee, which injects a venomous *antigen*.

[b] The *antigen* stimulates plasma cells to produce the *antibody* IgE (an immunoglobulin).

[c] The *antibody* attaches to the surface of the tissue basophil granulocytes (mast cells). Thus the individual is said to be sensitized.

[d] The next time the sensitized individual is stung and exposed to *antigen*, the coating IgE (on the tissue basophil granulocytes) binds the newly introduced antigen,

[e] causing the release of stored and unstored substances followed by a series of events known as *immediate hypersensitivity reaction* ranging from negligible to serious *anaphylactic shock*, which could result in death.

[2] The long-lived *tissue basophil granulocytes* (mast cells) are most numerous in the connective tissue surrounding blood vessels under the skin, digestive tract, and respiratory tree.

b. *Loose collagenous connective tissue*

Table 4-3 Tissue Basophil Granulocyte vs Blood
Basophil Granulocyte

	Tissues	Blood
Cell size:	20 to 30 μm	10 μm
Nucleus:	single, spherical, centrally located	bilobed or multilobed central or eccentric
Granules:	membrane bound	membrane bound
numbers:	+++++++	+++
stain:	basophilic metachromatic	basophilic metachromatic
contain:	heparin (type 1 cell) chondroitin sulfate (type 2) histamine leukotriene C ECF-A PAF serotonin	heparin chondroitin sulfate histamine heparan sulfate dermatan sulfate

Heparin (stored) is a powerful anticoagulant.

Histamine (stored) induces vascular permeability, stimulates contraction of bronchiolar smooth muscle, and assists in decreasing blood pressure.

ECF-A (stored) *e*osinophil *c*hemotactic *f*actor of *a*naphylaxis. Attracts acidophil granular leucocytes (eosinophils) and neutrophils.

Leukotriene-C (unstored) (formerly SFC-A) increases vascular permeability and induces slow contraction of smooth muscle.

PAF *p*latelet-*a*ctivating *f*actor. Aggregates thrombocytes and stimulates release of serotonin.

Serotonin constricts blood vessels and assists in increasing blood pressure.

(1) Formerly was called "areolar" connective tissue. Early investigators would inject substances such as india ink into a fragment of loose connective tissue and find that the ink remained confined in a space. This finding led to the name areolar.

(2) The current nomenclature specifies that the predominant fibers are loosely arranged, with no apparent orientation.

(3) Intertwined with these fibers are reticular fibers and refractile branching elastic fibers.

(4) An abundant extracellular matrix provides the proper milieu for a variety of cells reflecting its physiological condition or pathology. Fibroblasts and macrophages predominate.

(5) Loose collagenous connective tissue forms the packing around blood and lymphatic vessels: in the **lamina propria mucosae** (under various epithelia), **lamina propria serosae** (under mesothelium), and in skin. For student laboratory study, fragments for staining with metachromatic dyes are easily obtained from the axilla of

rats. Examination of fresh tissue provides an excellent medium for comprehending this well-vascularized connective tissue which is quite pliable and doesn't resist stress very well.

2. *Compact* (dense) *collagenous connective tissue* is similar to loose collagenous connective tissue except that the amount of collagen increases substantially, while the amount of ground substance decreases. Fibroblasts are the predominant cell type. Other cell types occur in fewer numbers than in the loose variety. Depending on fiber orientation, two types of compact connective tissues are distinguished. Between these two extremes are intermediate forms that frequently can cause classification problems. There should never be such great emphasis on precise classification that significance of the tissue is lost. Students should describe what is seen, rather than force a classification.

a. *Compact irregular collagenous connective tissue* has bundles of fibers arranged in no specific pattern, apparently to provide a medium that resists stress from multiple directions. It is easily recognized in several places — in the thick padding of the dermis (skin), capsules of lymphatic organs, and muscle and nerve sheaths.

b. *Compact regular connective tissue* is the same except that the fiber bundles are oriented in one direction to provide tremendous resistance to prolonged stress.

(1) An excellent example is the *tendon*, which joins muscle to bone. So dominant are the collagen bundles that tendons appear white and glistening in the fresh state. *Fibrocytes* no longer producing fibers lie outside the fibers, compressed along the length of the fibers. Their elongated nuclei are arranged like a line of boxcars.

(2) Binding each fiber, each bundle, and the entire tendon are loose collagenous connective tissue sheaths, which also provide the protective packing for pervading nutrient blood vessels, nerves, and lymphatic vessels.

c. *Intermediate forms* between compact regular and compact irregular connective tissue:

(1) *Ligaments*, groups of collagenous fiber bundles that form capsules joining bone to bone. Localized thickenings strengthen the capsules to prevent hyperextension or hyperflexion of the joint.

(2) *Lamellar fibrous connective tissue*, composed of inseparable interwoven layers of collagen fibers (also called *fasciae* or *aponeuroses*). The layers are interconnected by fibers of compact collagenous irregular connective tissue. Examples are superficial fascia, deep fascia, and the fascia lata (on the lateral thigh).

(3) Also **periosteum, perichondrium,** and the **sclera.**

3. *Reticular connective tissue* consists of an argyrophilic reticular fiber network that provides attachment sites for *reticulocytes* and *fixed macrophages*. The reticular fibers in lymphatic organs are directly continuous with the collagenous bundles that form septae and capsules. Certainly the other cells found in the loose connective tissue will be found here, as well as occasional elastic fibers.

4. *Elastic connective tissue* is characterized by a larger number of highly refractile, branching elastic fibers forming net-like units. Elastic fibers appear homogeneous, but TEM reveals a composition of finer, spirally wound fibrils. The spiraling may account for the fiber's ability to be stretched and return to its original form.

a. Elastic fibers occur almost everywhere to some degree. Where dominant over collagen or reticular fibers, the connective tissue is termed *elastic connective* tissue.

b. *Elastic connective tissue* forms major portions of the fasciae covering the anterior abdominal wall, the aorta and arterial walls, trachea and bronchi, vocal cords, the suspensory ligament of the penis and the intestinal wall.

B. *Specialized connective tissue*

1. *Adipose connective tissue* is composed of masses of *adipocytes* (fat cells) that also occur in every connective tissue either alone or in small groups. Individual adipocytes are ensheathed in a network of reticular fibers. Groups of adipocytes are bound by an intermingling of reticular fibers. Small blood vessels and nerves course freely through the reticulum. Two forms are recognized:

a. *White adipose connective tissue:* The adipocytes reach diameters from 25 μm to 200 μm according to the amount of lipid in the cytoplasm. Aggregates of adipocytes compose lobules that are separated by connective tissue septae of reticular and collagen fibers. Elastic fibers are relatively few.

(1) While adipose tissue exists almost everywhere, abundant deposits concentrate in specific areas. The *subcutaneous tissue* immediately beneath the skin is a repository of white adipose connective tissue. In adult females about 23% of the body weight is adipose tissue, which is well developed in the subcutaneous tissue of the breasts, gluteal region, hips, and thighs. Adult males, with 18% of the body weight as adipose tissue, have a thick layer in the shoulders, neck areas, and gluteal region. Infants and children show no significant sex differences until puberty, when the uniform layer of subcutaneous tissue, the **panniculus adiposus**, acquires a distribution characteristic of men and women. Distribution is regulated by sex hormones and adrenocortical hormones.

(2) In the abdominal cavity, adipose connective tissue is deposited in the greater omentum and around the kidney; in the orbit of the eye it serves as a protective padding.

(3) Adipocytes develop from the same mesenchymal cells that give rise to fibroblasts. The adipoblast (progenitor of adipocytes) resembles the fibroblast except for tiny lipid droplets accumulating in the cytoplasm. Coalescence of the tiny droplets forms one single *unilocular* droplet, surrounded by a thin rim of cytoplasm (signet ring shape). The massive lipid droplet squeezes the cytoplasmic structures (nucleus, mitochondria, etc) to the periphery.

b. *Brown adipose connective tissue* (brown fat) appears brown because the deep red of the rich vascularization combines with the yellow of the cytoplasmic lipid droplets (Lindberg, 1970). It occurs primarily in hibernating animals. The *multilocular adipocytes*, averaging 60 μm in diameter, contain small cytoplasmic lipid droplets that failed to coalesce. Though rare in adult humans, something resembling brown fat occurs in the human embryo and fetus (Merklin, 1973). This *fetal fat* occurs primarily in the posterior cervical, axillary, suprailiac, perirenal, and suprarenal gland regions. With advancing age, brown fat is replaced by white adipose tissue. In certain pathological conditions, brown adipose tissue may develop. The major function of brown fat is heat production.

2. *Pigmented connective tissue* possesses cells containing large quantities of *melanin* pigment. The pigment cells, called *melanophores*, occur in the pigmented connective tissue of one of the eye layers, the *choroid*.

3. *Mesenchyma* or *mesenchymal connective tissue* (in the embryo) differentiates from mesodermal cells to form a network of stellate-shaped *mesenchymal cells* bathed in a thick ground substance of gel-like consistency. The mesenchymal cells in the embryo and fetus develop into fibroblasts that produce a few reticular fibers plus a large amount of ground substance that reacts positively for *mucin* (in histochemical tests). Lymphoid cells and free macrophages also reside in this tissue.

a. In the fetal umbilical cord, mucin-containing connective tissue is called *embryonic* or *mucous connective tissue*.

b. In the adult, mesenchymal connective tissue occurs in the *vitreous body* (humor) of the eye.

Questions

DIRECTIONS: For each of the items in this section, one or more of the numbered options is correct. Select
- **A** if only *1, 2, and 3* are correct
- **B** if only *1 and 3* are correct
- **C** if only *2 and 4* are correct
- **D** if only *4* is correct
- **E** if *all* are correct

---

1. Examples of structural glycoproteins are
   1. fibronectin
   2. keratan sulfate
   3. laminin
   4. heparan

2. The fibroblast, in contrast to the fibrocyte,
   1. is in the quiescent phase
   2. has a large bulbous golgi complex
   3. is attached to a substrate
   4. has a moderate cytoplasmic basophilia

3. Which of the following are present in basement membrane?
   1. Type IV collagen
   2. Laminin
   3. Entactin
   4. Type I collagen

4. Plasma cells
   1. possess a cartwheel, eccentric nucleus
   2. possess a rich basophilic cytoplasm
   3. possess a juxtanuclear area, devoid of rER
   4. are derived from B lymphocytes

5. The tissue basophil (mast cell), in contrast to the blood basophil,
   1. is larger
   2. possesses a single spherical nucleus
   3. has more granules
   4. contains leukotriene C, ECF-A, PAF, and serotonin

		Directions Summarized		
A	**B**	**C**	**D**	**E**
1,2,3	1,3	2,4	4	All are
only	only	only	only	correct

6. Monocytes
   1. are precursors of macrophages
   2. aggregate to form epithelioid cells
   3. live only 4 days in circulating blood
   4. store histamine

7. Intermediate forms of compact connective tissue occur(s) in
   1. lamina propria mucosae
   2. tendons
   3. choroid
   4. periosteum

8. Elastic connective tissue
   1. stains black with silver stains
   2. has highly refractile branching fibers
   3. is predominant in ligaments
   4. occurs in the arterial walls

9. Brown adipose connective tissue
   1. exists in hibernating animals
   2. consists of unilocular adipocytes
   3. may occur in human embryos and fetuses
   4. contains large quantities of melanin pigment

10. The reticulocyte
   1. manufactures reticular fibers
   2. is derived from mesenchyme
   3. forms the stroma of lymphoid organs
   4. is an immature erythrocyte

Explanatory Answers

1. B. 1 and 3 are correct. Fibronectin and laminin are two structural glycoproteins distinguished from the proteoglycans by their greater amounts of proteins and differing polysaccharide side chains. Fibronectin (*fibra*, fiber; *nectere*, to bind) binds to other proteins such as collagen and fibrin. Fibronectin is found in connective tissues and on the surface of many cell types. Laminin is localized in basement membranes where it helps epithelia attach to type IV collagen. Keratin sulfate and heparan are glycosaminoglycans of proteoglycans.

2. C. 2 and 4 are correct. A large bulbous golgi complex characterizes active, productive cells. Together with moderate amounts of rough endoplasmic reticulum (moderate basophilia) the cell manufactures tropocollagen molecules that will be assembled into collagen fibrils and fibers. Answers 1 and 3 reflect the fibrocyte. The golgi complex and rER are diminished, so minimal energy is consumed.

3. A. 1, 2, and 3 are correct. Basement membranes contain type IV collagen, laminin, entactin, and heparan sulfate proteoglycan. Connective tissue in the dermis of the skin ranges from a loose variety to a dense irregular form. Mesenchymal connective tissue is composed of stellate mesenchymal cells in a large amount of a gel-like ground substance, with minimal amounts of fiber types. It does occur in the umbilical cord of the fetus and newborn, but certainly not in the adult umbilical cord. The vitreous body of the adult eye is the best representation of the embryonic type of mesenchymal tissue. The panniculus adiposus is a subcutaneous layer of fat.

4. E. All answers are correct. The eccentrically placed nucleus has a cartwheel appearance with heterochromatin clumps forming the spokes. The basophilia of the cytoplasm results from the large amount of rough endoplasmic reticulum that may be distended with its product. An area devoid of rER is occupied by the cytocentrum, which houses the centrioles. The B lymphocyte is stimulated to become a plasma cell when it contacts a macrophage. As a plasma cell is produces specific antibodies against specific antigens.

5. E. All answers are correct. The granules in the tissue basophil are more uniform and may number several hundred, while the blood basophils have far fewer granules of varying shape and size. The nucleus of the tissue basophil is singular and oval while that of the blood basophil is lobed.

6. A. Answers 1, 2, and 3 are correct. In circulating blood, monocytes live for only 4 days, but on entering the connective tissue ground substance they may begin a new life as macrophages. In chronic inflammation, aggregates can form epithelioid cells. A coalescence of epithelioid cells, the foreign body giant cells, may attempt to phagocytize immense indigestible foreign particles. Histamine is stored in tissue basophil granulocytes (mast cells) and blood basophil granular leucocytes.

7. D. The answer is 4. The periosteum and perichondrium are connective tissue sheaths surrounding bone and cartilage, respectively. These sheaths carry vasculature, nerves, and lymphatics. They exist between compact regular and compact irregular in fiber orientation. Pigmented tissue forms the choroid layer of the eye; tendons form the most compact regular connective tissue in the body; the lamina propria mucosae of the intestine is composed of loose connective tissue.

8. C. Answers are 2 and 4. The fibers that stain black with silver stains are the reticular fibers. Elastic fibers do not stain with silver. Elastic fibers are highly refractile and branch. While present in all connective tissues, they form the greatest number in elastic connective tissue (hence the name). Collagen fibers predominate in ligaments. In arteries, elastic fibers contribute to the elasticity of the walls.

9. B. Answers are 1 and 3. Brown adipose connective tissue occurs primarily in hibernating animals. It is rare in adult humans, but may exist in human embryos and fetuses. The component adipocytes are filled with multiple lipid droplets and hence are called multilocular adipocytes. The brown color does not come from melanin, but from the rich vascularization surrounding each of the adipocytes. The blending of the yellowish lipid droplets and the dark red color of capillary blood is responsible for the brownish color. Unilocular adipocytes form the white adipose connective tissue.

10. A. Answers 1, 2, and 3 are correct. This question emphasizes the necessity to remove the confusion between reticulocyte and reticular cell. The latter term has been deleted and reticulocyte is the preferred term for the cell that manufactures reticular fibers. It is derived from the embryonic mesenchymal cell and shares many of its properties and characteristics.

5 Blood and Lymph

I. *Introduction: Blood* is designated a connective tissue composed of cells suspended in a liquid (sol) intercellular medium. The absence of reticular, collagen, and elastic fibers does not alter the designation. Blood and lymph are conveyed in vessels lined by endothelium.

II. *Blood cell development* (**hemocytopoesis,** cf Chapter 8)

A. Blood, lymph, and the conveying vessels are mesodermal derivatives.

B. In a 2-week embryo, small groups of pluripotential cells, in yolk sac *mesenchyme*, develop into *hemocytoblasts,* the stem cells for all red and white cells. Developing cells are transported by new vessels to other hemocytopoetic sites. In the fetus, sequential sites of development are the liver, spleen, and finally the bone marrow, which continues as the major site throughout life. In some hematological conditions, blood cell development may reoccur in the spleen, liver, or sites other than bone marrow.

III. *Statistical data*

A. Blood comprises 7% of the total body weight.

B. *Sedimentation:* If a freshly drawn sample of blood stands in a test tube, the heavier formed elements (cells) settle to the bottom. The component *cells* compose 45% of the volume, while the remaining 55% is intercellular liquid *plasma.* From the bottom of the tube upward, the following percentages are recorded:

1. *Erythrocytes* (red blood cells, RBC) = *40%* and, as the heaviest cells, settle at the bottom.

a. The packed cell volume (PCV) of erythrocytes is called the hematocrit (H) measured in cubic millimeters of blood.

b. The normal number of erythrocytes/mm^3 = 10×10^6.

2. *Leucocytes* (white blood cells, WBC) = *1* to *3%* and form a thin white "buffy" layer on the surface of the sedimented erythrocytes. The total normal number of leucocytes, 5000 to 13,000 per milliliter of blood, is broken down as follows:

    a. *Neutrophils* = 3000 to 6000/mm³

    b. *Lymphocytes* = 1000 to 4000/mm³

    c. *Monocytes* = 200 to 600/mm³

    d. *Acidophils* (eosinophils) = 120 to 350/mm³

    e. *Basophils* = up to 40/mm³

3. *Thrombocytes* (platelets) are the lightest elements and form on the surface of the leucocyte layer. Their total number, 200,000 to 400,000/mm³, surpasses the concentration of leucocytes.

4. *Blood plasma*, the straw-colored fluid above the packed cells, comprises 52 to 55% of the total blood sample and consists of:

    a. water = 91.5%

    b. proteins = 7%. Separated by electrophoresis into:

        (1) albumin = 55%

        (2) globulins = 38%

        (3) fibrinogen = 7%

    c. other = 1.5%: inorganic salts, lipids, enzymes, hormones, vitamins, and carbohydrates.

C. Using these statistics, tissue culturists attempted to duplicate plasma to develop synthetic plasmas. However, the most successful tissue and cell growth has required natural plasma in the culture medium. Apparently, more needs to be learned about the nature and components of plasma.

IV. *Erythrocytes* (red blood cells) (Fig. 5-1): In man and most mammals, the lack of nuclei, nucleoli, mitochondria, golgi complex, centrioles, and ribonucleic acid is probably the ultimate in cell differentiation and specialization. However, their absence not only reduces the life span of erythrocytes (120 days), but also renders them incapable of self-propagation. New blood cells are constantly supplied from the bone marrow to transport oxygen from the lung to the body tissues and carbon dioxide from the tissues to the lung for exhaling (Harris and Kellermeyer, 1970).

A. Certain essential *average data* is necessary to appreciate the role of erythrocytes (Platt, 1969):

    1. Volume: 35 ml/kg of body weight

    2. Count: Females: 4.5 million/ml; Males: 6.2 million/ml

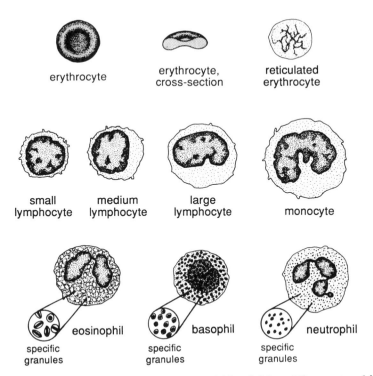

Figure 5-1 Mature cells of the peripheral blood. Note: The neutrophil is depicted with a "drumstick" appendage.

3. Size: 8 μm in diameter

4. Surface area: 3500 square meters (for total cells)

5. Specific gravity: 1.02 to 1.08

6. Color: Individual cells: pale green-yellow; A thick film: reddish, due to the content of hemoglobin

B. *Permeability* of the erythrocyte plasmalemma has been studied more than any other cell membrane (Cohen, 1983).

1. Erythrocytes suspended in balanced salt solutions (BSS) retain their characteristic shape. The concentration of salts within the erythrocyte are *isotonic* with the salts in the BSS.

2. *Crenation:* If the concentration of salts (especially sodium

chloride) in the BSS is increased *(a hypertonic solution),* water escapes through the plasmalemma, resulting in *crenation* where the cells resemble thistles.

3. *Hemolysis:* Decreasing the concentration of salts in the BSS (a *hypotonic* solution) by increasing the water content initiates an opposite reaction. Water enters through the erythrocyte plasmalemma until the cell bursts. Escaping hemoglobin gives the BSS a reddish hue, while the empty erythrocyte shells become *erythrocyte shadows* or "ghosts."

C. *Aggregation:* If a fresh drop of blood is placed on a glass slide, erythrocytes tend to adhere like stacks of poker chips in *erythrocyte aggregates* (columns of Rouleaux). Occasionally, this poorly understood phenomenon may occur in the living subject, when blood circulation is sluggish.

D. *Agglutination:* In some diseases, agglutination or clumping of cells results by the action of *agglutinin,* a nonspecific protein.

E. *Cell forms:* Deviation in cell shape = *poikilocytosis.*

1. *Normocytes:* the normal cell, 7.5 to 8.5 μm in diameter.

2. *Macrocytes:* 9 to 12 μm in diameter.

3. *Microcytes:* 6 μm in diameter or smaller.

4. *Sickle cells:* shaped like sickles, these erythrocytes occur in the disease *sickle cell anemia.*

F. *Staining characteristics*

1. Romanowsky-type stains: hematoxylin, eosin-azure II, and methylene blue tinge erythrocytes a reddish hue, attesting to their *acidophilia.* Hemoglobin has an affinity for the acidic portion of the stains.

2. *Reticulated erythrocytes* (Fig. 5-1) in the peripheral circulation acquire an even bluish tint with most blood stains. The residual polyribosomes are responsible for this *basophilia.*

a. When immature erythrocytes are stained with brilliant cresyl blue, the residual polyribosomes form fine strands resembling a reticulum. The name reticulated erythrocyte given to immature peripheral blood erythrocytes emphasizes this characteristic.

b. Reticulated erythrocytes, forming 1 to 2% of the circulating erthrocyte population provide a rough index of erythrocyte formation. A higher percentage would signal that erythrocytes are being released too rapidly in response to a need for oxygen. Such a condition occurs at high altitudes.

G. EM characteristics (Tanaka and Goodman, 1972)

1. TEM: The mature erythrocyte is recognized by the lack of a nucleus and the uniform distribution of the electron-dense hemoglobin pigment. This unique density is attributed to the high content of hemoglobin-bound iron.

2. TEM: Reticulated erythrocytes exhibit profiles of polyribosomes and occasional mitochondria in addition to the hemoglobin.

3. SEM: (Elgsaeter et al, 1986). The three-dimensional biconcave disk shape of the erythrocyte is appreciated best in scanning electron micrographs. Crenated erythrocytes appear smaller than normal erythrocytes with finger-like protrusions covering the surface.

IV. The *leucocytes* (Fig. 5-1). [Please note the spelling. In the current Latin-based *Nomina Histologica*, the spelling is leuco- instead of leuko- since there is no "k" in Latin.] The blood leucocytes (white blood cells) are recognized by characteristic nuclear configurations and the reactions of cytoplasmic granules to Romanowsky-type stains.

A. Two categories of leucocytes are distinguished: *agranular leucocytes* and *granular leucocytes* based on the presence of *specific granules* in the cytoplasm. Percentages refer to the leucocytes in the "buffy layer or coat." Numbers may vary according to the time of day, presence of food in the digestive tract, site of removal of a blood sample, and the influence of disease. The latter may reduce the total number of leucocytes below 5000/mm³ or increase it far above 13,000/mm³.

1. *Agranular leucocytes:* Although these cells are classified as agranular, it should be realized that some azurophilic (affinity for azure dyes in blood stains) nonspecific granules occur in their cytoplasm.

a. *Agranular lymphocytes* occur in gradient sizes from the *small lymphocyte* to the *medium-sized lymphocyte* to the *large lymphocyte* to the largest *monocyte*. In the small lymphocyte, the cytoplasm forms a thin rim around the nucleus. Progression through the several sizes reflects the increasing amounts of cytoplasm. The largest agranular cells are indigenous to lymphatic tissues and bone marrow, where they are recognized as *stem cells* or *hemocytoblasts*.

b. *Lymphocytes:* Three sizes — small, medium, and large — comprise 20 to 40% of the total leucocyte (granular and agranular) count.

(1) *Small lymphocytes*, 6 to 8 µm in diameter, are mostly nucleus with a thin rim of cytoplasm. In preparations stained with

Wright's stain or Giemsa stain, nuclear details are obscured. In tissue culture, lymphocytes move in a "hand mirror" fashion, with the nucleus advancing while the cytoplasm trails behind (Amenta, 1967). Nucleoli, a cytocentrum nidating in a nuclear indentation, and heterochromatin associated with the nucleolemma can be visualized. Via TEM, mitochondria and azurophilic nonspecific granules are resolved with great clarity and definition.

(2) *Medium* and *large lymphocytes*, up to 18 μm in diameter, possess a slightly larger nucleus, but the quantity of cytoplasm is markedly increased. Cytoplasmic structures present in the smaller lymphocytes also occur in these larger cells, in addition to the azurophilic granules, which are probably *lysosomes*.

(3) Lymphocytes are involved in the immune responses of the body where they regulate the production of antibodies. Functionally, at least three categories of lymphocytes are distinguished by immunofluorescent surface markers, *T lymphocytes, B lymphocytes* and *null lymphocytes* (Greaves et al, 1974).

(a) *T lymphocytes* (forming several subclasses) play a significant role in cell-mediated immunity by screening out antigenic foreign cells and interacting with the macrophages to destroy foreign cells. T lymphocytes produce a group of factors, the *lymphokines*, that stimulate macrophages to initiate phagocytic functions (Yoshida and Kobayashi, 1985). T lymphocytes, accounting for 80% of the circulating lymphocytes, have a relatively long life span (Bevan and Fink, 1978).

[1] *"Helper" T lymphocytes* literally "help" the other category of lymphocytes, the *B lymphocytes*, to produce antibodies.

[2] *"Suppressor" T lymphocytes* suppress the production of antibodies by B lymphocytes. The mechanisms involved in "helping" and "suppressing" are not quite clear.

[3] *"Killer" T lymphocytes* produce a variety of cytotoxic substances with the ability to destroy cancer cells or grafts of foreign tissue.

(b) *B lymphocytes* account for about 10% of the circulating lymphocytes. These specialized cells can be stimulated to divide a number of times prior to differentiating into the *plasma cell*, which produces immunoglobulins. (The plasma cell will be considered in Chapter 6.) One group of immunoglobulins, the *opsonins*, invest foreign invaders (ie, bacteria) with a delicious substance that encourages phagocytosis by macrophages.

(c) *Null lymphocytes*, comprising about 5% of the circulating lymphocytes, are so named because they possess neither of the immunofluorescent surface markers that distinguish T lymphocytes or B lymphocytes. Some investigators consider null lymphocytes as pluripotential cells comparable to the stem cell or hemocytoblast. Indeed, it was the great histologist Alexander Maximow (1930), followed by his protege William Bloom, who expounded the *unitarian theory* of blood cell formation at a time when all others claimed that there were two or more stem cells (*dualistic theory*). Maximow proposed the small lymphocyte as a totipotent cell equivalent to the hemocytoblast, while others claimed the small lymphocyte was a terminal cell with no further potential. Modern immunological studies appear to support the proposals of Maximow and Bloom.

(4) Lymphocytes display a remarkable capacity for *immunological memory*. Immunological surface markers on lymphocytes are so numerous that for each *antigen* there is one specific responsive lymphocyte. It appears there are as many lymphocyte types as there are antigens. Upon exposure to a supposed invading foreign *antigen "X,"* a lymphocyte is stimulated to undergo numerous mitotic divisions to produce a clone of similar lymphocytes.

(a) Immediately some of these, the *B lymphocytes*, differentiate into plasma cells that produce *antibodies* against that specific *antigen "X."* The plasma cell, in this instance, is called an *effector cell*.

(b) The remaining lymphocytes in the pool, termed *memory lymphocytes*, become inactive until *antigen "X"* reappears on the scene. Whenever this time arrives, and it may take years, the memory lymphocytes "remember" and respond more rapidly and more aggressively than did the first effector cells.

c. *Monocytes*, the largest of the agranulocytes, (10 to 20 μm in diameter) comprise 2 to 8% of the total leucocytes in the circulating blood. Their morphological characteristics are virtually impossible to distinguish from the hemocytoblast (stem cell) in the bone marrow.

(1) The early name, *the macrophage*, has been well earned. In circulating blood it is a dormant cell in its short life span (up to 100 hours), but upon gaining access to the connective tissues, the monocyte can become a voracious macrophage. Most probably it dies there, for no evidence has been forthcoming that it reenters the circulation.

(2) Nuclear chromatin is dispersed widely as euchromatin, rather than the heterochromatin clumps seen in lymphocytes. Two to three nucleoli are characteristic of this nucleus.

(3) The faint basophilia of the cytoplasm is attributed to some free ribosomes and polyribosomes, minimal profiles of granular endoplasmic reticulum, and some lysosomal azurophilic granules. Elongated mitochrondria are distributed evenly throughout the cyto-

plasm. The cytocentrum, housing the centrioles, nidates in the in-dented, eccentrically placed *nucleus*. Associated with this region is a well-developed golgi complex. Fanning out from the centrosome are microfilaments and microtubules similar to "astral rays" in mitosis.

   2. *Granular leucocytes:* Three types of granular leucocytes are distinguished via staining properties with Romanowsky-type stains. The granules characterizing these cells are termed *specific granules* as opposed to *nonspecific* azurophilic granules. The three types are neu-trophils, acidophils, and basophils.

   a. *Neutrophils* (polymorphonuclear leucocytes or polys), com-prise 50 to 70% of peripheral blood leucocytes. Consequently, in a "normal" blood smear, this leucocyte cell type should predominate (Murphy, 1976).

   (1) They measure from 10 to 15 μm in diameter and have an extremely short life span of up to 4 hours in peripheral blood. If they are successful in gaining entrance to the connective tissues, their life span is extended up to 4 days.

   (2) The *neutrophil nucleus* in peripheral blood, with one to five lobes, provides invaluable information to the hematologist. A cell with one lobe in a horseshoe shape, the *"band-neutrophil,"* is consid-ered immature, while one with five lobes is mature. Peripheral blood smears provide evidence of bone marrow activity. If most neutrophils possess one or two lobes, there is a "shift to the left," that is, too many immature cells are being produced. The hematologist must determine whether this shift is a transient or a sign of pathological problems. Likewise, a "shift to the right" (too many five-lobed nuclei) signals that the bone marrow is failing to replenish the supply of neutrophils. This explanation of lobulation is not quite that simple, for in some diseases, *immature five-lobed nuclei* appear. In females, a *"drumstick"* appendage to one of the lobes represents the inactive heterochromatic *X chromosome*. This characteristic is not always obvious, because the appendage may have been folded under one of the lobes during preparation of the smear.

   (3) The *neutrophil cytoplasm* contains two thirds specific granules and one third *azurophilic granules* (Bainton et al, 1971).

   (a) Membrane-bound *specific granules* are spherical in shape and measure about 0.1 μm in diameter. Some elongated ones appear via TEM. While difficult to resolve with the light microscope, the variation in staining from a faint blue to a delicate pink acknowl-edges their presence. The term *neutrophil* aptly characterizes their staining properties. Via TEM, the specific neutrophil granules are membrane bound. Several substances have been localized in these granules: lysozyme, lactoferrin, alkaline phosphatase, and collagenase. The azurophilic granules are primary lysosomes. Mitochondria, a golgi complex, some free polyribosomes, and liberal amounts of glycogen round out the cytoplasmic structures.

(b) *Azurophilic granules*, in addition to lysozyme, alkaline phosphatase, and collagenase, also contain the antibacterial myeloperoxidase and several other substances (Bainton and Farquhar, 1970).

(4) Neutrophils are scavenger phagocytes in connective tissues, maneuvering about by ameboid movement as they develop cytotoxins to destroy phagocytized bacteria. The lysozymes in the azurophilic granules hydrolyse dead bacteria, which then diffuse out of the plasmalemma into the surrounding connective tissues. These cells are so voracious that they will confront any and all comers: carbon particles, bacteria, whole cells, and even slivers. The white pus of an infection is an accumulation of neutrophils that died in the line of duty. The attraction of neutrophils to dead or dying cells is termed *necrotaxis*, a form of *chemotaxis*.

(5) Ameboid movement is studied readily in tissue culture (Ramsey, 1972). Whereas lymphocytes traveled in a "hand-mirror" fashion with the nucleus leading, the neutrophil does the opposite: the nucleus tails behind a leading flow of cytoplasm in the advancing pseudopodium.

b. *Acidophils* (eosinophils) (Beeson and Bass, 1977) [The prefix acido- replaces the more limited prefix eosino-, avoiding dye reference in preference to general staining affinity.]: The *acidophils* number from 1 to 5% of the circulating blood. In a fresh drop of blood, the spherical acidophil measures about 9 μm in diameter, but in a smear preparation it may flatten to 15 μm in diameter. The golgi complex, rER or sER, and mitochondria are poorly developed, but cytoplasmic glycogen is abundant.

(1) *Specific granules* (Bainton and Farquhar, 1970): In humans, highly refractile membrane-bound granules (about 200 per cell) exhibit an affinity for the acidic portion of Romanowsky-type stains. They range from 0.5 to 1.5 μm in length and 0.3 to 1.0 μm in width. Each granule is composed of an *internum* and an *externum*.

(a) The *internum* is the elongated, laminated, crystalline, electron-dense core composed of a protein. The many arginine residues in the protein are responsible for the acidophilia of the granules. This proteinaceous material is deadly to helminthic parasites (schistosomes).

(b) The *externum* is the electron-lucent material surrounding the core. It provides the proper environment for the following enzymes: acid phosphatase (capable of causing lysis), myeloperoxidase, RNAase, and about five others. The myeloperoxidase of acidophils does not exhibit the great antibacteriocidal activity as does that of neutrophils. Ultraviolet microbeam irradiation of acidophils in tissue culture may release some of the enzymes that cause nuclear pyknosis (Amenta, 1962).

(2) The eccentric bilobed *nucleus* is united by a thin strand of chromatin. The cytocentrum in the clear cytoplasmic area between the lobes is partially surrounded by acidophil granules that appear to push the nuclear lobes to the periphery of the cell.

(3) Eosinophils display an ameboid motion with the nucleus trailing behind the granules in the advancing pseudopodia.

(4) The complete role of acidophils is not quite clear, but they do increase in total numbers in allergic conditions and parasitic infections. In these conditions, elevated numbers occur in the mucosa of the respiratory tract, digestive tract, and reproductive tract. Invading parasites are usually coated with actively phagocytic acidophils.

(5) Some drugs exhibit an influence on the acidophil population. Corticosteroids, for example, cause a decrease in peripheral blood acidophils, but not in those of bone marrow. Speculation exists that corticosteroids interfere with the release of acidophils from bone marrow.

c. *Basophils* (Dvorak, 1978), measuring about 10 – 15 μm in diameter, make up no more than 1% of the total leucocyte count in circulating blood, which accounts for the difficulties experienced by students in locating basophils. This problem may be alleviated by examining dry blood smears toward the edges of the slide. When a drop of blood is dragged across the slide, the basophils usually are swirled outward by the created currents. In tissue cultures, the gently phagocytic ameboid basophil moves about with the nucleus first, dragging the granular cytoplasm.

(1) The bilobed *nucleus* does not have as much heterochromatin as the acidophil or the neutrophil, but in smears this is difficult to discern because the large nonuniform basophilic granules tend to obscure nuclear details.

(2) That the *basophilic-specific granules* exhibit metachromasia is attributed to their high content of the anticoagulant heparin. In addition, the granules contain histamine, which generates *leucotrienes* responsible for slow contraction of smooth muscle. To preserve these large, irregularly shaped granules, alcohol fixatives must be

used, because the granules are soluble in aqueous fixatives. With Romanowsky dyes, they stain a deep purple. Electron microscopy reveals that the granules are membrane bound and filled with "mini-granules" of uniform size.

    d. *Thrombocytes* (White and Clawson, 1980): In circulating blood are small plasmalemma-bound fragments detached from bone marrow megacaryocytes. These are the *thrombocytes* (platelets), which are variable in size and shape and average about $3\mu m$ in width. They may contain any of the basic cytoplasmic structures found in megacaryocytes: microtubules, mitochondria, peroxisomes, lyso-somes, alpha granules, delta granules, and glycogen. In dry smears, clumped thrombocytes stain pink along with some dark basophilic granules. Thrombocytes present two recognizable parts under the light microscope: a dark central *granulomere*, surrounded by the lighter blue stained *hyalomere*.

    (1) *Thrombocytopenia* is a condition of thrombocyte defi-ciency associated with hemorrhage.

    (2) Attached thrombocytes in tissue culture exhibit a re-markable rigidity that can deform the plasmalemma of passing eryth-rocytes or other cells.

    (3) Thrombocytes

        (a) assist in the clotting of blood,

        (b) participate in stimulating contraction of injured blood vessels to control hemorrhage,

        (c) plug defects in vascular endothelium by adhering to each other and almost any available surface (because of a glycocalyx rich in glycosaminoglycans and glycoproteins).

V. *Lymph* is an ultrafiltrate of blood plasma.

    A. Lymph originates in the connective tissue interstices where cap-illary networks release fluid from the arterial side of the capillary bed and recapture it on the venous side of the capillary bed. Excess fluid crosses the endothelium of "blind" unidirectional lymphatic capil-laries, which flow into larger vessels of the lymphatic system. Blockage of the lymphatic capillaries results in *edema* (accumulation of fluid) in the connective tissues.

    B. The composition of lymph fluid (water, electrolytes, and from 2 to 5% of proteins) varies in different parts of the body. For example, the lymph fluid in the *lacteals* (blind-ended capillaries of the intestinal villi) differs from that in the connective tissue of the dorsum of the hand. Lymph fluid in lacteals is usually filled with *chylomicrons* that were transported from the intestinal lumen through the absorptive cells of the digestive tract and then into the lacteals.

C. Lymph flows centrally toward larger vessels and eventually to the largest lymphatic vessels that empty into the blood vascular system.

D. During this journey, lymph nodes are encountered, through which the lymph fluid percolates and *small lymphocytes* are added. Rarely, and usually in pathological conditions, *larger lymphocytes* could be added.

E. In the largest lymphatic vessels, lymph resembles blood plasma and may even clot to form a soft gelatinous mass.

F. Before entering the circulation, lymph fluid is found to contain (1) tissue fluids, (2) lymphocytes, (3) lipids, and (4) occasionally some blood cells.

Questions

DIRECTIONS: For each of the items in this section, one or more of the numbered options is correct. Select

    A if only *1, 2, and 3* are correct
    B if only *1 and 3* are correct
    C if only *2 and 4* are correct
    D if only *4* is correct
    E if *all* are correct

1. In a freshly drawn sample of blood, the greatest percentage of all the sedimented cells belongs to
   1. basophils
   2. neutrophils
   3. acidophils
   4. erythrocytes

2. Blood plasma contains a number of substances. Which of the following are among them?
   1. Water
   2. Proteins
   3. Inorganic salts
   4. Hormones

3. If the concentration of salts within erythrocytes is greater than the concentration of salts in the solution in which they are suspended, then which of the following pertain?
   1. The cells become microcytes
   2. The solution is hypotonic
   3. The cell membrane becomes impermeable.
   4. Hemolysis occurs.

4. Lymphocytes
   1. move in a hand mirror fashion, nucleus first
   2. are involved in regulation of antibody production
   3. form three distinct groups based on surface markers
   4. possess specific granules in their cytoplasm

5. The monocyte
   1. dies in the connective tissues
   2. has an intense cytoplasmic basophilia
   3. becomes a macrophage
   4. morphologically resembles no other cell

6. Neutrophils
   1. live only 4 hours in peripheral blood
   2. with "band" nuclei are considered immature
   3. with a "drumstick" nuclear appendage are from females
   4. have 2/3 specific granules and 1/3 azurophilic granules in the cytoplasm

7. Acidophil (eosinophil) granules
   1. are highly refractile
   2. have an electron-dense core with substances that are deadly to parasites
   3. have an electron-lucent layer containing several enzymes.
   4. are azurophilic

8. Basophil granules
   1. are preserved with aqueous fixatives
   2. contain heparin and histamine
   3. have a uniform morphology
   4. exhibit metachromasia

		Directions Summarized		
A	**B**	**C**	**D**	**E**
1,2,3	1,3	2,4	4	All are
only	only	only	only	correct

9. Thrombocytes
   1. possess several basic cytoplasmic structures
   2. move with the nucleus advancing and cytoplasm trailing
   3. assist in the clotting of blood
   4. are derived from B lymphocytes

10. Lymph
    1. is an ultrafiltrate of blood plasma
    2. is derived from connective tissue fluid
    3. contains water, electrolytes, and proteins
    4. acquires lymphocytes as it passes through lymph nodes

Explanatory Answers

1. D. The answer is the erythrocytes, which form 40% of the total sedimented cells. Because the neutrophil makes up to 50 to 70% of the total leucocyte count, one might be tempted to include neutrophils and erythrocytes as the answer. The question specifically asks for the greatest percentage of all the sedimented cells.

2. E. Blood plasma contains all the components listed in the question. Among the proteins are albumins, globulins, and fibrinogen. In addition to the hormones, there are lipids, enzymes, vitamins, and carbohydrates.

3. C. In a hypotonic solution, water crosses the plasmalemma, causing the cell to swell, first resembling a macrocyte and ultimately bursting to release the hemoglobin. The erythrocyte shell is called a *shadow* or a *ghost*. Answer 1 is incorrect because the microcyte is smaller than the normocyte. Answer 3 is incorrect because the plasmalemma increases permeability to permit water to enter in an attempt to equalize the concentration of salts.

4. A. The first three are correct. Answer 4 is incorrect because specific granules are characteristic of the granular leucocytes. The granules in lymphocytes are the azurophilic lysosome granules. Characteristic movements of leucocytes in tissue culture assist with identification in experimental conditions. Lymphocytes and basophils move with the nucleus at the head trailing a tail of cytoplasm. Neutrophils and acidophils move with pseudopodia advancing while the nucleus trails behind.

5. B. 1 and 3 are correct. 1. There is no evidence that the monocyte ever returns to the circulation once it enters the connective tissues. 3. In the connective tissues it becomes a macrophage with a voracious phagocytic appetite. 2. The abundant cytoplasm stains faintly basophilic because there are only minimal amounts of ribosomes, polyribosomes, and azurophilic granules. 4. The monocyte in the peripheral blood can be identified, but in bone marrow it can not be distinguished from the hemocytoblast or stem cell.

6. E. All are correct. 1. If neutrophils leave the peripheral blood they may live up to 4 days in connective tissue. 2. The band or stab neutrophil possesses one elongated nucleus that may be formed into a horseshoe shape or may fold upon itself to resemble a dagger, hence the name "stab" cell. The more nuclear lobes the older the cell, or in certain diseases more immature multilobulated nuclei appear. 3. The drumstick is the inactive heterchromatinized X-chromosome. 4. This is true.

7. B. The granules in human acidophilic granulocytes are all rather uniform and large enough to be resolved. They are specific granules in contrast to the nonspecific azurophilc granules.

8. C. 2 and 4 are correct. Heparin is an anticoagulant. Histamine generates leukotrienes, which are responsible for the slow contraction of smooth muscle. Basophil granules are not uniform in size, but they are filled with mini-granules of uniform size.

9. C. 2 and 4 are correct. There is no nucleus in the thrombocyte, since it is a cytoplasmic fragment of the bone marrow megacaryocyte. The B lymphocyte gives rise to the plasma cell and not the thrombocytes.

10. E. All are correct. Lymph fluid is derived as an ultrafiltrate of blood plasma. After traversing the capillary endothelium, it enters the connective tissue spaces. Some of the fluid returns to the venous side of the capillary bed, while the rest enters the blind lymphatic capillaries and flows through successively larger lymphatic channels until it enters the circulatory system. On its journey lymph passes through lymph nodes, which add lymphocytes to change the composition of the lymph.

6 Cartilage Tissue

I. *Introduction*: Cartilage, as a structural connective tissue, provides exceptional qualities of support, firmness, plasticity, elasticity, and resiliency. In the embryo these qualities are advantageous in providing a provisional skeleton. Various forms of cartilage persist in the adult where the uniqueness of cartilage cannot be substituted by bone or other tissues (Hall, 1983).

A. The *chondrocyte*, the singular resident *cell type*, nestles in a soft but firm matrix cavity, the *cartilaginous lacuna*.

1. Each *chondrocyte* may divide (by mitosis) several times to form an isogenous group of chondrocytes.

2. Several isogenous groups form *chondrocyte aggregates*, consisting of *cell matrix territories* and *interterritorial matrix*.

3. Ultrastructure of chondrocytes

a. The nuclear chromatin is distributed as

(1) Heterochromatin attached to the inner leaf of the nuclear membrane, and

(2) active euchromatin in the extended form.

b. A prominent nucleolus is located eccentrically.

c. An irregular nucleolemma (nuclear membrane) shows pores where inner and outer leaves fuse.

d. Granular endoplasmic reticulum (rER) characterizes active chondrocytes. The cisternae are dilated with product to be packaged by the golgi complex.

4. The external surface of the plasmalemma is populated by microvilli, which anchor the chondrocyte in the matrix.

5. Inactive chondrocytes contain cytoplasmic lipid droplets that coalesce to form unilocular droplets similar to those in white adipocytes.

B. The *interterritorial matrix*

    1. Biochemical substances (Chakrabarti and Park, 1980)

    a. sulfated glycosaminoglycans (chondroitin-4-sulfate and chondroitin-6-sulfate)

    b. keratan sulfate

    c. some hyaluronic acid

    d. others

    2. Three zones around the cartilage cell territories are distinguished on the basis of staining characteristics:

    a. an inner zone of basophilia immediately around each lacuna and cluster of lacunae defining areas of greatest concentration of the strongly acidic sulfated groups.

    b. an outer zone of acidophilia surrounds the rim of a basophilic proteoglycan matrix.

    c. interterritorial zones, with minimal to no apparent staining.

    3. *Matrix fibers* (which assist in classification of cartilage) are collagen types I and II and elastic fibers.

II. *Classification:* While three types of cartilage, *hyaline cartilage*, *fibrous cartilage*, and *elastic cartilage* can be distinguished, it must be emphasized that gradations from one type to another occur normally and pathologically (Fig. 6-1).

    A. *Hyaline cartilage* presents a "glassy," homogeneous, bluish-white appearance in the fresh condition. Its smooth slippery external surface is suited for smooth movements in joint surfaces (Kuettner et al, 1986).

    1. Only type II collagen fibers are distinguished in the interterritorial matrix. These randomly oriented fibers have the same refractive index as the matrix, and hence are difficult to resolve with light microscopy (Minns and Stevens, 1977). Type II collagen fibers

    a. are very thin (about 10 to 20 nm),

    b. consist of tropocollagen molecules composed of three alpha chains,

    c. appear to have no definable banding patterns, (apparently there is less polymerization than in other types of collagen).

    d. are absent from zones surrounding each lacuna.

    2. Hyaline cartilage occurs in the

    a. embryo as a provisional skeleton,

    b. fetal and neonatal developing long bones,

    c. adult

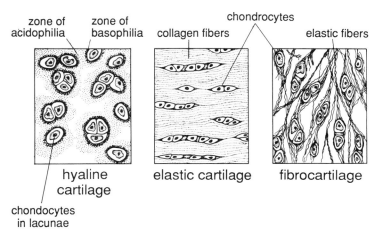

Figure 6-1 Three types of cartilage.

(1) articular surfaces of long bones,
(2) epiphyseal plate of growing long bones,
(3) ends of ribs articulating with the sternum,
(4) nose, larynx, and tracheobronchial tree.

B. *Elastic cartilage* is similar to hyaline cartilage in structure and development, except that in addition to type II collagen fibers, there are scattered *elastic fibers* that are packed more densely around the lacunae. The similarity is emphasized in some areas where the two types coexist. The number of elastic fibers decreases peripherally toward the perichondrium. Elastic cartilage, yellowish in its natural state, provides flexible support in the

1. external ear,

2. epiglottis,

3. auditory tube (Eustachian tube),

4. corniculate and cuneiform cartilages of the larynx.

C. *Fibrous cartilage* (fibrocartilage) is distinguished by massive numbers of cationic type I collagen bundles, which confer a distinct acidophilia to the sparse extracellular matrix. In contrast to hyaline or elastic cartilage, the perichondrium is absent. Chondrocytes exist singly, in pairs, in clusters, or assembled in columns between the collagen fiber bundles. Fibrous cartilage is found where tensile strength, ability to withstand shocks, firm support, and resilience are required, particularly in the

    1. Intervertebral disks that are interposed between individual vertebral bodies. The upper and lower surfaces of each intervertebral disk are coated with thin layers of hyaline cartilage, which anchors into the corresponding vertebral bodies. Around the sides, the disk attaches to the anterior longitudinal ligament and the posterior longitudinal ligament. A perichondrium is lacking. Each disk consists of two major components:

    a. an **annulus fibrosus** of concentric lamellae of fibrous cartilage extending obliquely from one vertebra to another. The alternating patterns of fiber bundles form a characteristic herringbone pattern.

    (1) The lamellae are thinner and less numerous posteriorly than anteriorly.

    (2) Peripheral parts of the annulus fibrosus may be supplied by adjacent blood vessels.

    b. an oval **nucleus pulposus** (a remnant of the embryonic notochord), enclosed in the center by the concentric lamellae of the annulus fibrosus. It is the annulus fibrosis that acts as a shock absorber, and not the nucleus pulposus.

    (1) The nucleus pulposus is composed of a few notochordal spherical cells dispersed in a semiliquid, gelatinous matrix rich in hyaluronic acid and keratan sulfate.

    (2) With increasing age (starting at age 10), the nucleus pulposus regresses (dehydration and degeneration) and is replaced by fibrous cartilage.

    (3) After age 20, injury to the fibrous cartilage may result in herniation of the mucoid substance, which impinges on nerves exiting the spinal cord. This injury, commonly called a dislocated or "slipped" disk, compresses adjacent spinal nerve roots, causing leg pain or low back pain.

    2. Symphysis pubica joining the pubic bones. The bone ends are coated with hyaline cartilage into which the midline fibrous cartilage anchors. A slit-like, fluid-filled cavity in the fibrous cartilage enlarges during pregnancy to permit the increased movement required during parturition.

    3. And in a few areas where it might appear as a *transitional form* between hyaline cartilage and compact connective tissue, such as *menisci*. (In the adult, compact connective tissue may readily transform to fibrous cartilage.)

4. Fibrous cartilage also is associated with
   a. joint capsules (example: the rim of the glenoid fossa of the scapula),
   b. insertions of tendons into bone, where compact connective tissue may form fibrous cartilage.

III. Chondrohistogenesis (development of cartilage) of all forms of cartilage follows a similar sequence commencing with the mesenchyme (Fig. 6-2).

A. In the embryo, mesenchymal cells round up and assemble into clusters of *prechondral tissue*. Cells hypertrophy (enlarge) and differentiate into *chondroblasts*.

B. Chondroblasts synthesize the metachromatic sulfated glycosaminoglycan matrix. Continued production of the pericellular matrix isolates and segregates clusters of cells. Chondroblasts multiply to form isogenous groups of chondrocytres.

C. As the matrix density increases, it becomes increasingly difficult for cell multiplication to occur; there just is no more room.

D. While the matrix is relatively soft, cartilage grows from within by *interstitial increments* (interstitial growth). This *proliferation status* occurs only in the early embryo. The progeny from a single chondroblast increase by mitoses with every cell contributing to the intercellu-

Figure 6-2 Chondrohistogenesis.

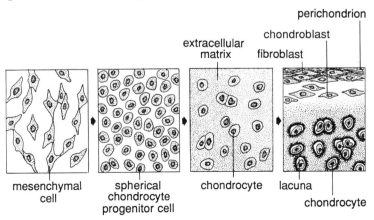

lar matrix. Interstitial growth increases cell numbers, which produce the increasing amount of matrix in the center of the growing cartilage.

E. Aging matrix hardens to the extent that interstitial growth becomes impossible. Therefore, continued growth in width and length is feasible only by *appositional increments* at the cartilage periphery. In appositional growth, fibroblasts originating from the inner layer of **perichondrium** differentiate into chondroblasts that will synthesize additional matrix and provide new cells.

1. The **perichondrium** is a dense fibrous collagenous sheath surrounding the cartilage matrix.

2. The **perichondrium** is continuous with the cartilage it surrounds and with the loose connective tissue surrounding it.

3. Two layers form the perichondrium:
   a. **stratum fibrosum,** resembling compact connective tissue with flattened fibroblasts.
   b. **stratum cellulare,** a cellular layer with the cartilage progenitor cells.

4. Fibroblasts in the perichondrium are flattened by the density of the collagenous fibers, but those closer to the cartilage matrix, in the *stratum cellulare*, assume the characteristics of *chondroblasts*.

5. Chondroblasts are the generative cells of cartilage.
   a. They actively form sulfated glycosaminoglycans.
   b. The nuclei are spherical with one or two small nucleoli.
   c. The cytoplasm contains lipid droplets that provide nourishment to isolated chondrocytes.

6. The vascular supply is abundant in the connective tissues surrounding the cartilage, but in more mature cartilage there are no blood vessels, nerves, or lymphatics in the cartilage matrix. Consequently, chondrocytes isolated from the blood vessels by the matrix depend upon the nutritional value of stored lipid. In the early embryo, cartilage developing in the mesenchyme is highly vascularized. In later stages, the degree of vascularization decreases. In mature avascular cartilage, nutritional demands are met by *cartilage canals* in the matrix and by *diffusion*. When cartilage becomes too thick, the increased diffusion distance (3 mm) is too great, and after depletion of the lipid content, the chondrocytes perish from lack of nutrition.

F. Injury to cartilage is followed by activation of the normally quiescent perichondrium. Fibroblasts differentiate into chondroblasts, which are capable of repairing and replenishing the injured cartilage.

If damage is too extensive, compact connective tissue forms instead of cartilage.

Questions

DIRECTIONS: For each of the items in this section, one or more of the numbered options is correct. Select

    A if only *1, 2, and 3* are correct
    B if only *1 and 3* are correct
    C if only *2 and 4* are correct
    D if only *4* is correct
    E if *all* are correct

1. The active chondrocyte
    1. resides in a cartilaginous lacuna
    2. has a prominent golgi complex
    3. produces cartilage matrix
    4. has an acidophilic cytoplasm

2. The interterritorial martrix of cartilage contains
    1. proteoglycans
    2. a rich vasculature
    3. fibers
    4. sensory nerve fibers

3. Hyaline cartilage possesses
    1. elastic fibers
    2. type I collagen fibers
    3. reticular fibers
    4. type II collagen fibers

4. Fibrous cartilage (fibrocartilage)
    1. has a two-layered perichondrium
    2. contains type I collagen fibers
    3. is well vascularized
    4. forms the annulus fibrosis of intervertebral disks

		Directions Summarized		
A	**B**	**C**	**D**	**E**
1,2,3	1,3	2,4	4	All are
only	only	only	only	correct

5. Elastic cartilage
   1. has a two-layered perichondrium
   2. contains type II collagen fibers
   3. provides a flexible form of support
   4. contains elastic fibers

6. The intervertebral disk
   1. anchors into hyaline cartilage
   2. forms the concentric layers of annulus fibrosus
   3. contains the nucleus pulposis
   4. surrounds a slit-like, fluid-filled cavity

7. The perichondrium
   1. is required around all forms of cartilage
   2. consists of concentric layers of the annulus fibrosus
   3. is composed of compact collagenous connective tissue
   4. consists of two layers

8. The interterritorial matrix of cartilage contains
   1. sulfated glycosaminoglycans
   2. histamine
   3. keratan sulfate
   4. heparin

9. Cartilage grows by
   1. decreasing the vascular supply
   2. interstitial increments
   3. invasion of connective tissue elements
   4. appositional increments

10. On the basis of staining characteristics, cartilage matrix
    1. is metachromatic
    2. has a zone of acidophilia surrounding zones around lacunae
    3. has little to no stain in interterritorial zones
    4. has a zone of basophilia around each lacuna

Explanatory Answers

1. A. 1, 2, and 3 are correct. 4 is wrong. The cytoplasm is basophilic because of the presence of granular endoplasmic reticulum. The matrix is synthesized in the rER, packaged in the prominent golgi complex, and discharged through the plasmalemma. Each chondrocyte resides in a lacuna of cartilaginous matrix.

2. B. 1 and 3 are correct. The proteoglycans form the embedment for the various fibers that characterize the cartilage types (I, II, and elastic). Only in the early embryonic mesenchyme are blood vessels found. Once the mesenchyme coalesces to form small islands of chondroblasts, the vasculature remains peripheral. Generally, cartilage is avascular and asensory.

3. D. 4 is correct. Only type II collagen fibers occur in hyaline cartilage. These are delicate fibers with no apparent banding patterns. The other fibers are not found in hyaline cartilage in normal conditions.

4. C. 2 and 4 are correct. Fibrous cartilage contains type I collagen fibers in the annulus fibrosus of the intervertebral disk. Only at the very periphery is fibrous cartilage sometimes vascularized, otherwise it receives nutrition as do the other two forms of cartilage. Fibrous cartilage lacks a perichondrium.

5. E. All are correct. In addition to elastic fibers, there are many type II fibers. The flexible support required of the external ear and the epiglottis, for example, is provided by elastic cartilage. Like hyaline cartilage, a perichondrium covers the elastic cartilage.

6. A. 1, 2, and 3 are correct. The slit-like fluid-filled cavity is found in the symphysis pubis. The disk has the nucleus pulposis, derived from the embryonic notochord, to act as a shock absorber.

7. D. Only 4 is correct. Perichondrium does not form around fibrous cartilage, only hyaline and elastic cartilage. The perichondrium consists of two layers, an outer compact collagenous connective tissue and an inner vascular with chondrogenic potencies.

8. B. 1 and 3 are correct. In addition to the sulfated glycosaminoglycans and keratan sulfate, there also is some hyaluronic acid. Heparin and histamine are mediators produced by tissue basophils and blood basophils.

9. C. 2 and 4 are correct. In early chondrohistogenesis, the softer cartilage grows from within by adding increments of cartilage matrix (interstitial increments). After formation of the perichondrium, and after the matrix hardens, continued growth in width and length occurs only by adding increments at the periphery (appositional increments). Decreasing the blood supply to the perichondrium will cause immediate death. Invasion of connective tissue elements will begin to form bone.

10. E. All are correct. There is a gradual gradation of metachromasia from one territory of cells to another. These are artificially designated into three zones: the zone surrounding the lacunar embedded cells is strongly basophilic. As the distance increases away from the lacunae, the degree of basophilia decreases until it is acidophilic. About midway between two territories, substances that diffuse from chondrocyte are minimal to none, and hence there is little to no stain to the lacunae.

7 Osseous Tissue

I. *Introduction:* The concept of *osseous tissue* as a static organ was superseded by one of dynamism, in which bone is recognized as a living tissue constantly undergoing remodeling. *Bone* serves as a mineral depot, particularly for regulation of calcium homeostasis. The turnover of bone occurs via two essential remodeling processes: bone formation and bone resorption. *Bone* density and strength, reaching its peak between 30 and 35 years of age, is attributed to an orderly calcification of the extracellular matrix. Its structural integrity, hardness, and ability to withstand stress are attributed to the unique organization of *organic* and *inorganic* components in the extracellular matrix (Bourne, 1972; Hancox, 1972).

A. *Organic components* in the extracellular matrix

1. Collagenous proteins: 95% are *type I collagen fibers*

2. Noncollagenous proteins: 5%

a. *glycoproteins* which bind calcium and promote calcification, examples:

(1) *osteopontin*, a bone sialoprotein, is synthesized by osteoblasts and appears to function in cell – matrix adhesion interactions (Oldberg et al, 1986; Mark et al, 1987).

(2) *osteonectin*, synthesized by osteoblasts, is found in high concentrations in bone extracellular matrix and in thrombocytes (platelets) (Termine et al, 1981; Bolander et al, 1988).

b. *glycosaminoglycans*

(1) chondroitin-4-sulfate

(2) chondroitin-6-sulfate

(3) keratan sulfate

c. *phosphoproteins*

d. *bone Gla protein* (BGP, osteocalcin), a small protein isolated from the extracellular matrix. BGP, synthesized by osteoblasts, has proved useful for clinical analysis of bone metabolism (Nishimoto and Price, 1980).

3. Extraction of the organic components leaves the bone (example: fibula) hard and looking every bit like the original bone. However, it is as brittle as chalk and will, in fact, write on a blackboard. This observation leads to the conclusion that bone hardness is attributed to inorganic salts.

B. *Inorganic components*

1. 75% of the dry mass of the extracellular matrix is composed of several *inorganic salts* with the following percentages:
   a. 85% calcium phosphate
   b. 10% calcium carbonate
   c. 5% total of calcium fluoride, magnesium fluoride, and also several other ions, especially citrate, potassium, and sodium

2. The combination of calcium and phosphorus to form *hydroxyapatite crystals* (shaped into slender rods about 50 nm long $\times$ 4 nm thick) is responsible for the hardness and firmness of bone.
   a. The hydroxyapatite crystals occur at about 65-nm intervals alongside the collagen fibers. Surrounding this complex is the extracellular matrix.
   b. Surface ions of the hydroxyapatite crystals are hydrated as a shell of water around the *crystal + collagen* combination, thus permitting an efficient exchange of liquids with the extracellular matrix.

3. Treatment of a long thin *fibula* with a weak acid or a chelating agent extracts the inorganic salts, leaving only organic components (collagen and extracellular matrix). So flexible is this *decalcified bone* that it can be tied into a knot. Preparations of this type can be sectioned, stained, and mounted for microscopic study.

II. *Macroscopic structure*

A. *Long bones:* An adult long bone possesses two knobby ends, the **epiphyses** (singular = epiphysis), united by a long shaft, the **diaphysis** (Fig. 7-1).

1. As the diaphysis approaches the epiphysis, it widens into the **metaphysis**.

2. During development, the **epiphysis** consists of cartilage, but later is replaced by **os spongiosum** or *spongy bone*. A section through this area reveals a myriad of bony lines crisscrossing the area like bridge struts or buttresses. Each bony line is a **trabecula ossea**, translated = a *trabecula* of *trabecula* of *bone*.

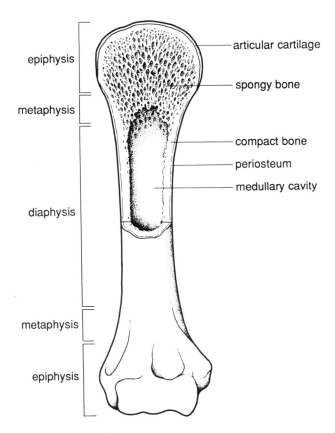

Figure 7-1 Parts of a long bone.

3. A cross (horizontal) section through the diaphysis forms a ring of *compact bone* surrounding the *medullary cavity* which houses the *marrow*.

    a. The **periosteum**, a compact collagenous connective tissue surrounding the periphery of bone and attached to it, is endowed with **osteogenetic** (bone-forming) potential.

    b. The **endosteum**, a compact collagenous connective tissue surrounding the medullary cavity but attached to the compact bone, is likewise endowed with *osteogenetic* potencies.

4. A longitudinal section through an entire long bone cuts from one epiphysis to the other. The following are noted:

a. *Compact bone* (**os compactum**) forms the *diaphyseal* shaft surrounding the medullary cavity.

b. The **epiphysis** is covered by a thin layer of compact bone to protect the delicate bony *trabeculae* making up *spongy bone.* The trabeculae are oriented in distinct functional stress lines. Throughout most of an individual's life, the thin epiphyseal compact bone layer is coated on the outer articular surface with hyaline cartilage.

B. *Flat bones* differ in morphology and in development (cf *membranous ossification* below).

1. A section through a "flat" parietal bone reveals two layers of *compact bone* (**os compactum**) sandwiching a core of *spongy bone* named as follows:

a. **lamina externa** (upper table), the outer layer of compact bone, which is covered by scalp,

b. **lamina interna** (lower table), the inner layer of compact bone facing the cranial cavity,

c. *diploe*, the middle layer of spongy bone between lamina externa and lamina interna.

2. **Periosteum** adheres to the lamina externa of the flat bones of the skull, just as periosteum attaches to the outer surface of the diaphyseal shaft.

3. **Endosteum**, however, does not adhere to the lamina interna as it does in the diaphyseal medullary cavity. Instead, the free **endosteum** is represented by the **dura mater**, one of the three layers covering the brain (and spinal cord).

III. *Microscopic structure*

A. Preparation of a ground bone section (Gray, 1973). Sections of compact bone are cut to desired a thickness of about 5 mm, using commercially available saws. Well-fixed sections of bone are ground individually on optical or metallurgical grinding wheels. The grinding powder could be powdered carborundum, jeweler's rouge, household cleanser, or even tooth powder. After polishing both sides of the ground section, it is dehydrated, dried, and mounted on a slide. The mounting medium prevents the escape of air from lacunae and anastomosing canaliculi, so that when light passes through the microthin section, these appear black as if stained (no stain is used). Viewing sections of ground bone via Nomarski interference provides a dazzling spectrum of colors in an otherwise colorless fragment.

B. A decalcified specimen is prepared as outlined above. The decalcified bone may be sectioned on a microtome, stained, and mounted per usual.

C. These techniques reveal the following morphology (Fig. 7-2):

   1. Periosteum is composed of the two definitive layers:

     a. an external **stratum fibrosum** (= *fibrous layer*) composed of compact collagenous connective tissue. Fibroblasts are flattened between collagen fibers. The surrounding connective tissue as well as collagenous fibers of tendons and ligaments anchor into the stratum fibrosum.

     b. an internal **stratum osteogenicum** (= *osteogenic*) *layer* containing fibroblast derivatives, the **osteoprogenitor cells**, that can differentiate into *osteoblasts* (bone-forming cells). Collagenous fibers emanating from this layer anchor the periosteum to the compact

Figure 7-2 3-D diagram of a microscopic bone section.

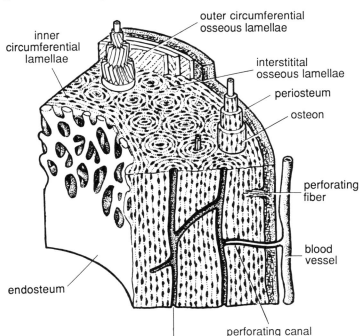

inner circumferential lamellae

outer circumferential osseous lamellae

interstitital osseous lamellae

periosteum

osteon

perforating fiber

blood vessel

endosteum

perforating canal

osteon canal

bone. These are the **fibra perforans** (= *perforating fibers*) (formerly Sharpey's fibers).

2. Lamella ossea are sheets of compact calcified collagenous connective tissue making up compact bone. Each of the sheets are interwoven in precise, determined, structurally sound patterns. The collagen fibers of one sheet spiral in a left-hand helix, while the next spirals in a right-hand helix and so on. *Osseous lamellae* exist as

a. *external circumferential lamellae,* covered by periosteum, form several outer layers of compact bone.

b. *internal circumferential lamellae,* covered by endosteum, form several inner layers of compact bone adjacent to the medullary cavity.

c. *osteons* (formerly Haversian systems) (Cohen and Harris, 1958; Cooper et al, 1966) are formed of concentric osseous lamellae encasing longitudinally coursing capillaries, postcapillary venules, and loose connective tissue. Some *osteons* may be composed of 4 to 20 lamellae. In all, the innermost lamella forms the narrow 30–70-μm-diameter *central canal.*

(1) Where one lamella adheres to another, there is a *cement line,* the **linea cementalis,** composed of mineralized adhesive substances but deficient in collagen fibers.

(2) Resorption of lamella does not usually occur at the **linea cementalis,** but across several lamellae. The *line* of *resorption* is termed **linea resorptionis.**

(3) Osteons, in the adult, form at the rate of 1 μm per day and are complete in 4 to 5 weeks.

d. *interstitial lamellae* are remnants of older osteons eroded during bone growth. They reside between the newer osteons. Usually only a quarter or half the diameter of a whole osteon is found, but there is no central canal.

e. endosteum is the collagenous connective tissue attached to the internal circumferential lamellae which forms a lining around the marrow cavity. Endosteum exhibits the same functional and structural characteristics as those of periosteum.

D. *Bone structure*

1. *Blood vessels* course in and along the periosteum to provide a rich vasculature to its **stratum osteogenicum.** Many of these branches perforate the external circumferential lamellae, interstitial lamellae, and osteon lamellae to supply the osteon canals as capillaries. *Perforating canals* (Volkman's) provide access to the *osteon central canals* and ultimately to the *medullary* (marrow) cavity for the *perforating blood vessels* (Ebner's).

2. Compressed between the concentric osseous lamellae are small spindle-shaped *lacunae* molded by *osteoblasts* that transform to *osteocytes* when encased. Osteocytes play an important role in the release of calcium to blood. When released, the osteocyte is capable of modulation with other bone cell types.

3. Radiating in three dimensions from one lacuna to the next are minute canals, the *osseous canaliculi*, which facilitate a "bucket brigade" type of metabolic exchange from the osteon central canal capillary outward for a distance of up to 15 osteocytes.

a. During **osteogenesis** (bone formation), the *osteoblasts* (bone-forming cells) extend peripheral cellular processes in three dimensions until they contact processes of neighboring *osteoblasts*.

b. Following calcification of the extracellular matrix around their cell bodies and processes, the osteocytes form gap junctions to assist in ion transfer and communication. These processes may be partially withdrawn or rejoined at any time. In old age they are completely withdrawn, making intercellular communication difficult. Aged osteocytes also have greatly diminished cytoplasmic structures.

c. The canaliculi remain patent, providing readily accessible avenues for metabolic exchange via tissue fluid flowing around the osteocyte processes and cell bodies.

IV. Osteogenesis

A. Prior to considering the process of **osteogenesis**, four essential points must be established and emphasized.

1. *Bone is a vascular tissue.*

a. For proper functioning of bone, osteocytes must be as close as possible to the blood vessels.

b. Osteon canal capillaries bring oxygen and nutrients toward the osteocytes via tissue fluids flowing through the canaliculi. Carbon dioxide and cellular wastes are removed in the reverse direction.

2. *Bone increases in size only by* adding new layers in *appositional increments.* Bone grows by deposition of mineral salts on surfaces of connective tissue elements, but never by interstitial increments. Cartilage, it is recalled, grows not only by *appositional increments,* but also by *interstitial increments.*

3. Once the *osteoblast* is encased in its lacuna, it ceases to exhibit the structural characteristics (golgi complex, rER, and abundant euchromatin) and differentiates into an *osteocyte*. If released from the lacuna, the osteocyte could resume its osteoblast (bone-forming) functions and morphology.

4. Throughout life, bone is continually molded and reshaped. Molecular, microscopic, and macroscopic modifications occur by adaptations to occupational stresses, aging, some disease processes, and hormonal imbalances.

B. Osteogenesis (bone development) is categorized into **osteogenesis cartilaginea** and **osteogenesis membranacea.**

1. Osteogenesis cartilaginea is the process of bone formation using a cartilage model that is gradually replaced by bone. For convenience only, this is presented in two phases, *perichondrial ossification* and *endochondral ossification.*

a. *Phase 1: Perichondrial ossification.* Formation of an *osteogenic stratum*, the **annulus osseous perichondrialis**. This is literally a *ring of bone around the cartilage* model. The perichondrium of the diaphyseal cartilage model assumes a new role in laying down the bony ring.

(1) First fibroblasts differentiate into *osteoblasts* (bone-forming cells), which deposit bone salts directly on the collagen fibers of the perichondrium (adjacent to the diaphyseal cartilage). This initial growth process, classified as *membranous ossification,* produces the **os periosteale reticulofibrosum** or *reticulofibrous periosteal bone.*

(2) Once the osseous annulus forms, the perichondrium is referred to as **periosteum**, although no obvious morphological differences are apparent.

b. *Phase 2: Endochondral ossification* (Fig. 7-3). Formation of a *primary ossification center* in the diaphysis. While the osseus annulus under the periosteum continues to be formed, chondrocytes in the center of the diaphyseal cartilage *hypertrophy* (swell). Interlacunar and interterritorial extracellular matrix is thinned by compression until adjacent lacunae break through and become confluent. Chondrocytes that do not die in the process are transformed into *osteoblasts* concerned with synthesis of osseous extracellular matrix and calcification of cartilage spicules.

(1) Invasion by *periosteal buds* of *mesenchymal connective tissue* and accompanying small *blood vessels* are provided access to the primary ossification center by *foramina* (small openings) in the periosteal osseous annulus.

(2) Attraction to this area of hypertrophied dying chondrocytes and enlarged lacunae suggests a *chemotactic* or *necrotactic* influ-

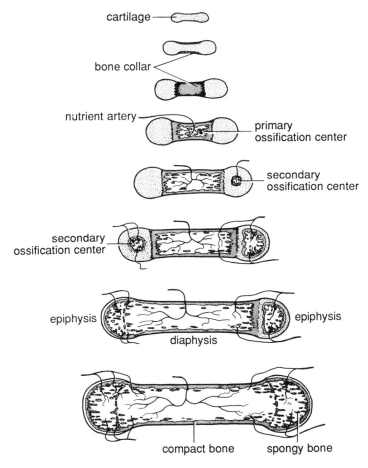

cartilage

bone collar

nutrient artery

primary
ossification center

secondary
ossification center

secondary
ossification center

epiphysis

epiphysis

diaphysis

compact bone   spongy bone

Figure 7-3 Endochondral ossification.

ence; that is, the dying cells emit a chemical substance that diffuses outward to the periphery. When the connective tissue cells "read" the chemical message, the invasion process commences. Mesenchymal connective tissue cells move toward the distressed area, dragging extracellular matrix, other cells, and capillaries. Characterization of the **glycocalyx** via immunohistochemical and viral receptor site studies gives credence to the concept of attraction and repulsion of cells.

(3) The osseous annulus provides the necessary rigidity to

the cartilage model that is being hollowed out in its center, thereby preventing collapse.

(4) *Bone deposition:* Invading mesenchymal connective tissue cells in the primary ossification center differentiate into

(a) *hemocytopoetic cells* (blood-forming cells). The primary ossification center at this point can be called a *primary marrow cavity.*

(b) *osteoprogenitor cells* that transform into the *osteoblasts* (bone-forming cells). The latter deposit the initial bony lamellae on calcified cartilage, forming an array of spicules that resemble *spongy bone (trabecular bone).* Subsequent deposition of inorganic salts in the trabecular interstices converts the mass into compact bone.

(5) *Enlargement* of the *primary ossification center*

(a) While the cartilage model continues growth, the primary ossification center of the diaphysis progressively enlarges as more lacunae become confluent and more mesenchymal connective tissue invades.

(b) Invading vessels assist in further enlargement of the *primary ossification center.*

(c) Concurrently the osseous annulus increases in size to provide greater support.

(6) Formation of *secondary ossification centers:* The epiphyses remain cartilaginous until birth, when *secondary centers of ossification* appear in the epiphyses, followed by a sequelae of events similar to those that form the primary centers of ossification. Almost all of the epiphyseal cartilage is eroded, except at two functionally significant sites:

(a) the *articular cartilage* (**cartilago articularis**) of the epiphyses, which provides a smooth articular surface.

(b) the *epiphyseal cartilage* (**cartilago epiphysialis**) provides a growth zone at the interface with the **diaphysis**. This epiphyseal cartilage is frequently called the "epiphyseal disk" or "epiphyseal plate." Recently introduced by some orthopedic authors is the term "physeal cartilage."

(7) *Zones of osteogenesis* (Fig. 7-4), in the *epiphyseal cartilage* of a developing long bone, characterize growth in length. To follow the description below, commence microscopic study at the epiphyseal side of the cartilage and work toward the diaphysis.

(a) **Zona reservata** is a quiescent area with no apparent activity. Resident chondrocytes divide periodically (over a 20-year period) to form columns of differentiating cells.

(b) **Zona proliferativa** is an active zone of chondrocytic

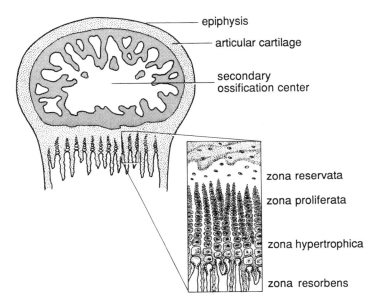

epiphysis

articular cartilage

secondary
ossification center

zona reservata

zona proliferata

zona hypertrophica

zona resorbens

Figure 7-4 Zones of osteogenesis in the epiphyseal cartilage.

mitoses immediately below the zona reservata. Mitotic growth accounts for lengthening the cartilage model by forming **columellae chondrocyti** (*chondrocyte columns*) parallel to the longitudinal axis of the humerus.

(c) **Zona hypertrophica**, closer to the diaphysis, has almost no mitotic figures. As maturing chondrocytes undergo hypertrophy (**chondrocytus hypertrophicus**) they compress the interlacunar matrix. The confluence of stacked lacunae in parallel columns resembles a honeycomb.

(d) **Zona resorbens** is a zone of calcification in which differentiating osteoblasts line up like epithelial cells along the cartilaginous spicules. When connective tissue fibers and calcium salt deposits imprison osteoblasts and their cytoplasmic processes, they are designated *osteocytes*.

(8) Transformation of *osteoblast* to *osteocyte*

(a) TEM reveals an abundance of rER in the *osteoblast*. The osteoblast does not undergo cell division but performs as a fully differentiated secretory cell secreting procollagen and extracellular matrix components of bone. The density of polyribosomes on the ER membranes is responsible for the basophilia of the cytoplasm.

(b) ER cisternae (swollen with secretory material), a prominent golgi complex, and numerous large mitochondria provide ample morphological evidence that the *osteoblast* is a functionally active cell.

(c) Embedment of the osteoblast by extracellular matrix (collagen + bone salts + amorphous substance) somehow signals cessation of its secretory activity.

(d) The rER and golgi complex gradually recede until the transformation from *osteoblast* to *osteocyte* is complete.

(9) Fate of the *epiphyseal cartilage*

(a) Hormones and vitamins influence the epiphyseal cartilage to produce extracellular matrix and chondrocyte columns at measured rates equivalent to the deposition of bone.

(b) The result of this activity is

[1] increase in bone length,

[2] maintenance of a relatively constant thickness to the epiphyseal cartilage.

(10) In x-ray films, the epiphyseal cartilage appears as a narrow translucent band that may be interpreted as a fracture line

(11) Bone ceases to grow in length when the chondrocytes of the epiphyseal cartilage no longer divide to produce new cells. In effect, the cartilage is "used up." Osseous tissue replaces the epiphyseal cartilage and continuity is established between the epiphyses and diaphysis. A radiopaque line appears in place of the translucent line of cartilage. Radiologists refer to this event as "fusion of the epiphysis."

(12) The epiphysis is occupied by **os spongiosum** or spongy bone (trabecular bone) surrounding red bone marrow spaces. The bony trabeculae are arranged in structural patterns adapted to resist local strains and stresses.

2. **Osteogenesis membranacea:** In this form of ossification, bone is deposited directly onto connective tissue extracellular matrix components. To best appreciate *membranous osteogenesis*, one should study the early development of the flat bones of the skull, the mandible, or clavicle. These bones, called *membrane bones*, develop in regions consisting only of primitive mesenchymal tissue. No cartilage model is required. The process of *membranous osteogenesis* involves

a. *vascularization* of the mesenchymal tissue

b. *differentiation* of mesenchymal cells into *osteoblasts*

c. *condensation* of extracellular matrix into dense acidophilic bars, the uncalcified *osteoid tissue*

    d. *encasement* of osteoblasts in the osteoid tissue

    e. *calcification* of osteoid tissue by osteoblastic activity lays down the **os membranaceum reticulofibrosum [primarium]**. This is the primary membrane bone in a network of fibers forming *osseous trabeculae*, or spicules of bone.

    f. *formation of lacunar* and canalicular *molds*, by the osteoblast body and its cytoplasmic processes

    g. Growth continues as layer upon layer of calcified matrix is added. This is the **os membranaceum lamellosum [secundarium]**, or secondary lamellar membrane bone, forming typical *osseous lamellae*. At first the bone appears spongy with spicules of trabecular bone. Growth of lamellated concentric osteon systems on either side of the spongy bone gives rise to compact bone (in the flat bone of the skull the compact bone forms **lamina externa** and **lamina interna**).

    (1) There is no difference in the microscopic comparison between thinly ground fragments of adult *compact bone* from

        (a) the diaphysis of the humerus and

        (b) the lamina externa or interna of the parietal bone of the skull

    (2) nor can the method of development be distinguished (endochondral osteogenesis vs membranous osteogenesis).

    h. Primitive mesenchymal tissue filling the spaces between trabeculae of spongy bone differentiate into the hemopoetic tissue of red marrow.

V. *Proportional growth of bone*

    A. Endochondral bone grows in length by activity of the epiphyseal cartilage. Periosteal osteogenesis permits growth in width via *appositional increments*. Likewise, in flat bones of the cranium, appositional increments add successive layers of bone as the overall size increases.

    B. It is apparent that the developing marrow cavity increases in size proportionately to the thickness of the diaphyseal shaft and that the flat bones of the skull do not get thicker and thicker. Should this be allowed to occur, dense bone would acquire a mass that would be excessively heavy for the fetus. Instead, bone growth in length and width is regulated proportionately to keep pace with a growing fetus.

    C. *Resorption of bone:* Deposition of bone in one region is followed by resorption and remolding at another region. Resorption is associated with the appearance of a specialized phagocytic cell, the multinucleated *osteoclast*.

    1. *Osteoclasts* ("bone breakers") appear on the surfaces of bone undergoing active resorption of the bone matrix.

a. During life, an intricate relationship between *osteoblasts, osteocytes,* and *osteoclasts* is required to remodel, reshape, and reconstruct bone in response to a variety of stresses and strains.

b. In the disease osteoporosis (DeLuca et al, 1981), bone is resorbed at a faster rate than it is laid down. In this situation, the *osteoclasts* increase in number far beyond those found in the normal condition.

2. *Osteoclasts* in the process of resorbing bone reside in eroded pits, the *lacunae* of *erosion* (Howship's lacunae). In longitudinal sections of the growing ends of long bone, adequate numbers may be found for student study.

3. The *osteoclast* via *light microscopy* appears as a multinucleated cell detached from the bone lining the *lacuna* of *erosion*, apparently resulting from the trauma of "fixation."

a. Depending on the plane of section, there may be 5 to 10 individual nuclei. In the whole cell there are about 20, although numbers up to 200 have been reported.

b. Nuclei are commonly seen on the side of the cell furthest from the bony surface of the lacuna of erosion.

4. The *osteoclast* via *electron microscopy* (Holtrop, 1972), is characterized in three regions:

a. *Region I:* The surface in contact with the bone undergoing erosion shows

(1) a *ruffled border.* It is hypothesized that this border is concerned with anchoring the *osteoclast* in the lacuna of erosion. Movement of the osteoclast, via ameboid activity, to another site is characterized by withdrawal of the ruffled border, which does not reappear until it is anchored again.

(2) *microprojections, microfolds,* and *microvilli* in contact with the erosion areas, which apparently make up the active resorption surface. Inorganic calcium phosphate crystals are solubilized and removed by osteoclastic activity.

(3) a *"clear band"* surrounding the fimbriated border that is devoid of mitochondria, endoplasmic reticulum, golgi complex, and lysosomes.

b. *Region II:* A region of *vesicles* appears behind the clear band. Although the nature of these vesicles has not been completely clarified, it appears that they may have pinched off the plasmalemma at the base of the ruffles to enclose phagocytosed material. Fusion with lysosomes would initiate the process of cellular digestion.

c. *Region III:* The region opposite the ruffled border contains *cytoplasmic structures* (mitochondria, golgi complex, etc) and the *multiple nuclei.*

5. *Origin* of the *osteoclast* (Fishman and Hay, 1962): Osteoclasts were thought to arise from cells of bone lineage via fusion of osteogenic cells and/or osteoblasts. Indeed, controversy over the origin of the osteoclast resulted in widespread research efforts. Transplantation of bone tissue into nonosseous tissues, vital staining, parabiotic studies, labeling specific cell types with tritiated thymidine, and many other important studies point to the *monocyte as the precursor* of the osteoclast. Knowledge of the origin is required to combat those diseases that actively resorb bone faster than it can be formed.

VI. *Joints:* Three major types permit the articulation of bones.

A. *Types*

1. *Synarthrosis:* These are relatively immovable joints characteristic of

a. fibrous sutures of the skull,

b. articulations of the roots of teeth with the mandible and maxilla,

c. the cartilaginous articulation between epiphysis and diaphysis.

2. *Amphiarthrosis:* Capable of slight movements, these joints occur in articulations where fibrocartilage is the interosseous medium:

a. between vertebrae,

b. between pubic bones at the symphysis pubis.

3. *Diarthrosis* (Fig. 7-5): Joints of this type are freely movable. Age changes subject the individual to various joint diseases. With increasing age these changes become more prominent. Diarthrotic joints have the following basic structure:

a. The *articular cartilage* is hyaline cartilage that coats the epiphyses, which articulate against one another. It differs from hyaline cartilage in other areas in lacking a perichondrium. Apparently, the chondrocytes depend on diffusion of substances in the synovial fluid for sustenance. With aging, articular cartilage exhibits tears, cracks, and fissures. The collagen fibers present a unique disposition, delineating three definitive zones:

(1) zona superficialis, a tangential zone in with the fibers are oriented in a plane horizontal to the surface.

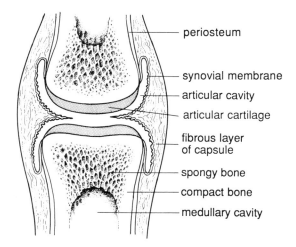

Figure 7-5 Joint, diarthrosis.

(2) **zona intermedia**, a transitional zone with the fiber orientation changing from horizontal to perpendicular fibers.

(3) **zona profunda**, the deep zone with fibers arranged at right angles to the surface. The collagen fibers are anchored in this zone and extend upward into the zona intermedia, then arch into the zona superficialis where the arch peaks as fibers parallel the surface. Multiple arching fibers give the articular cartilage its ability to withstand tremendous stress changes such as those that occur in the quick starting and stopping of basketball players.

(4) **lamina ossea subchondrialis** is a layer of mature bone to which the articular cartilage fuses and anchors.

b. An *articular capsule* surrounding the joint complex, is composed of two layers:

(1) a **stratum fibrosum**, the outer fibrous layer, may be thickened at some sites to form *ligaments*.

(2) a **stratum synoviale**, the internal layer facing the joint cavity, is commonly referred to as the "synovial membrane." The **stratum synoviale** encloses the entire joint except over the articular cartilage. The stratum synoviale rests on a loose connective tissue layer, the **lamina propria synovialis**. *Three parts* may be distinguished:

(a) **pars plana** is the smooth glistening surface of the greater part of the stratum synoviale.

(b) **pars villosa:** Numerous villi (**villi synovialis**), increasing the surface area, are supplied with nerves and are highly vascularized with blood and lymphatic capillaries.

(c) **plica synovialis:** These synovial folds vastly increase the surface area of the "synovial membrane" and provide an appropriate milieu for two special cells of the "synovial membrane," the **cellulae synovialis**, which lie among the connective tissue fibers:

[1] **synoviocytus phagocyticus:** These cells are phagocytic in character and are responsible for maintaining a clean environment.

[2] **synoviocytus secretorius:** These are the cells that are responsible for producing the synovial fluid.

c. The *synovial fluid*, a lubricating fluid filling the joint cavity, is produced by the synovial secretory cells of the **stratum synoviale**. Highly polymerized hyaluronic acid imparts a thick viscous quality to the fluid and promotes its lubricating properties. Practically all blood cell types can be found in synovial fluid, especially monocytes. With aging, the synovial membrane exhibits fibrosis, accumulation of mononuclear leucocytes (lymphocytes and monocytes), and a gradual increase in viscosity. After age 35, the fluid becomes more viscous, and athletes (eg, baseball catchers) find a more limited movement.

Questions

DIRECTIONS: Select the best answer to the question or incomplete statement. There may be other options that are partially correct, but there is only one best answer.

1. Which of the following statements does not pertain to osseous tissue?
   A. Type II collagen fibers predominate.
   B. Calcium phosphate has the greatest percentage of all the inorganic salts in bone.
   C. Osseous tissue contains glycoproteins that bind calcium and promote calcification.
   D. Calcium and phosphorus contribute to the formation of hydroxyapatite.
   E. Extraction of the organic components of osseous tissue leave bone as brittle as chalk.

2. The humerus (of the arm) has two ends and a long piece attaching each of the ends. Listed below are the names and positions applied to the parts of this bone. Which statement below does not pertain?
   A. Epiphysis is the articular part related to the shoulder joint.
   B. Metaphysis is the expanded part related to the epiphysis above in A.
   C. Diploe is the spongy layer situated between two layers of compact bone.
   D. Epiphysis is the articular part related to the elbow joint.
   E. Metaphysis is the expanded part related to the epiphysis above in D.

3. In perichondrial ossification, all the following are true EXCEPT
   A. the perichondrium first lays down a ring of bone around the diaphysis
   B. the initial growth process is membranous ossification
   C. fibroblasts of the perichondrium first must differentiate into osteoblasts
   D. the perichondrium of flat bones of the skull is immediately under the scalp
   E. the internal layer of the perichondrium is the osteogenic layer

4. The statements below pertain to epiphyseal cartilage EXCEPT
   A. it participates in the process of increasing bone length
   B. it is involved in condensation of extracellular matrix into osteoid tissue
   C. it maintains a relative thickness during bone growth
   D. it is eventually "used up" and is replaced by osseous tissue
   E. it is under the influence of hormones and vitamins especially during the active period of growth

5. In the disease osteoporosis, bone is resorbed at a faster rate than it is laid down. Which cells increase in number?
   A. Osteoblasts
   B. Fibroblasts
   C. Osteocytes
   D. Mesenchymal cells
   E. Osteoclasts

6. The best evidence to date implicates which cell as the immediate progenitor of the osteoclast?
   A. Fibroblast
   B. Osteocyte
   C. Monocyte
   D. Osteoblast
   E. None of the above

7. The articular capsule possesses all the following layers EXCEPT
   A. stratum fibrosum
   B. lamina propria synovialis
   C. stratum synoviale
   D. stratum osteogenicum
   E. none of the above

8. An arterial vessel approaching the periosteum to an osteon canal travels through all of the following EXCEPT
   A. an inner zone of basophilia
   B. periosteum
   C. external circumferential lamellae
   D. interstitial lamellae
   E. osteon concentric lamellae

9. All the following steps occur in membranous osteogenesis EXCEPT
   A. vascularization of mesenchymal tissue
   B. differentiation of mesenchymal cells into osteoblasts
   C. formation of osteoid tissue
   D. calcification of osteoid tissue
   E. formation of the zona proliferative

10. Which of the following statements is incorrect concerning age changes in the skeletal system?
    A. Osteocytes withdraw their cell processes.
    B. Synovial fluid becomes less viscous.
    C. There is increased incidence of intervertebral disk pathology.
    D. Articular cartilage shows tears, cracks, and fissures.
    E. Inflammatory joint disease increases.

Explanatory Answers

1. A. Type II and type I collagen bundles occur in cartilage. **B.** Osseous tissue contains only type I collagen bundles, which calicify. Whereas that of cartilage does not. Calcium phosphate constitutes 85%, the greatest percentage of all the inorganic salts in bone. **C.** These glycoproteins are sialoprotein and osteonectin. **D.** Hydroxyapatite in the form of crystalline rods associates with the collagen fibers.

2. C. The diploe is the name applied to the os spongiosum of flat bones, which contains red marrow. In the humerus, the epiphyses possess os spongiosum, but the diaphysis is composed of compact bone surrounding the medullary cavity, which contains bone marrow.

3. D. The flat bones of the skull develop by membranous osteogenesis. There is no cartilage involved and hence there is no perichondrium. From the time bone forms in the skull, the osteogenic tissue is periosteum. In the diaphysis of a long bone, as soon as the first bone is formed, the perichondrium is renamed periosteum.

4. B. The condensation of extracellular matrix into dense acidophilic bars, the uncalcified osteoid tissue, occurs in membranous osteogenesis. The other statements are correct for the epiphyseal cartilage.

5. E. The osteoclast is associated with active bone resorption. In osteoporosis these cells increase dramatically.

6. C. The osteoclasts were thought to arise from cells of bone lineage. The current information points to the monocyte as the precursor of the osteoclast.

7. D. The articular capsule has the first three layers (A, B, C). The stratum osteogenicum (osteogenic layer) is a layer of the periostium. It contains fibroblasts that can differentiate into osteoblasts.

8. A. The inner zone of basophilia surrounds the lacuna of a chondrocyte. The arterial vessels do not penetrate the extracellular matrix in cartilage, thus chondrocytes depend on diffusion of nutrients from peripheral vessels. In bone the capillary must be close enough so that the 15th osteocyte away from the central canal can be nourished.

9. E. The zona proliferativa is one zone of osteogenesis in the epiphyseal cartilage. Since cartilage is involved, this is cartilaginous osteogenesis. In membranous osteogenesis bone is deposited directly on connective tissue.

10. B. All the changes listed to occur with progressing age, except that the synovial fluid becomes *more* viscous due to the decrease in hyaluronic levels.

8 Myeloid Tissue, Hemocytopoesis

I. Hemocytopoesis (also *hemopoesis*), the process of *blood cell formation*, occurs in

A. *lymphatic tissue*, which produces lymphocytes.

B. *myeloid tissue* or *bone marrow*, which produces all blood cell types.

II. *Myeloid tissue* is a specialized tissue consisting of *vascular* and *extravascular compartments*. The latter houses the several blood cell lines in varying developmental stages. Bone marrow accounts for 3.5 to 5.9% of the adult body weight (1600 gm to 3700 gm), approximately the weight of the liver (Wintrobe, 1962). There are no lymphatic vessels in the bone marrow (Tavassoli and Yoffey, 1983).

A. *Vasculature* (DeBruyn, 1981): The *marrow cavity* (**cavitas medullaris**) of bone is supplied by one or more *nutrient arteries* that gain entrance through a small opening in the compact bone, the *nutrient foramen*.

1. In the marrow cavity, *nutrient arteries* divide into central arteries that send arterioles to

    a. the *sinusoidal vessels* (Fig. 8-1), which are classified as modified blood capillaries. They form radially arranged plexuses around a *central marrow vein*. [n.b. Some textbooks refer to these vessels as "venous sinuses." The *Nomina Histologica* states: the "**vas capillare sinusoideum** is a modified blood capillary occurring in the liver, bone marrow, and various endocrine organs."]

        (1) The *lumen* of a sinusoid, varying in width from 50 μm to 75 μm, is surrounded by a nonfenestrated endothelium specialized to

            (a) store large quantities of blood under low pressure,

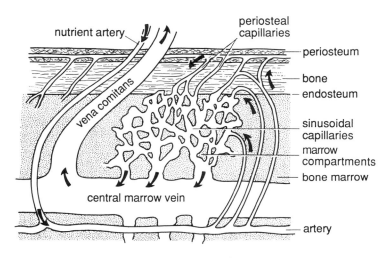

Figure 8-1 Bone marrow vasculature (after DeBruyn, 1981).

    (b) facilitate the entrance of newly matured blood cells into the circulation.

    [1] The endothelial cells develop transient openings to allow new blood cells to enter the circulation via *diapedesis*. Some blood cells insinuate at junctional sites.

    [2] The endothelial cells normally permit only cells that have matured to reach the bloodstream.

    [3] Most blood cells in the blood stream are prevented from gaining access to the hemocytopoetic compartments.

    (2) The endothelial cells, held together by circumferential zonulae adherens and probably gap junctions, possess small vesicles in the cytoplasm and scattered micropinocytotic vesicles along the luminal and abluminal surfaces. [As such they clearly resemble capillary endothelium rather than venous endothelium.]

    (3) The peripheral parts of the sinusoidal plexuses attach to the endosteum to prevent damaging movements.

    b. and back to *periosteal capillaries* to supply the periosteum.

    2. A poorly defined *basement membrane* of discontinuous flocculent material surrounds the sinusoidal capillaries. This material preserves so poorly that earlier investigators considered the basement membrane to be absent or negligible (Weiss, 1976).

    a. A closely applied *adventitial coat* of delicate reticular fibers (surrounding the basement membrane) contains branching *reticulocytes* with the ability to

(1) *accumulate lipids,*

(2) *develop* new *adipocytes* (Tavassoli, 1976).

(a) In the marrow of long bones, adipocytes contain saturated fats and hence do not convert easily to hemocytopoetic cells.

(b) In bones that normally contain red marrow, the adipocytes contain unsaturated fats. Thus they can revert easily to hemocytopoetic cells if needed.

(3) *hypertrophy* (but appear empty). As such they contribute to the white gelatinous appearance of aging marrow.

b. The *adventitial coat* generally covers 40% to 60% of the abluminal (external) endothelial surface areas.

(1) In response to toxic substances

(a) the adventitial coat and flocculent basement membrane *spread* to cover most of the sinusoidal surface, in an effort to shield the developing blood cells.

(b) the *reticulocytes* become fatty and may generate many more *adipocytes* turning red marrow into yellow marrow. This reduces the hemocytopoetic capacity of bone marrow and results in *anemia.*

(2) In response to some diseases (eg, leukemia), the reticular cells lose their lipids to provide more space for hemocytopoesis.

3. Blood from the sinusoidal capillaries drains into the large *central marrow vein,* which then conveys it to a **vena comitans** (the vein that accompanies the nutrient artery to exit through the *nutrient foramen*).

B. *Extravascular compartments.* The sinusoidal capillaries provide the **stroma medullae** (framework of the medullary cavity) to protect and support foci of developing blood cell lines. While stromal fibers occur around the sinusoidal vessels, they are scarce in the surrounding compartments.

1. *Adipocytes* are numerous and an easily identified cell type, often occupying a volume far greater than that of the blood-forming cells.

a. *Red bone marrow* (**medulla ossium rubra**) (actively producing blood cells) may have up to 75% of the volume occupied by adipocytes. Generally, the amount of *red marrow = yellow marrow.*

b. *Yellow bone marrow* (**medullar ossium flava**) (relatively inactive), with adipocytes exceeding 75% of the volume, develops the distinctive yellowish color. Thus, when the percentage of adipocytes exceeds 75%, **hemocytopoesis** decreases. An increase in temperature causes replacement of yellow marrow by red marrow (Huggins and Blocksom, 1936).

2. Primitive bone marrow occurs in the second fetal month when bones first begin to ossify.

    a. Bone marrow is the major blood-forming organ in the last three fetal months.

    b. In neonates and small children, only red marrow is found in all the bones.

3. About age 5, a gradual transformation from red to yellow marrow is initiated until both forms are equal.

4. In the adult, red marrow occurs only in the flat bones of the skull, the vertebrae, ribs, sternum, clavicles, pelvic bones, and in the epiphyses of long bones.

5. In old age, starvation, and in some diseases, the marrow becomes gelatinous: the **medulla ossium gelatinosum**.

III. Hemocytopoesis: *Blood cell formation*

    A. The *stem cell* for all blood cells is the *hemocytoblast* (*hemo-* = blood, *cyto-* = cell, *blast-* = primitive, formative).

    1. Investigators postulate only one pleuripotent *stem cell* for all blood cell types, the *hemocytoblast*, which exists in low numbers and has a low mitotic index.

    2. *Hemocytoblasts* differentiate into mitotically active stem cells that are unipotential for each peripheral blood cell type. These are morphologically unique and identifiable (eg, specific granules appear).

    B. The term "colony-forming unit" (CFU) has not received recognition in the *Nomina Histologica*, although all blood cell types in the mouse have been traced to it. Proponents cite experiments (in the mouse) to support the smaller CFU to the larger hemocytoblast as the true stem cell (Till and McCullough, 1980). In this text the term *hemocytoblast* will designate the stem cell.

    C. In the progressive series of changes associated with the differentiation of all blood cells, this text considers hemocytopoesis in three arbitrary stages:

    1. *Early:* cells derived from the hemocytoblast, with a few visible features that permit assignment to one of the cell lines.

    2. *Middle:* cells recognized by cytoplasmic and nuclear changes and an increased mitotic rate.

3. *Late:* cells that are almost mature.

D. *Theories of* **hemocytopoesis** (Maximow, 1930)

1. Dualistic (polyphyletic) theory: Some early authors postulated two morphologically distinct stem cells:
  a. for lymphatic tissue, the *lymphoblast,*
  b. for bone marrow, the *myeloblast.*

2. Unitarian (monophyletic) theory: Others pointed to one cell, the *hemocytoblast,* as the stem cell for all blood cell lines.

3. In addition to the several distinctions made in each of the theories, one specific point separated the two:
  a. *Unitarian:* the small lymphocyte is a premitotic cell; that is, it retains the potencies of its progenitors. Current immunological evidence supports this early proposal.
  b. *Dualistic:* the small lymphocyte is a postmitotic cell, ie, a terminal cell. This idea is no longer acceptable.

E. *Identification of the hemocytoblast:* While authors agree on a functional definition for the hemocytoblast, identification by morphological criteria is virtually impossible at the light or electron microscopic level. The best one could state is that the hemocytoblast or "stem cell" resembles a lymphocyte.

IV. **Erythrocytopoesis** (Harrison, 1976): *formation* of *erythrocytes* via a series of orderly nuclear and cytoplasmic events which produces specialized functional cells lacking a nucleus and a cytoplasm filled with hemoglobin. The entire process occurs over a period of one week. Islands of developing erythrocytes are arranged around one or more macrophages, whose charge is to phagocytose extruded nuclei and defective erythroblasts. The staining properties of the developing erythrocytes account for nomenclature of stages (Fig. 8-2):

A. *Early stages* in **erythrocytopoesis**

1. *Proerythroblasts* are spherical cells
  a. about 14 μm to 19 μm in diameter, with rims of basophilic cytoplasm,
  b. with large nuclei with uniformly distributed chromatin, and two or more nucleoli,
  c. undergoing several mitotic divisions to produce:

2. *Basophilic erythroblasts* (smaller in size):
  a. cytoplasm is deeply basophilic (polyribosomes fill the cytoplasm),

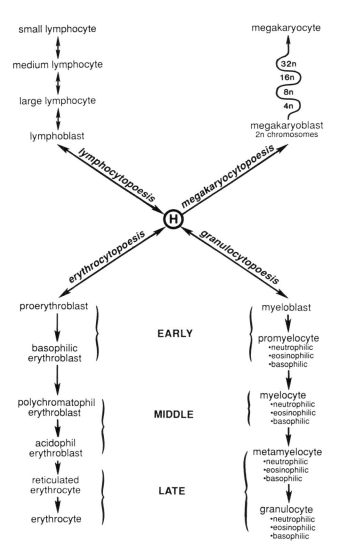

Figure 8-2 Hemocytopoesis. The circled H represents the hemocytoblast.

    b. nuclear chromatin is condensed into small heterochromatic clumps, and nucleoli disappear. Loss of nucleoli is correlated with a loss of ribosomal production,

    c. basophilic erythroblasts divide to produce:

B. *Middle stages* in **erythrocytopoesis**

    1. *Polychromatophilic erythroblasts*:

        a. overall size continues to decrease.

        b. *hemoglobin*, with recovered *iron*, begins to be synthesized.

        (1) Iron is recovered from old or damaged erythrocytes (phagocytosed by macrophages in the spleen).

        (2) Iron is transported from the spleen via the iron-binding globulin *plasma transferrin* to the bone marrow where it is taken up by specific transferrin receptors on the plasmalemma of developing erythrocytes. Ultimately it is brought into the erythropoetic cell and incorporated into the hemoglobin molecule.

        (3) The old degraded hemogloblin (sans iron) is transported to the liver for excretion as the bile pigment *bilirubin*.

        c. *acidophilic hemoglobin*, synthesized on resident polyribosomes, continues to accumulate, resulting in a spectrum of colors from the *basic* blue through purple to the *acidic* salmon pink.

        d. nuclei lack nucleoli and are reduced in size.

    2. *Acidophilic erythroblast* (old names: eosinophilic erythroblast, normoblast, orthochromatic erythroblast):

        a. size: 8 μm to 14 μm.

        b. the cytoplasm is distinctly acidophilic, with a tinge of basophilia resulting from residual polyribosomes.

        c. the cytoplasm is filled with hemoglobin.

        d. no other cytoplasmic structures are encountered except for scattered mitochondria.

        e. nuclear chromatin is clumped in darkly stained blocks (resembling a checkerboard).

        f. the nucleus is positioned eccentrically and extruded with a thin coating of cytoplasm, enclosed in a portion of the plasmalemma (Campbell, 1968).

    C. *Late stages* of **erythrocytopoesis**

    1. Erythrocytus reticulatus (*hemoreticulocyte*) or *reticulated erythrocyte* (the name reticulocyte for this cell has been deleted from the *Nomina Histologica*)

        a. average size 7.5 μm to 8 μm.

        b. enucleated cells have almost the full complement of hemoglobin.

c. residual polyribosomes give cells a slight greenish tint. If the cells are stained with brilliant cresyl blue, the residual polyribosomes clump into a network. Hence the name "reticulated" erythrocyte.

d. *reticulated erythrocytes* may enter the circulation in small numbers and account for 1% of the peripheral erythrocyte population.

(1) An increase above 1% indicates an increased demand for mature erythrocytes,

(2) and with the mature erythrocytes, immature reticulated erythrocytes will follow.

2. The mature *erythrocyte* (red blood cell, rbc) ready to be introduced into the circulation occurs in large numbers close to the sinusoids.

a. Since these cells are incapable of ameboid motion, they reside next to the sinusoidal endothelium to facilitate entrance into the circulation.

b. This position, however, is detrimental to the developing erythrocytes, since they are the first cells to be exposed to invading toxic substances, hence the anemia that usually follows exposure to toxic substances.

D. *Regulation* of *erythropoesis* (Rifkin and Marks, 1975). When increased erythrocyte formation is required, the hormone *erythropoetin* occurs in the blood in higher titers than normal. This hormone, probably formed in the kidney, maintains adequate numbers of erythrocytes in the circulation. Erythropoetin targets the bone marrow.

V. **Granulocytopoesis** is the process that gives rise to the granulocytes. It takes approximately 10 days from the time any one cell line differentiates from the hemocytoblast to the mature granulocyte.

A. *Early stages* in **granulocytopoesis** are not distinguished from one another (*neutro-* vs *acido-* vs *baso-*)

1. *Myeloblasts*, derived from the hemocytoblast, are cells committed to form a line in the granulocytic series.

a. It is a small cell with a basophilic cytoplasm devoid of azurophilic or specific granules.

b. Three or more nucleoli may assist in distinguishing the *myeloblast* from the *erythroblast*. However, the phenomenon of nucleolar fusion cautions against placing much confidence in this morphological characteristic.

2. *Promyelocytes* are designated when the first small metachromatic azurophilic granules appear in the cytoplasm. Promyelocytes in

all three series cannot be distinguished morphologically from one another.

    a. The nucleus has several nuceloli and a dispersed chromatin. Later the chromatin begins to condense to inactive heterochromatin and the nucleoli begin to recede and become inconspicuous.

    b. *Azurophilic granules* (membrane bound) arise from the concave face of the golgi complex and are considered to be *lysosomes* (Bainton and Farquhar, 1966).

       (1) Early promyelocytes accumulate a few membrane-bound azurophilic granules around the cytocentrum. They measure 0.1 μm to 0.25 μm in diameter.

       (2) Granules form by activity of the rER and are packaged as dense core vacuoles by the golgi complex.

       (3) Several dense core vacuoles fuse to form dense bodies.

       (4) Dense bodies coalesce with others to form the azurophilic granules.

       (5) As *lysosomes*, they contain peroxidase, acid phosphatase, and several other enzymes.

    c. The total size of the promyelocytes may increase up to 24 μm in diameter, as the number of azurophilic granules increase, indicating continued correlated activity of the nucleoli + rER + golgi.

    d. This stage is followed by several mitotic divisions resulting in progressively smaller cells, with regressed cytoplasmic structures.

  B. *Middle stages* in **granulocytopoesis**

    1. *Myelocytes* are so designated when a second type of granule forms, the *specific granule*, at the convex surface of the golgi complex (Bainton and Farquhar, 1966).

    a. *Neutrophilic myelocytes:* more numerous than other granulocytes.

       (1) smaller than the promyelocyte counterparts.

       (2) chromatin is condensed to form a kidney-shaped nucleus.

       (3) the *specific granules* have little affinity for acid or basic moiety of routine blood stains.

       (4) contain the enzyme alkaline phosphatase and the antibacteriocidal protein *phagocytin*.

       (5) The number of mitochondria decrease and other cytoplasmic structures recede or disappear, but small amounts of glycogen appear.

    b. *Acidophilic myelocytes:* less numerous than neutrophilic myelocytes.

(1) The nucleus shows clumps of chromatin accumulating along the plasmalemma.

(2) The cytoplasm has azurophilic granules and much larger *specific granules* that have an affinity for the acidic moiety of the blood stains. These are less dense than the azurophilic granules.

(a) *Specific granules* are rich in peroxidase.

(b) Cytochemical reactions for peroxidase occur in the rER cisternae, pericisternal cytoplasm, golgi complex, and forming golgi vesicles.

(c) Acid phosphatase and arylsulfatase have the same cellular distribution as peroxidase, which indicates that the cell is capable of synthesizing and packaging several enzyme proteins at the same time.

c. *Basophilic myelocytes* are difficult to find in routine bone marrow preparations, because of their normally low numbers and because the few specific granules fail to preserve well.

(1) The nucleus does not stain as darkly as the other myelocytes.

(2) A few metachromatic azurophilic granules are found in the cytoplasm.

(3) Metachromatic specific granules vary in size.

2. *Metamyelocytes (juvenilis)*

a. *Neutrophilic metamyelocytes*

(1) have a deeply indented nucleus with condensed heterochromatin,

(2) the nucleus continues to be reshaped, forming an elongated nucleus that could

(a) appear as a "band form" or

(b) fold on itself to appear as a dagger or a "stab cell."

(3) specific granules comprise about 80% of the granules whereas azurophilic granules comprise 20%.

(4) in infections, immature forms may be released into the circulation. In peripheral blood smears, they serve as important indicators of apparent or "hidden" infections.

b. *Acidophilic metamyelocytes*

(1) possess an indented nucleus,

(2) crystallization of the contents of the specific granules is initiated.

c. *Basophilic metamyelocytes*

(1) The number of specific granules increases.

(2) The nucleus is indented.

C. *Late stages* in **granulocytopoesis** [refer to the chapter on blood for mature forms]

  1. *Neutrophilic granulocytes:* Maturation begins with nuclear segmentation. Generally, three lobes form before exiting the marrow. Circulating neutrophils may develop up to five lobes.

  2. *Acidophilic granulocytes*
   a. possess a bilobed nucleus and
   b. other characteristics, per chapter on blood.

  3. *Basophilic granulocytes*
   a. possess a nucleus with two or three lobes,
   b. contain heparin in the specific granules, important in lipoprotein metabolism and in hemostasis.

D. *Regulation* of **granulocytopoesis** (Golden and Cline, 1974): Myeloid tissue reserves *mature* granulocytes, equal to 10 to 15 times the number in peripheral blood, for release upon demand. Should the need continue, precursors in the *middle* or *early* stages step up production. The hormone *leukopoetin* (granulopoetin) has been cited as the chemical stimulus to commence production.

VI. Megacaryocytopoesis (n.b.: -*karyo*- now is -*caryo*-)

A. *Megacaryoblast (MCB)*

  1. This stage, derived from the hemocytoblast, differentiates progressively through a series of internal changes.

  2. Unlike other blood cells, this active mitotic precursor of megacaryocytes undergoes nuclear division and nuclear fusion without cytoplasmic division.

B. *Megacaryocyte (MCC)* (Pennington, 1979)

  1. Progressive changes in the *MCB* form mature *MCCs* with 8 to 16 times the DNA content of normal diploid cells.

  2. The mature *MCC* may achieve diameters up to 10 times the diameter of the mature erythrocyte.

  3. Tubular cytoplasmic channels permeate the *MCC* to form multiple "platelet demarcation membranes" (PDM) (Tavassoli, 1980).

  4. The cytoplasmic processes delineated by the PDM will give rise to the *thromobocytes* (platelets).

VII. Thrombocytopoesis (Becker and DeBruyn, 1976)

A. *Megacaryocyte (MCC)*

1. In lower vertebrates, whole cells involved in the clotting process are known as *thrombocytes.*

2. In humans, only cytoplasmic fragments of the *MCC* circulate to assist in the clotting mechanism.

B. *Thrombocyte formation* (DeBruyn, 1981)

1. Demarcation membranes form cytoplasmic channels that isolate thrombocytic processes.

2. The processes penetrate transient migration pores of the sinusoidal vessels.

3. Constrictions of intravascular processes fragment off as *thrombocytes* (platelets).

4. The hormone *thrombopoetin* stimulates megacaryocyte formation and release of thrombocytes.

VIII. Monocytopoesis (Nichols et al, 1971)

A. *Monoblasts* are derived from the same stem cell that can also give rise to granulocytes. This obviously is the hemocytoblast.

B. *Monocytes* (cf descriptions in chapter on blood)

1. Although the exact cellular events have not been ascertained morphologically, it is clear that monocytes are formed in myeloid tissue.

2. Monocytes leave the circulation, enter the tissues during inflammation and immune responses, and differentiate into macrophages or participate in several functions, some of which are associated with cell-mediated immune responses (van Furth, 1982).

3. Monocytes are the source of *osteoclasts.*

IX. Lymphocytopoesis (Osmond, 1975)

A. *Lymphoblasts* are derived from hemocytoblasts.

B. *Lymphocytes* from bone marrow form a sizable percentage.

1. *Lymphocytes* are reaffirmed as potential stem cells.

2. *Germinal centers* in bone marrow are scarce.

3. Some lymphocytes formed in the bone marrow migrate to other lymphatic tissues for further maturation.

a. Two general populations of lymphocytes are formed in the bone marrow:

(1) *T lymphocytes* migrate to the *thymus (T)* for further differentiation.

(2) *B lymphocytes* remain in the *bone (B)* marrow for full differentiation.

X. Fate of blood cells

A. *Erythrocytes* (Bessis, 1966)

1. After leaving the bone marrow, mature erythrocytes survive for 120 days. During this period they circulate continuously through the vascular system.

2. Their destruction occurs outside the vascular system, in tissues policed by *macrophages*

a. in the *spleen.* Erythrocytes escape between the elongated endothelial cells to the red pulp, where they may be

(1) phagocytozed if worn out or

(2) returned to the circulation if good.

b. in *bone marrow.* Developing erythrocytes surround a macrophage, which digests not only extruded nuclei, but improperly formed cells.

B. *Other blood cells*

1. *Leucocytes* serve limited life spans.

a. *Granulocytes* function and die in the connective tissues.

b. *Monocytes* retain sufficient mitotic capabilities to divide and form *macrophages* in the connective tissues.

c. *Lymphocytes* have two populations,

(1) one short lived and

(2) one long lived. Since immunological memory lasts for years, some lymphocytes must survive for at least this long.

2. *Thrombocytes,* unlike leucocytes, function entirely within the vascular system.

a. They are equipped with minimal cellular structures for survival.

b. Thrombocytes function for a maximum of 10 days after release from the bone marrow.

Questions

DIRECTIONS: Each of the questions or incomplete statements below is followed by suggested answers or completions. Select the single *best* answer for each question.

1. According to the *Nomina Histologica*, sinusoidal vessels of bone marrow are considered
   A. modified blood capillaries
   B. specialized veins
   C. fenestrated
   D. composed of reticulocytes
   E. to receive venous blood from the periosteum

2. The bone marrow basement membrane is composed of
   A. a lamina densa
   B. an incomplete layer of flocculent material
   C. a lamina rara
   D. a lamina fibroreticularis
   E. none of the above

3. The bone marrow adventitial coat
   A. is a modified endothelium
   B. covers a layer of circularly arranged smooth muscle
   C. covers between 40 to 50% of the endothelial surface
   D. is composed of fibroblasts and collagen fibers
   E. does not exist

4. Hemocytopoesis in bone marrow ceases
   A. when yellow marrow decreases in content
   B. at age 5
   C. when adipocytes exceed 75% of the volume of cells
   D. when the temperature increases
   E. only at death

5. All the following occur during erythropoesis EXCEPT
   A. production of hemoglobin increases acidophilia
   B. extrusion of nuclei
   C. increase of basophilia in earliest stage
   D. release of premature cells with residual polyribosomes
   E. production of specific granules

6. All the following occur during granulocytopoesis EXCEPT
   A. in early stages, several nucleoli are seen
   B. metachromatic azurophilic granules appear first
   C. maturing nuclei may be indented, bilobed, or segmented
   D. specific granules arise from the concave surface of the golgi complex
   E. 10 to 15 times the number of mature granulocytes as in the circulating blood are held in reserve in bone marrow

7. Neutrophil granulocyte-specific granules contain
   A. phagocytin
   B. peroxidase
   C. heparin
   D. acid phosphatase
   E. arylsulfatase

8. Megacaryocytopoesis produces all the following EXCEPT
   A. megacaryocytes
   B. cells with 8 to 16 times the DNA in diploid cells
   C. mature cells by nucleokinesis without cytokinesis
   D. mature cells 10 times the diameter of an erythrocyte
   E. monocytes

9. Granulocytopoesis is controlled by which substance?
   A. Erythropoetin
   B. Leukopoetin
   C. Phagocytin
   D. Diapedesis
   E. Hemoglobin

10. Erythrocytes are destroyed
    A. by diapedesis
    B. in the spleen and bone marrow
    C. in the thymus
    D. in the circulation
    E. in lymph nodes

Explanatory Answers

1. **A.** Sinusoidal vessels are considered to be modified blood capillaries per the *Nomina Histologica*. The literature is resplendent with

confusing terminology. Not only are there problems with the understanding of the capillary nature, but the terms sinusoid and sinus seem to be used indiscriminately.

2. B. The basement membrane is a poorly defined flocculent material that does not preserve very well. In fact, some of the older literature stated that there was no basement membrane.

3. C. The adventitial coat, composed of delicate reticular fibers and branching reticulocytes, covers 40 to 60% of the endothelial cell surface. The adventitial reticulocytes respond to toxic substances by becoming large and spreading the flocculent basement membrane plus reticular fibers over the remaining open surfaces.

4. C. When the amount of fat exceeds 75%, bone marrow is considered active or red. Below 75% the marrow is considered inactive or yellow. An increase in temperature causes yellow marrow to become active (red). It is true that death brings about a cessation of hemocytopoesis, but during life there are many pathological conditions that do so, even if temporarily. At five years of age, red marrow begins to change until red equals yellow.

5. E. Specific granules are formed in granulocytopoesis, not in erythrocytopoesis. The increasing cytoplasmic acidophilia of increasing hemoglobin content is responsible for the polychromatophilia of middle stages. The very earliest stages of development accumulate polyribosomes, which are responsible for the increased basophilia. Reticulated erythrocytes are prematurely released cells with residual polyribosomes.

6. D. The specific granules arise from the convex surface of the golgi complex, while the azurophilic granules arise from the concave surface. The statements are all correct.

7. A. Phagocytin is an antibacteriocidal protein. The specific granules also contain the enzyme alkaline phosphatase. The peroxidase-rich specific granules of acidophilic granulocytes also contain acid phosphatase and arylphosphatase. Heparin is found in basophil granulocytes.

8. E. Monocytes are produced by the process of monocytopoesis. The statements A through D are correct.

9. B. Leukopoetin (granulopoetin) controls granulocytopoesis by influencing the marrow to produce additional granulocytes. Erythropoetin controls erythropoesis. Diapedesis is a process and not a substance. Hemoglobin is produced in erythrocytes.

10. B. Aged erythrocytes are destroyed in the spleen, while imperfectly developed erythrocytes are destroyed at anytime during development, by macrophages, in the locus of formation in the bone marrow. T lymphocytes travel to the thymus for completion of maturation. Erythrocytes do not die in transit in the circulation. They may die accidental deaths, but not death from aging or developmental difficulties. The only blood that travels to the lymph nodes is the arteriole that feeds capillary plexuses surrounding germinal centers. Diapedesis is the process whereby blood cells enter the bloodstream through transient openings in the sinusoidal epithelium.

9 Muscle Tissue

I. *Introduction:* All living cells possess the fundamental property of *contractility*, but *myocytes* (muscle cells) have developed it to the greatest degree. Muscle tissue also transmits electrical impulses by depolarization of the plasmalemma in response to a neurotransmitter elaborated by nerve endings. Some myocytes conduct electrical impulses, but cannot contract. The best example is the **myocytus conducens cardiacus**, translated *cardiac conducting myocyte*.

    A. *Functionally,* two types of muscles are distinguished:

    1. *voluntary:* under the direct control of the central nervous system (striated skeletal).

    2. *involuntary:* under the control of the autonomic nervous system (nonstriated muscle tissue, striated cardiac muscle tissue, and some striated skeletal muscle tissue).

    B. *Structurally,* three muscle tissues are recognized:

    1. *Nonstriated muscle tissue* (smooth muscle) provides spiraled layers to the walls of *viscera* (digestive system, respiratory system, urinary system, and reproductive systems) and to the *vascular system* (arteries, veins, and lymphatics) (Somlyo and Somlyo, 1970).

    2. *Striated skeletal muscle tissue:* Striations are attributed to the longitudinal orientation of interdigitating *actin* and *myosin myofilaments*. Generally *voluntary*, this form is responsible for locomotion, maintenance of posture, and change in position.

    a. The following striated skeletal muscles are *involuntary:*

        (1) muscular wall (first part of esophagus),

        (2) tensor tympani (middle ear),

        (3) stapedius muscle (middle ear).

    3. *Striated cardiac muscle tissue, involuntary* in action, comprises the main mass of the heart musculature, or **myocardium**. Its myocytes present the same bands (striations) as skeletal myocytes.

II. Textus muscularis nonstriatus *(nonstriated muscle tissue, smooth muscle)* (Bolzer, 1962)

A. *Myogenesis:* the process of transforming a mesenchymal cell to a *myocyte* (muscle cell) (*myo-* is the Greek combining form meaning muscle).

1. Embryonic mesenchymal cells, derived from mesoderm, differentiate into several components:
   a. vascular endothelium,
   b. connective tissue elements,
   c. layers of *nonstriated muscle tissue* destined to function in visceral walls.

2. Not all muscle tissue is mesodermal in origin. Evidence exists that *nonstriated myocytes* of the *iris* differentiate from ectoderm of the developing optic cup.

3. *Myogenesis* involves elongation of the mesenchymal cell into a *myoblast* (precursor of the nonstriated myocyte) and differentiation of the *myoblast* into a spindle-shaped contractile *nonstriated myocyte*.

4. Primitive mesenchymal cells may differentiate into *reticulocytes* (old name: reticular cell). *Reticulocytes*, persisting in the adult, retain the mesenchymal potentiality to differentiate into *myoblasts* when needed. This is particularly evident in the pregnant uterus, where nonstriated myocytes increase in number *(hyperplasia).*

B. *Contraction depends on the relationship of nonstriated myocytes with the extracellular matrix.*

1. If a fragment of functional nonstriated muscle tissue is immersed in trypsin, the extracellular material is digested, leaving disassociated individual myocytes.

2. In this condition, myocytes may contract if stimulated, but they have nothing to act on. Hence isolated myocytes are useless.

3. The combination of nonstriated myocytes and associated connective tissue components functions to constrict the walls of tubular viscera.

C. *Light microscopy of nonstriated myocytes*

1. Isolated myocytes are elongated, spindle-shaped cells.

2. The larger cross-sectional diameter of the midportion is attributed to a *centrally located nucleus.*

3. In the relaxed state, the myocyte length ranges from 15 μm in blood vessels to 0.5 mm in hypertrophied nonstriated myocytes of the gravid (pregnant) uterus.

4. The **plasmalemma** encloses the acidophilic *cytoplasm* and a centrally located long oval *nucleus* and various cytoplasmic structures. [Older terms such as "sarcolemma" or "sarcoplasm" have been deleted from the *Nomina Histologica*. The International Nomenclature Committee considers such a specific application of the terms **plasmalemma** and **cytoplasma** to be tautologous.]

5. *Contraction* of nonstriated myocytes produces increased periodic accumulations (density) of cytoplasm resembling bands. The basophilic nucleus appears to be shortened during contraction by spiraling (Fig. 9-1).

6. Unstained conical areas at the polar ends of the oval nucleus of the myocyte result from myofibrils diverging over the nucleus. Cytoplasmic acidophilia is attributed to the fibrillar structures.

7. In *longitudinal sections*, nonstriated myocytes accommodate one another like brickwork. In *transverse (cross) sections*, the varia-

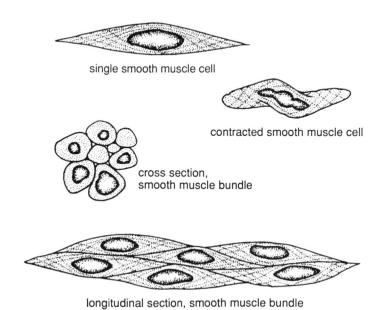

single smooth muscle cell

contracted smooth muscle cell

cross section, smooth muscle bundle

longitudinal section, smooth muscle bundle

Figure 9-1 Nonstriated (smooth) myocytes.

tion in cell diameters reflects this staggered pattern. The tapered myocyte *ends* have a small cross-sectional profile. The *middle*, bearing the central nucleus, displays the largest cross-sectional diameter. The *clear area*, devoid of nuclear material, is surrounded peripherally by acidophilic myofibrils. Between the clear area and the tapered end, cross sections are occupied by acidophilic myofibrils.

D. *Ultrastructure* of *nonstriated myocytes* (Somlyo et al, 1976)

1. Longitudinally oriented, slender **mitochondria** are interspersed singly or in clusters among the myofibrils. (Myofibrils are bundles of thin *myofilaments*.) Other cytoplasmic structures are centrioles, free polyribosomes, some granular ER, and glycogen.

2. The elongated *nucleus* has smooth contours and tapers at the ends to conform to the spindle shape of the myocyte.

3. Contractile *myofilaments*, although not in register as they are in striated myocytes, form a two-filament contractile system:

a. *Thick myofilaments* (**myofilamentum crassum**), 3 μm to 8 μm long, are composed of *myosin* molecules.

b. *Thin myofilaments* (**myofilamentum tenue**) are composed of *actin* molecules arranged in a ratio of 12 to 15 thin myofilaments to one thick myofilament. (Compare to striated skeletal myocytes, which have a ratio of one thick to six thin myofilaments.)

c. Although contractile mechanisms in nonstriated myocytes are not understood as well as those in striated skeletal myocytes, they appear to be dependent upon the interaction of myosin and actin (Schoenberg and Needham, 1976)

4. *Noncontractile* 10-nm-thick *filaments* contributing to the cytoskeleton appear to be associated with the dense bodies (Cooke, 1976).

5. The **plasmalemma** is distinguished by the

a. *caveoli*, numerous flask-like invaginations of the plasmalemma resembling micropinocytotic vesicles of capillary endothelium. *Caveoli* may bring extracellular substances into the cell, transmit impulses into the cell to initiate contractile mechanisms, and sequester calcium ions for transfer into the cytoplasm.

b. **area densa**, a unique characteristic of nonstriated myocytes. Fusiform *dense areas*, distributed throughout the cytoplasm and along the inner surface (PS) of the plasmalemma, resemble densities of desmosomes, zonulae adherens, and Z-lines of skeletal muscle. These may provide attachment sites for the contractile actin myofilaments and the noncontractile cytoskeletal filaments and contribute to cellular cohesiveness.

     c. nexus junctions occurring where intercellular spaces narrow to about 2 nm. Each **nexus** is a site of low electrical resistance for transmission of excitation stimuli from cell to cell (Dewey and Barr, 1962).

     6. A prominent *basement membrane*, synthesized by the myocyte, surrounds the plasmalemma. The interspace between the basement membranes of two adjacent myocytes is occupied by extracellular matrix and resident collagen fibrils.

III. Textus muscularis striatus skeletalis, *striated skeletal muscle tissue*

     A. **Striomyohistogenesis** (*strio-* Latin: fluted, striated, or striped; *myo-* Latin: muscle; *genesis:* formation) (Rhabdomyogenesis [*rhabdo-* equivalent Greek combining form])

     1. In the embryo, *dorsal somites* (segmented blocks of dense mesoderm) occur on either side of the midsagittal plane. Each somite is *innervated* by an adjacent nerve emanating from the developing spinal cord located in the midsagittal dorsal plane.

     2. Each somite gives rise to *dermatome* (which gives rise to connective tissue), *scleratome* (which gives rise to supporting tissues), and *myotome* (which gives rise to most skeletal muscle tissue). [Exception: striated skeletal muscles of the tongue, orbits, and branchial arch derivatives originate directly from mesenchyme.]

     3. *Myotome cells* differentiate into spindle-shaped *myoblasts* resembling the myoblasts that produced nonstriated myocytes.

     4. *Myoblasts* align in elongated bundles and undergo many mitotic divisions.

     5. *Myoblasts* fuse to form a multinucleated syncytium, the *myotube* that is an elongated cell with multiple centrally located nuceli.

     6. *Acidophilic myofibrils* accumulating in the cytoplasm during the fusion process soon extend through the lenghtening myotube.

     7. *Cross striations* developing in the myotube as the myofibrils profilerate are attributed to the myofilaments assembling in register.

     8. Central *nuclei* are pushed to the periphery of the myotube as the population of myofibrils increases.

     B. *Orientation* of *striated skeletal muscle tissue from the macroscopic to microscopic aspect* (Fig. 9-2)

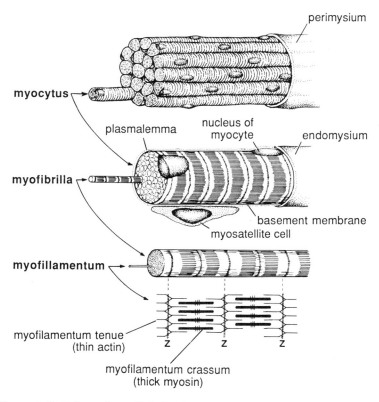

Figure 9-2 Orientation of skeletal myocytes.

1. Both the longest muscle (sartorius) and the shortest (stapedius) are invested with a thick layer of connective tissue called the **epimysium**, from which septae penetrate to divide the muscle into *fasciculi* (bundles). Each *fasciculus*, composed of individual myocytes, is ensheathed by a continuation of the epimysium, the thinner **perimysium**. Each striated skeletal myocyte and its basement membrane is coated by **endomysium**, a delicate loose connective tissue layer continued from the perimysium.

2. Blood vessels, lymphatic vessels, and nerves arborize throughout the connective tissue sheaths until capillary and nerve plexuses are formed around each cell.

3. In an average-size striated skeletal myocyte, *hundreds of nuclei*

are located in the peripheral cytoplasm immediately under the plasmalemma. Nuclei are flattened ovals, parallel to the longitudinal axis of the myocyte. One or two nucleoli are surrounded by a fair amount of chromatin.

4. Nuclei of associated *myosatellite cells*, with denser heterochromatin, depress the plasmalemma of the skeletal myocyte to the extent that it is difficult to define opposing cellular borders. Glycoprotein and reticular fibers invest the myosatellite cells.

5. Striated skeletal myocytes may regenerate after minor injuries if the surrounding basement membrane is intact. The *myosatellite cells* can differentiate into myoblasts and form the myocytes to replace injured ones. If damage to the muscle disrupts a significant amount of basement membrane, regeneration fails and the damaged area is filled with connective tissue to form a scar.

6. *Size* and *shape*: Striated skeletal myocytes range from 1 mm to 40 mm in length and may be up to 0.1 mm in diameter. They are cylindrical in shape and taper to a point at each end. The endomysium of each myocyte continues at the ends and joins the endomysium and perimysium to form strong tendons of origin and insertion.

7. Striated skeletal myocytes *usually do not branch*. One notable exception is the skeletal myocytes of the tongue, which branch from one side of the tongue to the other.

8. Polarization microscopy reveals two major repetitive bands along the length (up to 40 mm) of the myocyte: an *isotropic band*, *I-band*, which is doubly refractile and the *anisotropic band*, *A-band*, which is singly or less refractile.

    a. Stained with H & E, the *A-band* is *acidophilic* and hence appears darker than the I-band when viewed with conventional light microscopic lenses.

    b. the center of the *I-band* is *transected* by a narrow, darkly staining line, the **telophragma** or *Z-line* (Z from the German: Zwischen, literally, in between).

    c. The center of the *A-band* is *crossed* by a *light zone*, the **zona lucida** or *H-band* (H from the German: Heller, meaning bright).

    d. Within the **zona lucida** or *H-band* is the **mesophragma** or *M-line* (M also from the German: Mittlescheibe, the middle line)

    e. *Myomere* (old name, sarcomere): The *structural unit* of striated skeletal myocytes extends between two Z-lines, including the entire A-band and one half of the I-band on each side of the A-band. Events involved in contraction are referred to it.

C. *Ultrastructure of striated skeletal myocytes* (Fig. 9-3) (Huxley, 1960)

1. The *cytoplasm* (old name: sarcoplasm) of striated skeletal myocytes, containing a golgi complex, **mitochondria** (old name: sarcosomes), *agranular endoplasmic reticulum (sER)* (old name: sarcoplasmic reticulum), a few ribosomes, glycogen, and myofibrils, is confined in a **plasmalemma** (old name: sarcolemma) that extends the full length of the myocyte.

2. The *golgi complex* is reduced in size and relatively inactive in its juxtanuclear location.

3. Large *conspicuous mitochondria*, with closely packed parallel cristae, are abundant at the nuclear poles, under the plasmalemma and between the myofibrils. Paired bracelet-like mitochondria encircle individual myofibrils at the level of the *I-bands*, on either side of

Figure 9-3 Arrangements of skeletal myocyte myofilaments in relaxed and contracted longitudinal states and in cross sections. The numbers 1, 2, 3, and 4 under the cross sections correspond to the 1, 2, 3, and 4 of the relaxed longitudinal myofilament.

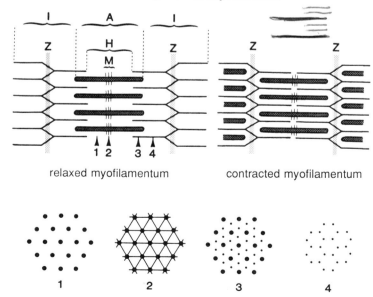

relaxed myofilamentum   contracted myofilamentum

each *Z-line* (Rambourg and Segretain, 1980). Their characteristics reflect the high energy requirements of contracting muscle.

4. The *endoplasmic reticulum* (Franzini-Armstrong, 1986) is devoid of associated polyribosomes, and hence there is no associated basophilia. The smooth *tubular elements* of the *sER* are oriented longitudinally and surround every myofibril. In the region of the *H-band*, **zona lucida**, the tubular elements anastomose freely to form the *reticular elements* of the *sER*. At the junction between the *A-band* and the *I-band*, the ends of the tubular elements enlarge to form *terminal cisternae*, which sequester the calcium ions for use during contraction.

5. The **plasmalemma** invaginates to form a complex *transverse tubular* or *T-tubular* system at the transition of every *A-band* and the *I-band*. Within the myocyte, *T-tubules* branch extensively at the transverse plane to surround each myofibril.

    a. The *T-tubules* do not communicate with the endoplasmic reticulum, but as invaginations of the plasmalemma, they communicate directly with the extracellular environment.

    b. The T-tubular system explains how central myofibrils at some distance from the plasmalemma contract at the same time as those close to the surface.

    c. Waves of depolarization may conduct rapidly, via the T-tubules from the surface plasmalemma to individual myofibrils, thus producing synchronous contraction of all myofibrils.

    d. The combination of *two terminal cisternae* sandwiching a *single T-tubule* is known as the *triad*.

6. *Myofibrils* are the major longitudinally oriented subunits of striated skeletal myocytes. In transverse (cross) sections, via LM, myofibrils appear as acidophilic dot-like densities about 100 to 200 nm in diameter.

7. At the EM level, each myofibril consists of an orderly arrangement of finer *myofilaments*, whose arrangement in register establishes the structural basis of the banding patterns. The *myofilaments* are subdivided into

    a. myofilamentum tenue: *thin myofilaments*, 5 nm in diameter, corresponding to the protein *actin*. In a relaxed myomere, thin actin myofilaments extend outward from the Z-line, across the I-band, and project between the thick myosin myofilaments without reaching the middle of the myomere.

    (1) Each *thin myofilament* is composed of a double-stranded helix of *actin molecules.* Each *strand* of the helix, termed *F-actin*, consists of a series of *G-actin* molecules.

(2) two regulatory proteins, *tropomyosin* and *troponin*, are reported to be associated with actin (Ebashi, 1974). *Tropomyosin* lies in a spiral groove along each side of the helix. *Troponin*, bound to specific sites along the tropomyosin molecule, consists of three components: *troponin-T* (*TnT*, which binds firmly to tropomyosin), *troponin-C* (*TnC*, binds calcium ions), and *troponin-I* (*TnI*, the inhibitor of actin – myosin interaction).

b. **myofilamentum crassum:** *thick myofilaments,* 10 nm in diameter, corresponding to the protein myosin. Thick myofilaments occupy the middle of the myomere and extend the entire length of the A-band (Fig. 9-6). The relatively dense A-band consists of both thick and thin myofilaments. Each *thick myosin myofilament* is composed of long molecules consisting of (Ganong, 1983)

(1) *light meromyosin* molecules, which are arranged parallel to each other in a staggered fashion, to form the "backbone" of the thick myosin myofilament.

(2) *heavy meromyosin* molecules, which can be separated into a *rod portion* and a *head portion.* Heavy meromyosin is believed to bind with actin molecules to initiate the sliding movements of the thin actin myofilaments.

c. The central lighter region of the *A-band*, occupied only by thick myosin filaments, corresponds to the *H-band.*

d. The **telophragma,** *Z-line,* forms the boundary between adjacent myomeres and interconnects thin actin myofilaments. Each thin actin myofilament on one side of the Z-line lies opposite the space between thin actin myofilaments of the adjacent side of the Z-line. Z-lines interconnect thin actin myofilaments of adjacent myomeres, creating a zig-zag appearance (Fig. 9-3) (Kelley and Cahill, 1972).

e. The **mesophragma,** *M-line,* occasionally visible with LM, is caused by transversely oriented filaments interconnecting the central region of adjacent thick myosin myofilaments (Luther and Squire, 1978).

D. *Mechanism of contraction* (Franzini-Armstrong et al, 1981)

1. During relaxation, troponin and tropomyosin form a complex that inhibits actin molecules from interacting with the heads of heavy meromyosin.

2. *Stimulation* of the muscle fiber by a nerve motor end plate produces a wave of *excitation* along the **plasmalemma** extending into

the *T-tubular system* causing a release of calcium ions from the agranular endoplasmic reticulum.

3. The released *calcium ions* enter the myofibrils and bind to troponin. This results in a change of conformation of the troponin–tropomyosin complex, thereby exposing the active sites of the actin molecules. *Actin* and *myosin* now are capable of reacting.

4. Although the precise mechanism requires further investigation, it is believed that the heads of heavy meromyosin attach to the active sites on thin actin myofilaments. A successive attachment, removal, and reattachment mechanism may explain how thin actin myofilaments are drawn along the thick myosin myofilaments into the *A-band*.

5. *Thick myosin myofilaments* remain relatively stable, while the *Z-lines* with attached *thin actin myofilaments* are approximated (Huxley, 1971). This sliding action of myofibrils is responsible for shortening the entire striated skeletal myocyte.

6. Upon relaxation, calcium ions return to the tubules of the agranular endoplasmic reticulum.

E. *Structural modifications resulting from contraction* of the striated skeletal myocyte results in the disappearance of all or most of the *I-band*. Approximation of the Z-lines as the thin actin myofilaments approach one another results in the disappearance of the *H-band* and hence shortening of the myomere. The bulging plasmalemma between the invagination points of the *T-tubules* fills with glycogen and cytoplasm.

F. *Striated skeletal myocyte types* (Gauthier, 1986)

1. Human striated skeletal myocytes are composed of two types, based on physiologic and biochemical properties:

   a. *Type I:* prominent in slow-contracting muscles,

      (1) characterized by small diameter, abundance of myoglobin, and high levels of oxidative enzymes.

      (2) mixed with type II in most striated skeletal muscle tissues, with some having one or the other predominate.

   b. *Type II:* prominent in fast-contracting muscles,

      (1) characterized by large diameter, lower myoglobin content, and high levels of glycolytic enzymes.

      (2) subdivided into *types IIA and IIB*.

         (a) *Type IIA* utilizes both oxidative and glycolytic enzymes.

         (b) *Type IIB* utilizes glycolysis for the production of ATP.

2. For nonhuman striated skeletal myocytes, utilize the following classifications, which do not necessarily correlate with the type I, types IIA and IIB classifications:
    a. slow-twitch oxidative (SO),
    b. fast-twitch oxidative-glycolytic (FOG),
    c. fast-twitch glycolytic (FG).

G. The *neuromuscular termination* (myoneural junction) (Heuser, 1976; Heuser et al, 1979) is the site of structural contact between a motor nerve ending and a striated skeletal myocyte. The following 10 points summarize the sequelae of events leading to concentration (Fig. 9-4).

1. Where the motor neuron terminus contacts a striated skeletal myocyte, several myocyte nuclei aggregate.

2. Several nuclei of *teloglial* cells, which ensheathe the motor neuron terminus, contribute to the entire complex forming the *motor end plate.*

3. The *axon terminus* divides into several branches that depress the myocyte plasmalemma into *synaptic troughs.* At the bottom of the synaptic trough, the myocyte plasmalemma forms leaf-like invaginations called *subneural clefts.*

4. The *myocyte basement membrane* separates the axon terminus (in the synaptic trough) from the myocyte plasmalemma.

5. Within the cytoplasm of the axon terminus, there are accumulations of *synaptic vesicles*, each of which stores approximately 10,000 molecules of the *neurotransmitter acetylcholine.*

6. The *myocyte plasmalemma* opposed to the axon terminus is characterized by *acetylcholine receptors.*

7. Via *exocytosis* the axonal synaptic vesicles release the acetylcholine into the space occupied by the basement membrane.

8. After filtering through the basement membrane, the acetylcholine combines with corresponding receptors on the myocyte plasmalemma to make the *plasmalemma more permeable* to *sodium ions.*

9. Sodium ions depolarize the myocyte plasmalemma to initiate an *action potential* that is transmitted over the plasmalemma and into the T-tubules.

10. Calcium ions sequestered in the *terminal cisternae* of the myocyte sER are activated and contraction is initiated.

A

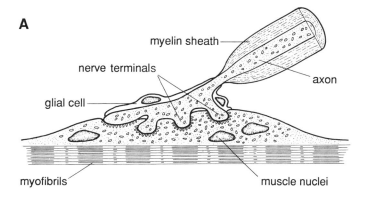

myelin sheath

nerve terminals

axon

glial cell

myofibrils

muscle nuclei

B

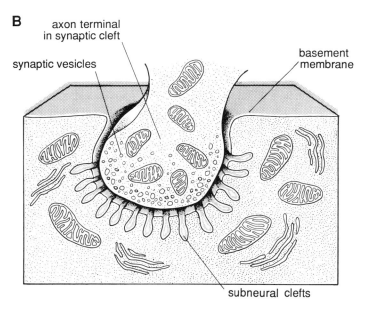

axon terminal
in synaptic cleft

synaptic vesicles

basement
membrane

subneural clefts

Figure 9-4 The neuromuscular termination.

IV. **Textus muscularis striatus cardiacus**, *striated cardiac muscle tissue* (The heart will be presented with the vascular system.)

    A. *Light microscopy of striated cardiac muscle tissue*

      1. Banding patterns and contraction mechanisms are similar to striated skeletal muscle. One additional "disc" is noted, the *intercalated disc* (see below). The unit of contraction is the *myomere* (old name, sarcomere).

      2. Each *cardiac myocyte* with one centrally located nucleus branches to form a cell with two, three, or four blunt ends (Fig. 9-5). Cross sections vary from cylindrical to oval depending on the plane of section. From blunted ends, finger-like processes interdigitate with those of adjacent cardiac myocytes. A *series* of interdigitating *cardiac myocytes* form a branching *myofiber* (Fig. 9-5). (The term *myofiber* is not a synonym for *myocyte*.)

Figure 9-5 Cardiac myocytes with two ends (A), three ends (B), and four ends (C), unite to form cardiac muscle branching fibers.

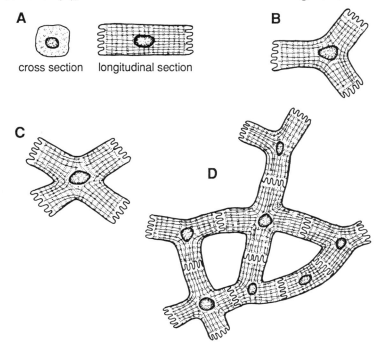

3. The cytoplasm contains *myofibrils* that extend from one end of the myocyte to the other, diverging over the *nucleus.* A *conical clear area* at the nuclear poles, resulting from the diverging myofibrils, contains a golgi complex and lipofuscin pigment granules. In aging humans this pigment increases to such an extent that it composes up to 20% of the dry myocardial weight! Abundant glycogen droplets and a few lipid droplets fill the interstices between myofibrils.

B. *Submicroscopic structure of striated cardiac myocytes* (McNutt and Fawcett, 1974)

1. *Intercalated discs* (Muir, 1975) are recognized as interdigitating junctional complexes, specialized for cohesion and transmission of electrical impulses. The *junctional complex* of an intercalated disc is characterized by three components:

a. macula adherens (the spot desmosome), the inner leaf of each opposing plasmalemma thickened for insertion of thin actin myofilaments of the I-band,

b. fascia adherens, an extensive cohesive area of variable outline. (In epithelial cells, the zonula adherens extends around the cell. In cardiac myocyte, extensiveness requires the term *fascia* rather than *zonula.*)

c. nexus *(gap junction)*, to conduct electrical impulses between cells.

2. *T-tubules* in human striated cardiac myocytes, residing at the Z-line, are distinctly larger than corresponding T-tubules of striated skeletal myocytes (at the junction of the I- and A-bands). They are lined by a thick glycoprotein layer continuous with that coating the plasmalemma. *T-tubules* are few or *absent* in the **myocardium** of *atria,* perhaps because these striated cardiac myocytes are much smaller than those of the ventricles. Interior myofibrils may be able to respond to waves of depolarization without the need for T-tubules.

3. *Agranular endoplasmic reticulum* (sER) is less complex than that of skeletal muscle. As it anastomoses freely around the myofibrils, occasional small dilatations of the terminals contact the T-tubules. Of special interest are the infrequent sER endings that abut the plasmalemma. A *diad* occurs where one dilated end of an sER tubule contacts a T-tubule. (Compare with the *triad* in skeletal myocytes.)

4. Mitochondria (old name: sarcosomes) of cardiac myocytes are occasionally larger than one myomere. Angular parallel cristae are closely spaced in zig-zag fashion, occasionally uniting to form a honeycomb appearance. Numerous mitochondria reside between the myofibrils.

5. *Specific atrial granules* (Jamieson and Palade, 1964), 0.3 to 0.4 μm, are present in the smaller striated cardiac myocytes of the atria, in the conical clear areas of the nuclear poles. Two polypeptide hormones have been extracted from the atrial myocytes: *cardionatrin* (deBold and Flynn, 1983), which produces diuretic and natriuretic effects, and *cardiodilatin*, which relaxes and dilates smooth muscle of the vascular system. The granule-containing cells are more abundant in the right atrium. Thus, the right atrium not only harbors the *sinuatrial node* (see below), but its *myoendocardial cells* place it alongside other endocrine organs (Forsmann et al, 1983; Metz et al, 1984).

6. *Myofibrils,* composed of *thin actin myofilaments* and *thick myosin myofilaments,* produce the same banding patterns as striated skeletal myocytes (except for the intercalated disc).

7. *Contraction* produces the same type of structural changes and

Figure 9-6 Electron micrograph of a contracting cardiac myocyte from the newt *Notophthalmus viridescens*. Note the disappearance of bands brought about by the interdigitation of actin and myosin myofilaments (×2000).

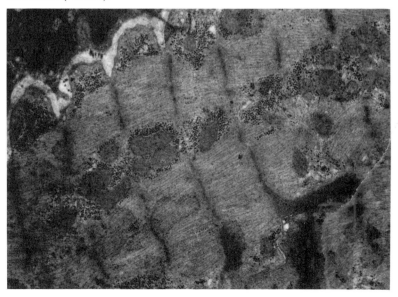

approximation of the Z-lines as striated skeletal myocytes and bulging plasmalemma with a glycogen-filled cytoplasm (Fig. 9-6).

8. Involuntary *cardiac myocytes* are innervated by the *autonomic nervous system (ANS)*, but at the same time receive a contraction stimulus from modified cardiac myocytes termed the *cardiac conduction myocytes* (old name: Purkinje fibers). Some *cardiac conduction myocytes* are specialized for initiating a stimulus for contraction, while the majority form *cardiac conduction myofibers*, which only transmit the stimulus to contract. *Cardiac conduction myocytes do not contract.*

a. The *parasympathetic* division *(vagus nerve)* of the ANS, the inherent beat of the heart.

b. The *sympathetic* division of the ANS releases norepinephrine from nerve endings to accelerate heart pulsations.

9. The *inherent cardiac beat* in the absence of autonomic innervation can be demonstrated by the following classroom procedure:

a. Expose the beating heart of the newt *Notophthalmus viridescens.* Separate the three-chambered heart from the large vessels and transfer it to amphibian Tyrode's solution and note that the heart pulsates in the absence of any connections with the nervous system.

b. Separation of the single ventricle from the two atria results in cessation of ventricular pulsations, while the atria continue to beat. This demonstrates that the ventricle has been separated from its source of excitation.

c. Careful dissection (under a dissecting microscope) of the tiny atria isolates the source of conduction to the right atrium.

10. Microscopic and submicroscopic structure of the *cardiac conduction myocytes* and the *myofibers*

a. *Cardiac conduction myocytes* are characterized by sparse myofibrils displaced toward the periphery, immediately under the plasmalemma. The myofibrils confer an acidophilia to the areas in which they are located.

b. The *interior cytoplasm* of the cardiac conduction myocytes, devoid of myofibers, is occupied by an abundance of glycogen and mitochondria, and hence does not take routine stains (H & E). With TEM, glycogen appears black.

c. Intercalated discs are not as pronounced as in cardiac myocytes. Instead, smaller interdigitations join the cells aided by typical desmosomes (no fascia adherens).

11. *Summary* of the *cardiac conduction system* (Truex and Smythe, 1964)

a. The heart possesses a conduction system.

b. Innervation by the autonomic nervous system increases or decreases the inherent beat.

c. An aggregation of modified cardiac myocytes, the *sinuatrial node (SA node)* (the pacemaker), initiates the cardiac beat from its location at the junction of the superior vena cava and right atrium.

d. The SA node transmits the impulse to another specialized node of cardiac conduction tissue, the *atrioventricular node (AV node)*, located at the junction of the coronary sinus, right atrium, and right ventricle.

e. From the AV node arise two large branches, the *antriventricular bundles*, which travel in the endocardium on each side of the interventricular septum as the *right limb* and the *left limb*. These huge myofibers, arborizing in the interventicular septum, decrease in diameter until they reach the apex of the heart. From here they ascend the ventricular and atrial walls, in the endocardium, as definitive *cardiac conduction myofibers* (composed of cardiac conduction myocytes).

f. Final impulses are transmitted to the striated cardiac myofibers of the myocardium, causing contraction.

Questions

DIRECTIONS: For each of the items in this section, one or more of the numbered options is correct. Select
    A if only *1, 2, and 3* are correct
    B if only *1 and 3* are correct
    C if only *2 and 4* are correct
    D if only *4* is correct
    E if *all* are correct

1. Myogenesis involves
    1. elongation of mesenchymal cells into myoblasts
    2. dedifferentiation of stem cells
    3. differentiation of a myoblast into a myocyte
    4. interactions with myeloid tissue

2. Nonstriated myocytes contain
   1. slender mitochondria interspersed among myofibrils
   2. contractile myofilaments
   3. noncontractile filaments
   4. dense areas throughout the cytoplasm

3. Connective tissue involved with striated skeletal muscle forms
   1. epimysium
   2. perimysium
   3. endomysium
   4. myomere

4. A *triad* consists of
   1. thin actin myofilaments
   2. two terminal cisternae
   3. a Z-line
   4. a T-tubule

5. Mitochondria of striated skeletal myocytes
   1. are abundant at the nuclear poles
   2. fit under the plasmalemma
   3. insert between individual myofibrils
   4. embrace individual myofibrils on each side of a Z-line

6. Thick myofilaments in striated myocytes are composed of
   1. tropomyosin
   2. light meromyosin
   3. troponin
   4. heavy meromyosin

7. The myoneural junction is characterized by
   1. an aggregation of myocyte nuclei
   2. the presence of a myocyte basement membrane
   3. an aggregation of teloglial cells
   4. a synaptic trough impressed with subneural clefts

8. Striated cardiac myocytes
   1. form myofibers
   2. are syncytial cells
   3. contain lipofuchsin pigment
   4. have few or absent T-tubules

Directions Summarized				
A	**B**	**C**	**D**	**E**
1,2,3	1,3	2,4	4	All are
only	only	only	only	correct

9. Striated cardiac myocytes of the right atrium are distinguished
   1. by massive T-tubules
   2. the absence of intercalated discs
   3. by the presence of triads
   4. by the presence of specific granules

10. Cardiac conduction myocytes are distinguished by
    1. intercalated discs that are not as pronounced as those of cardiac myocytes
    2. sparse myofibrils
    3. an abundance of cytoplasmic glycogen
    4. peripheral nuclei

Explanatory Answers

1. B. 1 and 3 are correct. These extracted steps pertain to all muscle tissue. Statement 2 is incorrect because differentiation is required. The term "myeloid" refers to bone marrow and not to muscle. The Greek *myos-* is the stem for muscle, the Greek *myelos-* is the stem for "fat-like," and in fact bone marrow contains well over 50% fat.

2. E. All are correct. The mitochondria occur singly or in clusters. The contractile myofilaments are composed of actin and myosin, which are not in register as are the actin and myosin of striated skeletal myocytes. Noncontractile filaments contribute to the cytoskeleton of the myocyte. Dense areas may provide attachment sites for both contractile myofilaments and noncontractile filaments.

3. A. 1, 2, and 3 are correct. The epimysium covers the entire muscle. Perimysium is formed by extensions of the epimysium, which form a sheath around fasciculi (bundles of striated skeletal myocytes). Endomysium, surrounding individual striated skeletal myocytes, originates from delicate extensions of the perimysium. The myomere is not a connective tissue sheath, but the unit of contraction.

4. D. 2 and 4 are correct. At the transition of every A-band and I-band the plasmalemma invaginates to form the T-tubular system. Terminal cisternae of the smooth endoplasmic reticulum abut the T-tubules. The combination of two T-tubules, one on either side of the T-tubule, comprises the *triad*. Actin myofilaments do indeed attach to either side of the Z-lines, but this is the area of the I-band.

5. E. All are correct. The disposition of mitochondria as stated in 1, 2, and 3 is not unusual. Unique are the paired bracelet-like mitochondria encircling individual myofibrils at the level of the I-bands, on either side of the Z-line.

6. D. 2 and 4 are correct. Thick myosin myofilaments are composed of the light meromyosin molecules forming the backbone of the thick myosin myofilament. The heavy meromyosin molecules, separated into a rod and head portion, initiate the sliding movements of the thin actin myofilaments. Tropomyosin and troponin are regulatory proteins associated with actin.

7. E. All are correct. The myoneural junction is specialized to facilitate exocytosis of synaptic vesicles containing the neurotransmitter acetylcholine and the acceptance of the neurotransmitter by acetylcholine receptors on the myocyte plasmalemma in the synaptic trough.

8. B. 1 and 3 are correct. A series of individual myocytes, united at interdigitations called the intercalated discs, form a branching myofiber. However, this is not a syncytium, nor are the individual myocytes a syncytium. The lipochrome pigment in humans increases until it composes 20% of the dry weight of an aged person's heart. T-tubules are larger than corresponding tubules in striated skeletal myocytes. However, in the atria the myocytes have a small diameter and need smaller or no T-tubules.

9. D. Only 4 is correct. Atrial myocytes containing specific granules are distinguished as myoendocardial cells producing two polypeptide hormones: cardionatrin and cardiodilatin. Granular leucocytes of the blood possess "specific granules." However, the specific granules of the atrial myocytes contain the hormones. Atrial myocytes possess not only smaller T-tubules than ventricular T-tubules, but they may be absent altogether. Triads usually exist only in striated skeletal myocytes. Intercalated discs are present in all cardiac myocytes. They are not as pronounced in cardiac conduction myocytes.

10. A. 1, 2, and 3 are correct. Intercalated discs have smaller interdigitations joined by desmosomes (macula adherens) instead of a fascia adherens. The sparse myofibrils are pushed to the periphery of the myocyte by the abundant glycogen. Each cardiac conduction myocyte has a single centrally placed nucleus.

10 Nerve Tissue

I. *Introduction*

A. *Nerve tissue*, one of the four basic tissues, is composed of highly differentiated nerve cells, the neurons, plus their associated supportive cells, the **neuroglia**. The *neuron*, the basic unit of the nervous system, is endowed with the special properties of *irritability* and *conductivity*.

B. Nerve tissue functions as the coordinating and integrating system of the body. *Neurons* possess cytoplasmic processes, which may extend great distances from the *neuron body* containing the nucleus.

1. External and internal environmental information in the form of specific stimuli (such as pain, temperature, pressure, and two-point discrimination) are conveyed to the *central nervous system (CNS)* by *afferent neurons* (carrying stimuli toward the CNS).

2. After this information is processed and recorded in the appropriate region of the CNS, motor commands are issued to *efferent neurons* (carrying stimuli away from the CNS) for coordinated responses of muscles, organs, glands, or visceral organs.

II. The nervous system is conveniently divided into three parts:

A. Pars centralis, *the central nervous system (CNS)*, consists of the brain and spinal cord.

B. Pars peripherica, *the peripheral nervous system (PNS)*, consists of cranial and spinal nerves that

1. relay sensory information from peripheral nerve endings (afferent neurons) back to the CNS. These endings are classified as

a. *exteroceptors*: from the skin,

b. *interoceptors*: from the viscera,

c. *proprioceptors*: from muscles, tendons, and joints.

2. convey motor stimuli (via efferent neurons) to an effector organ (eg, muscle).

C. Pars autonomica, *the autonomic nervous system (ANS),* consisting of portions of both systems above, is primarily concerned with regulation of visceral activities. Numerous small *ganglia* are included. Specialized areas are found in the thoracic aortic plexus, abdominal aortic plexus, and superior hypogastric plexus. Two subdivisions are distinguished: **pars sympathetica** and **pars parasympathetica.**

III. *Neurogenesis* (Fig. 10-1) (Levi-Montalcini, 1964; Jacobson, 1978)

A. The trilaminar embryo is composed of three germinal layers, an outer *ectoderm*, a middle *mesoderm*, and an inner *endoderm*.

B. The outer ectoderm gives rise to the nervous system.

    1. A flattened ectodermal sheet, the **lamina neuralis** (neural plate), forms an indentation in the midsagittal plane, the **plica neuralis.**

    2. The lamina neuralis creases the underlying mesoderm to form a groove, the **sulcus neuralis.**

    3. With progressive deepening, the edges of the **sulcus neuralis**

Figure 10-1 Stages in the formation of the neural tube from neural ectoderm.

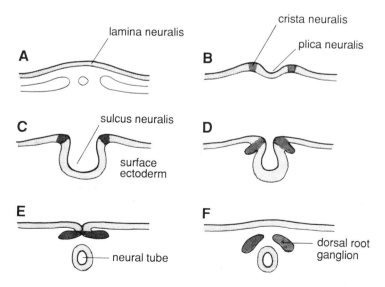

meet and fuse to form the *neural tube*, which separates from the outer ectodermal layer as if by a cephalic and caudal "zipping action." Thus, the brain and spinal cord are formed.

4. The midline fusing edges are composed of *neural crest cells*, which proliferate longitudinally to form columns of cells on the dorsolateral aspects of the *neural tube*. The parasagittal ridges of neural crest cells segment to become the anlage of *spinal ganglia, cranial ganglia, sympathetic ganglia, suprarenal medulla*, and *melanocytes* (pigment cells) (Weston, 1963).

C. Initially. the **lamina neuralis** is a single layer of cells, but during growth it develops (by mitosis) into a pseudostratified epithelium. The differentiated **lamina neuralis** produces

1. *neuroblasts*, progenitors of CNS neurons,

2. *spongioblasts*, progenitors of CNS neuroglia.

D. The *neural crest cells* differentiate to produce

1. *neuroblasts* that become neurons of PNS ganglia,

2. *spongioblasts* that give rise to PNS neuroglia.

IV. *Neurohistology*

A. The *neuron*, like other cells, possesses a nucleus and a typical complement of cytoplasmic structures (Peters et al, 1976). The major difference is that the plasmalemma and enclosed cytoplasm are drawn from the *neuron body* (nerve cell body) into elongated processes. Polarization of neurons is exhibited by cell processes called

1. *dendrities*, which convey stimuli *toward* the neuron body from a *receptor* (nerve ending),

2. *axons*, which carry impulses *away* from the neuron body to an *effector* structure (muscle).

B. *Neurons* are *classified* according to the number of axons and dendrites they possess (Fig. 10-2), exemplified by

1. *apolar neurons* seen in developing ellipsoidal cells of the neuroepithelium,

2. *unipolar neurons* are differentiating neuroepithelial cells with one leading process that invariabaly continues development through the bipolar phase. Occasional unipolar neurons may persist into the adult,

3. *bipolar neurons*, with one axon and one dendrite arising at opposite poles of the cell body, occur in

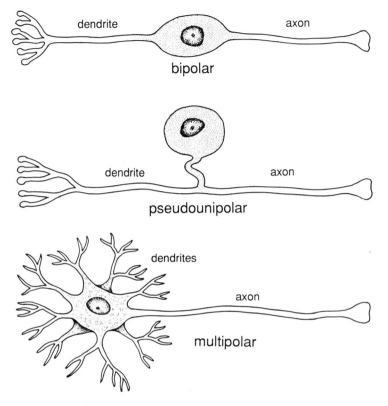

Figure 10-2 Principal types of neurons.

    a. *sensory ganglia*: cranial nerves V, VII, IX, X, XI,
    b. *dorsal root spinal ganglia*,
    c. *organs of special sense*, such as the eye and ear.

    4. *pseudounipolar neurons* begin as bipolar neurons whose processes come together and fuse. In *dorsal root spinal ganglia*, they are recognized by a smooth neuron body (no other processes). Around the neuron body are *ganglia gliocytes* (satellite cells) surrounded by a thin connective tissue capsule.

    5. *multipolar neurons*, with one axon and many dendrites, are most numerous in the CNS and autonomic ganglia. Examples: *motor neurons* of the ventral horn of the spinal cord, *pyramidal cells* of the cerebral cortex, and *piriform neurons* (formerly: Purkinje cells) of the cerebellum.

C. Each neuron component possesses characteristic features that facilitate identification via LM or EM.

1. The *neuron body* contains the nucleus. Great variation in the diameter of the neuron body exists throughout the nervous system, ranging from diameters of 4 μm for *granule cell* neurons to 100 μm for *giant pyramidal cells* of the cerebral cortex.

2. *Plasmalemma*: encloses the entire neuron (cell body, axon, dendrites).

3. The *nucleus* of most neurons is round and vesicular and contains a single large nucleolus. The greater portion of chromatin is euchromatin, suggesting a metabolically active cell. The intensely basophilic nucleolus contrasts with the paler staining chromatin.

4. *Cytoplasm* occurs around the nucleus (old name: perikaryon) and neuron body, in the axon (old name: axoplasm) and in the dendrites.

a. *Chromatophilic substance* (old name: Nissl substance) is the prominent clumped basophilic material in the neuron body and its dendrites. It is *absent* in the rim of cytoplasm of the neuron body immediately under the plasmalemma.

(1) TEM resolves parallel stacks of endoplasmic reticulum membranes studded with *polyribosomes* (rER). Free *polyribosomes* also populate the cytoplasm.

(2) The quantity, distribution, and size of the stacks varies from cell to cell, reflecting the activity of that particular neuron.

(3) *Axon reaction:* Any injury to the neuron body or its axon causes dissolution of the chromatophilic substance. It is important to observe that the chromatophilic substance is *absent* from the entire axon, including the *axon hillock* (where the axon joins the neuron body) (Palay et al, 1968).

b. A large, conspicuous *golgi complex* forms a half sphere capping one pole of the vesicular neuron nucleus. Flattened parallel cisternal membranes with bulbous ends are united by membranous tubules.

c. *Neurofibrils* are fibrous cytoplasmic constituents of the neuron cytoplasm.

(1) Stained by silver impregnation techniques for LM study, they form wavy threads coursing from dendrite to dendrite, dendrite to neuron body, and neuron body into the axon.

(2) Neurofibrils are *aggregates* of

(a) *neurofilaments:* rod-like structures composed of protein subunits approximately 10 nm in diameter. They contribute to the cytoskeleton of the neuron (Bray and Gilbert, 1981).

(b) *neurotubules:* hollow tubes 20 to 30 nm in diameter that may function in the *fast* component of cytoplasmic transport, ie, formation of synaptic vesicles.

d. **Mitochondria**, far smaller than those of other body cells, exist almost everywhere in the cytoplasm, particularly in the axonal synaptic terminals.

(1) Mitochondria, more than any other cytoplasmic structure, react to heat, carbon dioxide, osmotic changes, and fat solvents.

(2) The innumerable mitochondria reflect the great metabolic activity carried on by neurons.

e. A **cytocentrum**, containing the pair of centrioles, is prominent in dividing neuroblasts. Although difficult to resolve via LM, TEM resolves *centrioles* in fully differentiated neurons that do not divide.

f. *Vesicles:* Most neurons contain a variety of membrane-bound vesicles in the cytoplasm:

(1) lysosome vesicles,

(2) vesicles with inclusion granules,

(3) synaptic vesicles, scattered throughout the cytoplasm, seem to concentrate in the axon terminals where a synapse forms.

g. *Pigments*

(1) *Lipofuscin* is a lipochrome called the "wear and tear" pigment because it accumulates with advancing age. At the ultrastructural level, lipofuscin appears as electron-dense granules with an affinity for osmium.

(2) *Melanin* pigment is responsible for the black appearance of some neurons, especially those in the **substantia nigra** of the brain. Many neurons throughout the nervous system contain brown to black coarse pigment granules.

(a) Neurons containing more melanin have reduced amounts of lipofuscin, and vice versa.

(b) In Parkinson's disease and in senile degeneration, melanin pigment granules have a tendency to disintegrate with the neurons.

V. *Axons* and *dendrites*

A. The *axons* and *dendrites* are elongate cytoplasmic processes that originate from the cell body and that may travel long distances from the neuron bodies.

1. Nerves that provide motor stimuli to muscles in the foot have neuron bodies located in the ventral horn of the spinal cord. Axons must travel from this site to the foot to stimulate muscle contraction.

2. The structure and course of axons and dendrites have been studied most frequently via silver impregnation methods. Silver salts, which impregnate neuron processes, are reduced to metallic silver.

3. TEM distinguishes axons from dendrites by the presence of synaptic vesicles in the axon terminals.

4. The *neuropil*, the region surrounding the neuron body, is composed of what appears to be a haphazard arrangement of interlacing networks of axons, dendrites, glial cell processes, and capillary plexuses. Careful examination reveals precise structural and functional relationships between neurons and associated processes.

5. Axon and dendrite cytoplasm contains neurofilaments and neurotubules, but only dendrites possess chromatophilic substance.

6. *Myelin sheath.* Certain axons of the CNS and PNS possess an insulating sheath of "fatty" *myelin*, which greatly increases the conduction velocity of axons. *Neurolemmocytes* (old name: Schwann cells) are derived from neural crest cells. The *myelinization process* follows below (Fig. 10-3).

Figure 10-3 The process of myelinization.

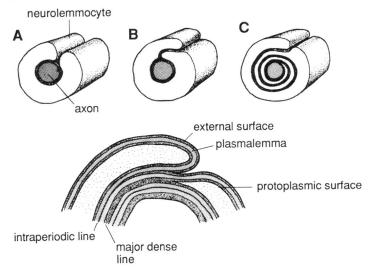

a. Stage one: shows the *axon* as a small circle embraced by the *neurolemmocyte* as if it were in the process of phagocytosis (Geren, 1956).

b. Stage two: the neurolemmocytes begin wrapping around the axon ("jelly-rolling") until several concentric layers of the plasmalemma are closely approximated. Their nuclei lie adjacent to individual nerve fibers in the peripheral nerve (Uzman, 1964).

c. Stage three: completion of the process shows the following identifiable layers or lines via TEM:

(1) *electron-dense intraperiodic lines*, 2 to 3 nm thick, formed from the fusion of the external surface of the neurolemmocyte plasmalemma (Revel and Hamilton, 1969).

(2) *electron-lucent spaces*, on either side of the dense lines, formed from the *lipid* component of the neurolemmocyte plasmalemma.

(3) *major dense lines* formed by the cytoplasmic surface of the neurolemmocyte plasmalemma.

7. One *neurolemmocyte* myelinates only one segment of an axon in the PNS. Many successive neurolemmocytes coat the axon, like a string of hot dogs. The intervals between neurolemmocytes are **nodus neurofibrae**, *node of the nerve fiber* (old name: node of Ranvier) (Peters, 1966).

VI. The *synapse* (Fig. 10-4) is essential in transmitting impulses from one neuron to another. Neurons of the CNS also maintain direct communication with one another via the **nexus** *(gap junctions)*.

A. The physical *discontinuity* between one neuron and another substantiates the neurone doctrine, which states that each neuron process is the outgrowth of a single nerve cell and not the result of fusion of many neurons. The region of physical discontinuity is referred to as the *synapse*.

B. The synapse is the site where the axon of one neuron terminates on another neuron (Gray, 1959):

1. body: *axosomatic synapse*.

2. axon: *axoaxonic synapse*.

3. dendrite: *axodendritic synapse*. These are most common and will be considered as the prototypes.

C. *Axodendritic synapses* have three main parts:

1. The *presynaptic part* is the axon terminal of the first neuron containing

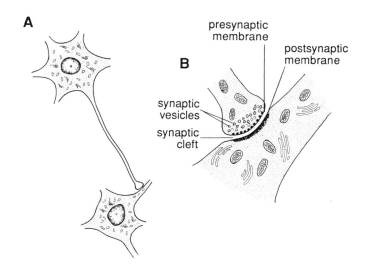

Figure 10-4 Principal features of the synapse.

a. *mitochondria*

b. *presynaptic membrane*, a thickened plasmalemma containing actin-like filaments. It presents a dense appearance called the **densitas presynaptica** (the presynaptic density).

c. *presynaptic vesicles*, 40 to 50 nm in diameter, containing neurotransmitter substances. Two types of vesicles have been identified based on the neurotransmitter released (Heuser and Reese, 1973): *dense vesicles* and *clear vesicles*.

2. The *synaptic fissure* (synaptic cleft) is a 20 to 30 nm interval between the presynaptic and postsynaptic parts of the synapse. The *fissure* is occupied by an electron-dense material, the **substantia intrafissuralis**, containing glycolipids and glycoproteins.

3. The *postsynaptic part* is a thickened region on the dendritic membrane of the second neuron, the *postsynaptic membrane*, with its own *postsynaptic density*.

VII. The **neuroglia** (Peters et al, 1976)

A. The term **neuroglia** literally means "nerve glue" and refers to those specialized cells with a supportive role in nerve tissue stroma. The CNS contains virtually no connective tissue, but the spaces between neurons are packed with cell bodies and processes of neuroglial cells. Neuroglia form an important constituent in the organization of the brain and spinal cord, but unfortunately they are a major source of CNS tumors. *Three glial cell types* (Fig. 10-5) are identified, with specific functions and relationships within the CNS (Glees, 1955):

1. *Astrocytes* are stellate cells with multiple radiating processes, occurring exclusively within the CNS. The outstanding EM feature of astrocytes is the presence of large (15 to 40 nm) glycogen granules in an electron-lucent cytoplasm. It is suggested that astrocytes play a role in nutrition of the CNS. Two forms exist:

a. *protoplasmic astrocytes* (Fig. 10-5A), localized in the gray matter of the brain,

b. *fibrous astrocytes* (Fig. 10-5B) in the white matter, located near neuron cell bodies and cerebral blood vessels.

2. *Oligodendrocytes* (Fig. 10-5C) are small cells with few processes, (Greek: *oligo-*, few or scanty). Although several functions have been proposed, that of myelin formation in the CNS is documented best. Oligodendrocytes myelinate several axons, in contrast to the neurolemmocytes of the PNS which myelinate only one axon.

3. *Microglia* (Fig. 10-5D), the only cellular elements of the nervous system derived from mesoderm, appear in development when blood capillaries enter the brain. They are evident in healthy nerve tissues, but become prevalent following injury to the nervous system. Microglia function as the "macrophages" of the CNS, clearing away debris of degenerating neurons and other cells at injury sites.

VIII. Terminationes nervorum, nerve terminations, are distinguished in two groups: *receptors* and *effectors* (Fig. 10-6).

A. *Receptors* receive sensory stimuli.

1. *Free nerve endings* (Fig. 10-6A), unmyelinated with no apparent modifications, except perhaps for a small knob, mediate sensations of pain and temperature. The endings, part of a network of terminal nerves, form the majority of sensory endings in the skin. Similar but less complex networks exist in the viscera. Free nerve endings on hair follicles, **terminatio folliculi pili**, form around hair follicles, qualifying the hair as a sense organ.

2. *Terminal nerve corpuscles* are modified sensory nerve endings that may be noncapsulated or capsulated.

a. *Noncapsulated tactile corpuscles*, possessing nerve terminals that are protected by other cells, are exemplified by

(1) *tactile epithelioid cells* (cells of Merkel) (Fig. 10-6B),

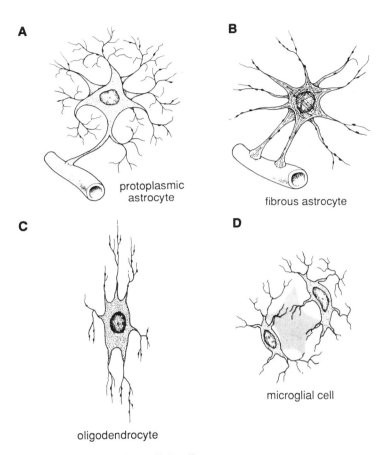

A

protoplasmic
astrocyte

B

fibrous astrocyte

C

oligodendrocyte

D

microglial cell

Figure 10-5 Principal glial cell types.

which are modified epidermal cells that form receptor complexes with sensory *nerve endings*. These specialized endings, usually excited by direct pressure in glabrous (hairless) and hairy skin, consist of

(a) *unmyelinated nerve terminals* that penetrated the epidermal basement membrane and maneuvered between cells of the epidermis to form cup-like discs that partially sink into a *tactile epithelioid cell*, so that the nerve ending is not exposed.

(b) *epithelioid cells*, characterized by many large, dense core vesicles (100 nm in diameter). These cells attach to adjacent epidermal cells via desmosomes, as do other epidermal cells.

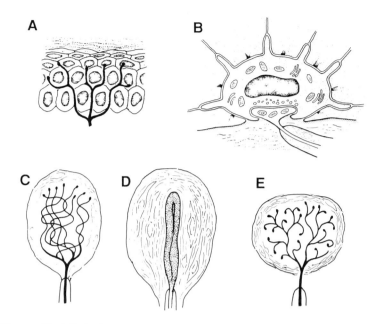

Figure 10-6 Principal nerve terminations. *A.* Free nerve endings. *B.* Tactile epithelioid cells. *C.* Tactile corpuscles. *D.* Lamellated corpuscles. *E.* Bulboid corpuscles.

    b. *Capsulated nerve corpuscles* have nerve endings enveloped in connective tissue lamellae.

    (1) *Tactile corpuscles* (old name: Meissner's corpuscle) (Fig. 10-6C) are elongated ellipsoids (about 150 μm long) of modified neurolemmocytes and some connective tissue. The tactile corpuscle encapsulates one or two nerve endings in the dermal papillae of glabrous (hairless) skin of fingertips, toes, palms, and soles, to mediate *touch*.

    (2) *Lamellated corpuscles* (old name: corpuscle of Vater-Pacini) (Fig. 10-6D) are the largest corpuscles (avg. 2 mm wide by 3 mm tall), specialized to respond to pressure, vibrations, and mechanical stimuli.

    (a) *Lamellated corpuscles* form white ellipsodial *external bulbs* composed of up to 30 or more concentric *lamellae* of white connective tissue cells and fibers. Between each lamella exists a fluid-filled space. The external bulb encapsulates an *internal bulb* covering the nerve ending. At least one or two myelin internodes are covered by the internal bulb composed of neurolemmocytes.

(b) *Lamellated corpuscles* occur in widely different tissues such as the dermis, cornea, heart wall, pancreas, mesentery, joints, and loose connective tissue.

(3) **Corpusculum bulboideum** (Fig. 10-6E) are smaller and simpler variations of lamellated corpuscles.

(a) *Genital corpuscles*, residing in the skin of the external genitalia and the nipple, react to touch or pressure.

(b) Other *bulboid corpuscles* (old names: corpuscles of Golgi-Mazzoni and end bulbs of Krause) occur in the capillary layer of skin, mucous membranes, ligaments, and tendons. Whether these are distinct entities or variations of the same structures in different tissues is unknown.

3. *Neurotendinous spindles* and *neuromuscular spindles*, reporting tension in tendons and stretching of muscles, are complex spirals of nerve endings encapsulated within lamellated connective tissue. They contribute to postural awareness and bilateral phasic adjustments. (The Latin for spindle is *fusi*, hence words such as *intrafusal* and *extrafusal myocytes*.)

a. *Neurotendinous spindles*, simple or encapsulated, respond to increased tension.

b. *Neuromuscular spindles* are complex elongated narrow structures consisting of the following (Fig. 10-7):

(1) *intrafusal myocytes:* thin, modified striated skeletal myocytes, 1 to 5 mm long in the center of the spindle. Myofibrils occupy the ends of the myocytes, while nuclei aggregate in the central segment.

(2) *extrafusal myocytes:* ordinary striated skeletal myocytes.

(3) *three types of nerve terminals:*

(a) *gamma efferents:* thin nerve terminals to ordinary, extrafusal, striated skeletal myocytes,

(b) *primary afferent:* thicker nerve terminals, forming *primary spiraled terminations*,

(c) *secondary afferents:* terminations that branch to form a "flowerspray."

B. *Effectors* evoke responses from the innervated structure. These specialized nerve endings are conveniently divided into two categories:

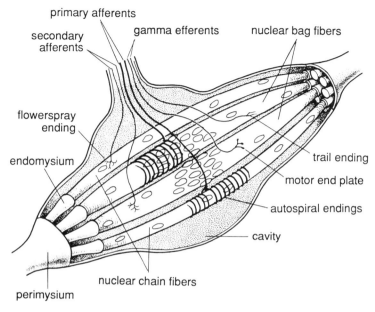

Figure 10-7 Neuromuscular spindles.

1. *neuromuscular termination* (Dennis, 1981)

a. *somatic efferent endings:* axons originate in the CNS and terminate in motor end plates of skeletal muscle.

b. *visceral efferent endings* originate in autonomic ganglion cells and terminate in branches that travel adjacent to individual myocytes. Numerous varicosities along the branches (boutons en passant) are filled with synaptic vesicles. Such nerve branch endings that do not form specialized junctions (as in skeletal muscle) occur in cardiac muscle (Fig. 10-8) and smooth muscle of viscera, blood vessels, and erector pili muscle associated with hair.

c. *visceral efferent endings: neuroepithelial terminations, neuroglandular terminations:* in exocrine glands, the terminations penetrate the basement membrane and associate closely with individual gland cells.

d. terminatio neurosecretoria (Scharrer and Scharrer, 1954): nerve cells that release hormones from their terminals. The hormones are transported to specific target organs, via the bloodstream, to effect a response. **Terminatio palisadica:** The word palisade is defined as a

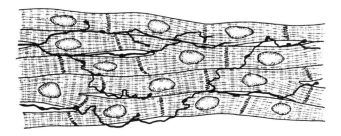

Figure 10-8 Visceral efferent endings in cardiac musle.

"long strong stake pointed at the top and set close with others as a defense." Such a situation is analogous to axons from neurosecretory cells in the hypothalamus passing in palisades into the posterior lobe of the hypothalamus (Fig. 10-9)

Figure 10-9 Neurosecretory terminations.

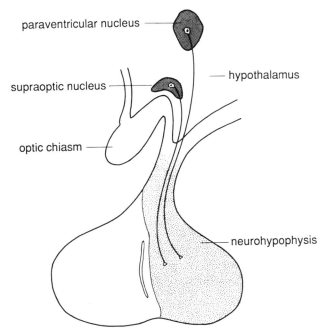

IX. *Peripheral nerve trunk*

   A. In histologic sections of a peripheral nerve trunk, certain characteristic features may be observed:

   1. The *neurolemma sheath* is the covering of individual axons by a series of neurolemmocytes, in which the outer plasmalemma is designated the *neurolemmal* sheath.

   a. Axons covered by a single layer of the neurolemmocyte plasmalemma are designated as *unmyelinated*.

   b. Axons surrounded by several layers of neurolemmocyte plasmalemma (the jelly roll) are *myelinated*.

   2. *Connective tissue coverings*

   a. Endoneurium: a delicate connective tissue layer surrounding individual axons and associated neurolemmocytes.

   b. Perineurium: a connective tissue layer of concentric, flattened fibroblasts and bundles of collagen fibers, organizing endoneurium-sheathed axons into *fasciculi*.

   c. Epineurium: a thick layer of connective tissue, surrounding fasiculi. The complex is referred to as a *nerve*. The epineurium, while ensheathing and protecting groups of fascicles on one nerve, may be joined to the epineurium of other nerves, the connective tissue surrounding arteries and veins, or the epimysium of muscles.

   3. A *nerve* consists of many axons or dendrites and their coverings arranged into several functional fasciculi. Variable degrees of myelinization may be found in a cross section of a single nerve. In a single *nerve*

   a. some fasciculi are made up of long *axons* carrying motor stimuli away from the CNS,

   b. some fasciculi are made up of long *dendrites* carrying sensory stimuli to the CNS.

Questions

DIRECTIONS: For each of the items in this section, one or more of the numbered options is correct. Select

  A if only *1, 2, and 3* are correct
  B if only *1 and 3* are correct
  C if only *2 and 4* are correct
  D if only *4* is correct
  E if *all* are correct

---

1. Neural crest cells during development send contributions to form
   1. cranial ganglia
   2. melanocytes
   3. suprarenal medulla
   4. spinal ganglia

2. Multipolar neurons are most numerous in the
   1. dorsal root ganglion
   2. ventral horn of the spinal cord
   3. sensory ganglion of the vagus nerve X
   4. autonomic ganglia

3. Chromatophilic substance (Nissl) is most prominent in
   1. cytoplasm surrounding the nucleus
   2. axon hillock
   3. dendrites
   4. cytoplasm under the plasmalemma

4. Lipofuscin is a pigment in neurons that
   1. accumulates with age
   2. has an affinity for osmium
   3. has electron-dense granules
   4. is responsible for the black appearance of some neurons

Directions Summarized				
A	**B**	**C**	**D**	**E**
1,2,3	1,3	2,4	4	All are
only	only	only	only	correct

5. The electron-dense intraperiodic lines in myelin surrounding axons results from fusion of neurolemmocyte plasmalemma
   1. cytoplasmic surfaces
   2. lipid component
   3. nodus neurofibrae
   4. external surface

6. The presynaptic part of an axon terminal is recognized by
   1. an accumulation of mitochondria
   2. a dense presynaptic membrane
   3. accumulation of presynaptic vesicles
   4. presence of chromatophilic substance (Nissl)

7. Oligodendrocytes
   1. are derived from mesoderm
   2. possess large glycogen granules
   3. function as macrophages
   4. can myelinate several axons

8. Lamellated corpuscles
   1. occur in the pancreas
   2. attach to epidermal cells via desmosomes
   3. possess an internal bulb over the nerve terminal
   4. encapsulate one or two nerve endings

9. Neuromuscular spindles consist of
   1. thin modified striated skeletal myocytes
   2. extrafusal myocytes
   3. three types of nerve terminals
   4. lamellated corpuscles

10. A single nerve
   1. is surrounded by endoneurium
   2. may be joined by connective tissue to an artery
   3. consists of axons carrying stimuli away from the CNS
   4. contains several fasciculi

Explanatory Answers

1. E. All are correct. Neural crest cells also provide neuroglia to the peripheral nervous system.

2. C. 2 and 4 are correct. The dorsal root ganglion and the sensory ganglion of the vagus nerve X (also VII, VIII, and XI) contain bipolar or pseudounipolar neurons. The ventral horn of the spinal gray matter contains the large multipolar motor neurons. The neurons of autonomic ganglia contain smaller multipolar motor neurons.

3. B. 1 and 3 are correct. Chromatophilic substance is absent from the rim of cytoplasm immediately under the plasmalemma, as well as the axon hillock and the entire axon.

4. A. 1, 2, and 3 are correct. Lipofuscin is the wear and tear pigment of the nervous system. The black appearance of some neurons in the CNS is attributed to melanin, a black pigment.

5. D. 4 is corret. Under the TEM, 1 produces a major dense line; 2 produces the electron-lucent space; and 3 is the node of the fiber (node of Ranvier) between successive neurolemmocytes.

6. A. 1, 2, and 3 are correct. 4 is incorrect because the chromatophilic substance does not occur anywhere in the axon or axon hillock. Injury to the axon will cause dissolution of this form of rER in the neuron body.

7. C. 2 and 4 are correct. Microglia, the only glial cells derived from mesoderm, function as macrophages. Astrocytes present the outstanding feature of large (15 to 40 nm) glycogen granules in an electron-lucent cytoplasm. Oligodendroglia are involved in myelin formation in the CNS.

8. B. 1 and 3 are correct. Large lamellated corpuscles (Vater-Pacini) respond to pressure, vibrations, and mechanical stimuli. Several layers (up to 30 or more) of connective tissue elements form an *external bulb* over the *internal bulb* (composed of neurolemmocytes). In addition to the pancreas, they occur in the dermis, cornea, heart wall, mesentery, joints, and loose connective tissue. The epitheliod cells form part of a noncapsulated tactile corpuscles (the old Merkel cells). The ellipsoid tactile corpuscles (Meissner's) encapsulate one or two nerve endings.

9. A. 1, 2, and 3 are correct. Lamellated corpuscles are not part of the neuromuscular spindle. Neuromuscular spindles consist of gamma efferent nerve terminals (motor), primary spiraled afferent terminals (sensory), and the flower-spray secondary afferent terminals (sensory). Extrafusal myocytes are ordinary striated skeletal myocytes; the intrafusal myocytes are modified striated skeletal myocytes.

10. C. 2 and 4 are correct. The epineurium surrounding a single nerve may fuse with the connective tissue surrounding an artery, vein, or lymphatic. It may also fuse with the epineurium of another nerve or the epimysium surrounding a muscle. Endoneurium surrounding only one nerve process (axon or dendrite) fuses with the endonerium of other nerve processes. Several endoneurium-bound nerve processes form a nerve fasciculus. One single nerve is made up of several fascicles with nerve processes carrying impulses to the CNS and from the CNS.

Organs and Systems
of the Body

11 The Cardiovascular System

I. *Introduction*: The cardiovascular system, by rhythmic contractions of the heart, circulates blood through a virtually closed system of vessels. In addition to blood cells, circulating blood transports

  A. oxygen, plus a variety of substances, to the body cells,

  B. cellular products away from body cells to other sites,

  C. carbon dioxide to the lungs.

II. *Histogenesis of blood vessels*

  A. The very first blood vessels develop within the mesenchyma of the human yolk sac. Stellate mesenchymal cells become spherical and aggregate as *blood islands*. As development progresses, scattered blood islands unite to form solid anastomosing cords of cells.

  1. The cells at the periphery of the cords flatten as *endothelioblasts* of the primitive blood vessels and later transform into *endothelial cells* of the definitive tubular vessels.

  2. Spherical cells in the center of the cords differentiate into *hemocytoblasts*, surrounded by extracellular *plasma* secreted by the blood island cells. Thus, formed *endothelial tubes* enclose the hemocytoblasts.

  3. *Endothelial tubes* proliferate by budding and fusing to form a vast *extraembryonic* plexus of primitive *capillaries* that envelop the entire yolk sac.

  4. Similarly, *intraembryonic* vascular plexuses form about the time somites form (20 days of gestation).

III. Vasa sanguinea, blood vessels: *Arteries* conduct blood away from the heart to *capillary* beds in tissues and organs. In the *capillaries*,

selected substances and cells exit the vessels, while others are permitted to enter the circulation. From the capillaries, blood is channeled
into *veins* for transportion to the heart, thus completing the circuit.
The following presentation begins with *capillaries*, which have the
simplest morphology, and proceeds to the *arteries, veins,* and the
heart.

A. **Vas capillare,** capillaries (Fig. 11-1)

1. Capillary endothelium consists of interdigitating, diamond-
shaped squamous cells (Fig. 11-1A).

   a. When two opposing corners of one endothelial cell are
brought together (Fig. 11-1B), a lumen is formed (Fig. 11-1C).

   (1) Several such interdigitating cells form a capillary *lumen*
large enough to allow one erythrocyte to pass through.

   (2) Opposing corners frequently overlap, leaving one end,
the *marginal fold*, protruding into the lumen (Fig. 11-1D).

   (3) Endothelial cell nuclei bulge into the lumen, the path of
least resistance.

   b. The luminal surface of the endothelium, *internal (luminal)
surface*, is usually smooth.

Figure 11-1 Capillary endothelium (follow text).

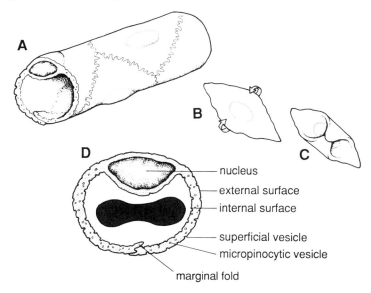

nucleus
external surface
internal surface
superficial vesicle
micropinocytic vesicle
marginal fold

c. the abluminal or *external (basal) surface* produces the basement membrane with which it is in contact.

2. Depressions (pits) on the luminal and abluminal plasmalemma surfaces form *superficial* vesicles (Fig. 11-1D).

a. The intervening layer of cytoplasm contains membrane-bound *micropinocytotic vesicles* derived from superficial vesicles.

b. *Micropinocytotic vesicles* serve as a transport mechanism across the capillary wall. Plasma proteins, antibodies, and other large molecules are exchanged across endothelial cell walls (Simionescu, 1981).

3. All capillaries have a total surface area about 1000 square meters, or 800 times that of the aorta.

4. Capillaries, with a reduced blood flow, have two zones: one attached to the arteriole and one attached to the venule (Fig. 11-2A):

a. vas capillare arteriale, the arterial capillary vessel, receives blood from an arteriole. A greater pressure (than that of the vas capillare venosum) forces some fluid out into the surrounding connective tissue.

b. vas capillare venosum, the *venous capillary vessel*, receives blood from the vas capillare arteriole. Because the venous capillary has a lower pressure than the arterial capillary, some connective tissue fluid reenters the circulation via the *venous capillary*.

5. The *basement membrane* secreted by the endothelial cells consists of two parts:

a. lamina densa, completely surrounding the *external [basal] surface*, leaving no discernible interruptions.

b. lamina lucida, interposed between the external [basal] surface and the lamina densa.

6. *Pericytes* (Rouget cells) (Fig. 11-2B) are pericapillary mesenchymal cells, frequently enclosed within a split lamina densa (Davson, 1967) (Fig. 11-2C). Several peripheral "arms" clasp the capillary wall. Elongated oval nuclei have a great proportion of euchromatin, reflecting developmental potencies in

a. wound healing, where *pericytes* develop into

(1) *fibroblasts*, which form scar tissue,

(2) *nonstriated (smooth) myocytes*, which generate the muscle layer (tunica media) of new vessels.

b. postnatal development, where *pericytes* function as precursors of contractile nonstriated (smooth) myocytes for developing vessels.

A   Capillary Plexus

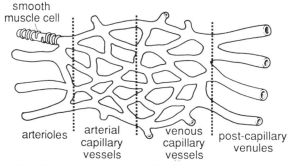

B   Capillary Pericyte – Whole

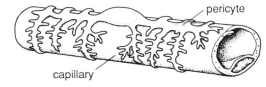

C   Section Through Pericyte Nucleus

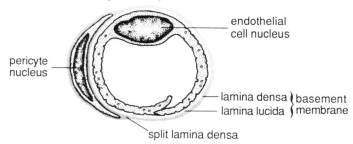

Figure 11-2 *A*. The plan of the capillary bed. *B*. 3-D relationship of pericyte to capillary. *C*. Cross-section relationship of pericyte to capillary.

7. *Capillaries function to*
    a. deliver blood (laden with oxygen, nutritional substances, and hormones) directly to stromal and parenchymal cells.
    b. receive wastes and synthesized cellular products for delivery to appropriate organs (example: CO_2 to the lung).

8. *Capillary types*: Because functional requirements of tissues differ, capillaries accommodate to tissue requirements. Thus, several capillary types exist (Fig. 11-3):

    a. *continuous capillaries*, consisting of uninterrupted plasmalemma surfaces. Two forms are recognized, *thick* and *thin*:

        (1) *thick continuous capillaries* (Fig. 11-3A) occur in striated

Figure 11-3 Capillary types.

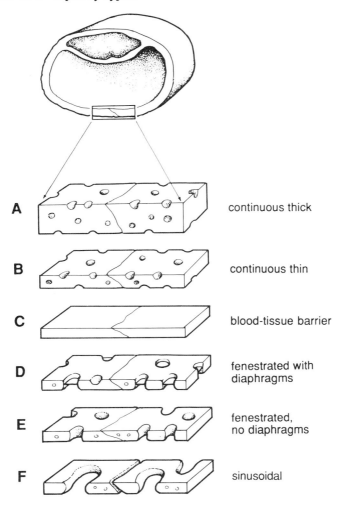

A   continuous thick

B   continuous thin

C   blood-tissue barrier

D   fenestrated with diaphragms

E   fenestrated, no diaphragms

F   sinusoidal

skeletal myocytes, nonstriated (smooth) myocytes, cardiac myocytes, and parts of the ovaries and testes. The following characteristics distinguish this type of capillary:

(a) 200-nm-thick endothelial cells, united by desmosomes and gap junctions,

(b) a complete basement membrane, surrounding the external (basal) surface,

(c) micropinocytotic vesicles, providing a dynamic hydrophilic transport system (Simionescu and Simionescu, 1981).

(2) *thin continuous capillaries* (Fig. 11-3B), in a few tissues, are similar to the thick variety, but are half the thickness (100 nm).

(3) Specialized *thin continuous capillaries* function as *blood–tissue barriers* (Fig. 11-3C), selecting only certain sized molecules to enter or exit the capillary.

(a) Two structural features distinguish blood–tissue barriers:

[1] **zonulae occludens** (tight junctions), which are impermeable to small ions and prevent materials from passing between endothelial cell junctions.

[2] *absence* (or rare occurences) of *micropinocytotic vesicles* eliminate micropinocytosis as a pathway for materials to exit or enter through the endothelial cell wall.

(b) Examples of *brain–tissue barriers*:

[1] *blood–brain barrier* (Brightman, 1977): The basement membrane, surrounding the endothelial cells, has 85% of its surface covered by glial cells (Maynard et al, 1957). Cerebral vessels in some sites have a minipore system to transport large molecules and proteins rather than a vesicular transport system.

[2] *blood–thymus barrier* (Raviola and Karnovsky, 1972) is remarkable in the character of its capillaries. Capillary segments just a few millimeters apart display different permeability properties. In the cortex of the thymus, the endothelial cells prevent circulating macromolecules from reaching lymphocytes. Medullary capillaries appear to be freely permeable to selected circulating macromolecules.

[3] *blood–ganglion* barrier (DePace, 1982) with capillaries possessing characteristics like those of the blood–brain barrier.

b. *Discontinuous capillary endothelium* features 60 to 100 nm *fenestrae* (Latin, windows) directly through the thickness of the endothelial cells. Selected fluids and certain sized molecules are permitted to enter or exit through these *fenestrae* (Maul, 1971). The following types are described:

(1) *fenestrated with diaphragms* (Fig. 11-3D):

(a) endothelial wall is 60 to 100 nm thick.

(b) The external (basal) surface of the capillary wall is surrounded by a continuous basement membrane.

(c) Like windows covered by thin panes of glass, fenestrae are occluded by *thin porous diaphragms* that facilitate interchange of certain molecules between the surrounding tissue and blood. The *diaphragm*, thinner than the 10-nm-thick plasmalemma, appears as a thin line in a TEM section. A small knob, 10 to 15 nm in diameter, occupies the center of the diaphragm. The chemical nature of the diaphragm and the manner by which molecules cross is still unknown.

(d) Fenestrated capillaries with diaphragms occur in sites requiring rapid fluid exchange between tissues and circulating blood, ie, gastrointestinal mucosa, choroid plexus in the ventricles of the brain, kidney peritubular plexuses, and the ciliary body of the eye.

(2) *fenestrated capillaries without diaphragms* (Fig. 11-3E) are found in renal glomeruli, where the basement membrane is three times thicker than in other capillaries.

B. *Sinusoid* (*sinus* + Greek *eidos* = "resemble") and *sinus* (Latin, "a hollow") **[vas capillare sinusoideum]** designate capillaries modified to retain large quantities of blood under low pressure.

1. The *sinusoid* **[vas capillare sinusoideum]** (Fig. 11-3F) conforms to its surroundings and presents a larger, irregular cross-sectional diameter than capillaries.

2. Desmosomes and other junctions may be missing, thus providing spaces between adjacent endothelial cells.

3. Basement membranes are sparse or absent, and connective tissue elements are minimal or lacking.

4. Variable sized fenestrae lack diaphragms.

5. Location of sinusoids:

    a. vas sinusoideum hepar (liver)

    b. vas sinusoideum medulla ossium (bone marrow)

    c. vas sinusoideum adenohypophysis (adenohypophysis)

    d. vas sinusoideum paraganglion sympatheticum (sympathetic ganglion)

C. The term *sinus* refers to *venous sinuses* only (with one exception, **sinus caroticus**, the dilated portion of the internal carotid artery). The following are correct usages for the term *sinus* in the cardiovascular system:

1. **sinus venosus**, the common venous receptacle of the embryonic heart.

2. **sinus venularis**, formerly "venous sinus" of the *spleen*, is a specialized postcapillary venule (with longitudinally arranged endothelial cells) connecting the *terminal capillary* and the **vena pulpa rubra** (vein of the red pulp) (cf section on spleen).

3. **sinus coronarius**, the coronary sinus of the heart.

4. **sinus dura matris**, the sinus of the dura mater in the brain, has several parts: **sinus transversus, sinus occipitalis, sinus sigmoideus, sinus sagittalis superior, sinus sagittalis inferior, sinus rectus, sinus petrosus inferior, sinus cavernosus, sinus intercavernosi,** and **sinus sphenoparietalis.**

5. **sinus venosus sclerae** is the venous sinus of the sclera of the eye.

D. *Arteries* are specialized vessels of the cardiovascular system that carry blood away from the heart.

1. The *aorta* (the largest artery) and its branches carry oxygenated blood from the left ventricle of the heart to the body tissues. The *pulmonary artery* and its branches deliver deoxygenated blood away from the right ventricle of the heart to the lungs.

2. From the aorta to the smallest capillaries in tissue beds, *arteries* branch dichotomously until the total cross-sectional diameters of all branches equals 800 times that of the aorta. With increased branching, there is a decrease in the rate of blood flow.

3. *General structure* of *arteries*. Every artery possesses three layers: the **tunica interna [intima]**, the **tunica media**, and the **tunica externa [adventitia]**. In arteries of different caliber, the **tunica media** presents the most varied changes.

   a. The **tunica interna [intima]** is composed of a luminal layer of endothelium (and basement membrane) resting on a *subendothelial stratum* of elastic fibers: the *internal elastic membrane*.

   b. The **tunica media** surrounds the tunica interna. Depending on the size of the artery, either circularly oriented nonstriated (smooth) myocytes or *fenestrated elastic membranes* predominate. The external boundary of the **tunica media** is demarcated by a loose ring of elastic fibers: the *external elastic membrane*.

[Editor's note: The term *circular* signifies a tight helix of muscle, directed clockwise on the right and counterclockwise on the left. Similarly, the term *longitudinal* signifies a helix, but one that is a long loose spiral.]

    c. The **tunica externa [adventitia]** consists of collagenous fibers and associated connective tissue cells.

    (1) The external limits are difficult to ascertain because the connective tissue elements intermingle with those of the surrounding connective tissue beds.

    (2) Because arteries and veins usually accompany one another, their united external layers are difficult to separate.

    (3) Vasa vasorum, lymphatic vessels, and nerves travel in the tunica externa and penetrate into the media.

    4. Three *types of arteries* are described below. The largest arteries have a preponderance of elastic connective tissue in the tunica media. Progressing from the largest to the smallest, the elastic tissue decreases gradually until it is negligible, while muscle predominates.

    a. Arteria elastotypica, *elastic-type arteries*: aorta, pulmonary trunk and arteries, brachiocephalic trunk, common carotids, and subclavian artery are large arteries.

    (1) Tunica interna [intima] (Schwartz and Benditt, 1972) is a layer 100 to 140 μm thick.

    (a) Endothelial cells, joined tightly by zonulae occludentes and gap junctions, rest on a thin continuous basement membrane.

    (b) Micropinocytotic vesicles may be involved in transendothelial transport of nutrients to the subendothelial layers.

    (c) A loose, subendothelial, connective tissue layer contains longitudinally oriented elastic fibers and nonstraited (smooth) myocytes.

    (d) The *internal elastic membrane*, demarcating the tunica interna from the tunica media, is distinguished better by TEM than LM.

    (2) Tunica media is a layer 500 μm thick. Large elastic-type arteries nearest the heart must accommodate to stretching by producing masses of elastic connective tissue in the tunica media.

    (a) Elastic tissue enables the artery to recoil, thus assisting the heart to propel blood.

    (b) Interlacing elastic fibers form 50 to 75 concentric sheets of *fenestrated elastic membranes*.

    (c) Intermingled with and inserted onto the fenestrated elastic membranes are spiraled branched bundles of nonstriated (smooth) myocytes coupled by gap junctions. Myocytes produce their own basement membranes plus variable amounts of collagen (types I, III, and IV) and elastic fibers.

(d) An *external elastic membrane* separating the tunica media from the tunica externa is better visualized via TEM.

(3) The **tunica externa [adventitia]**, the outer, relatively thin layer of connective tissue, is rather difficult to separate from surrounding connective tissues.

(a) collagen fibers are circularly arranged.

(b) **vasa vasorum** (vessel of vessels), **nervi vasorum** (nerves of vessels), and **vas lymphaticum vasorum** (lymphatic vessels of vessels) travel within the tunica externa to supply it and subjacent layers.

b. **Arteria mixtotypica** (medium arteries of the mixed type) are difficult to classify as elastic or muscular types. Two categories are considered, *transitional* and *specialized*.

(1) *Transitional* forms between elastic and muscular arteries have walls that resemble one or the other. Size alone can not classify these arteries. More importantly, the components of each layer, particularly the tunica media, must be examined. Examples:

(a) *Arteries to the head and extremities* (ie, internal carotid, axillary, common iliac, external iliac, and tibial) have nonstriated (smooth) myocytes in the tunica media disrupting the fenestrated elastic membranes in several places.

(b) *Visceral arteries arising directly from the aorta* (ie, superior mesenteric, renal, splenic, and celiac) may be distinguished by two layers in the tunica media:

[1] an inner muscular layer and

[2] an outer elastic layer (with typical fenestrated elastic laminae).

(2) *Specialized* forms adapt to special situations such as location or blood pressures. Examples:

(a) *Coronary arteries* have very thick walls to accommodate high pressures.

(b) *Pulmonary arteries* may have cardiac muscle extending for a short distance into the tunica media.

(c) *Lower extremity arteries* have a thicker tunica media than the upper extremity arteries.

(d) *Popliteal and axillary arteries*, subjected to excessive stretching, have increased numbers of longitudinal bundles of nonstriated (smooth) myocytes in the tunica interna and a tunica media resembling that of elastic arteries.

(e) *Arteries of the cranial cavity* (including the dura mater) possess

[1] a relatively thin tunica media lacking fenestrated elastic membranes,

[2] a pronounced external elastic membrane.

(f) *Umbilical arteries* (carrying blood to the fetus) possess a tunica interna lacking an internal elastic membrane.

[1] The intraabdominal portion of the tunica media possesses two layers of muscle:

[a] an inner longitudinal layer (which forms ridges in the lumen) and

[b] an outer circular layer.

[2] The extraabdominal portion of the tunica media possesses only a circularly oriented layer of muscle.

c. **Arteria myotypica** (muscular-type arteries) are distributing arteries of the extremities and the majority of arteries in the body down to a diameter of 0.5 mm.

(1) **Tunica interna [intima]** possesses

(a) an **endothelium** whose endothelial cells send long cellular processes through the fenestrae of the internal elastic membrane down to the nonstriated (smooth) myocytes of the tunica media.

[1] The *Gap junction* (**nexus**) and **zonula occludens** may be loosened, widened, or broken under various influences of disease (diabetes), drugs (nicotine), and hormones (epinephrine, serotonin, and angiotensin II), thus permitting blood to leak into the underlying layers.

[2] The *basement membrane* is thinner than that of elastic-type arteries but is continuous. In diabetes, the basement membrane may thicken as a result of reduced glycogen degradation (attributed to a change in glycosylation).

(b) a *subendothelial layer* of loose connective tissue and nonstriated (smooth) myocytes organized in longitudinal bundles. Where some arteries bifurcate (ie, coronary, renal, splenic, intracranial, nasal mucosa, and the thyroid), the subendothelial layer thickens into *intimal cushions* that bulge into the lumen. These cushions apparently assist in controlling blood flow.

(c) an undulating, prominent, birefringent *internal elastic membrane* demarcating the tunica interna from the tunica media.

(2) **Tunica media** of the **arteria myotypica** consists of

(a) 10 to 40 layers of circularly oriented, nonstriated (smooth) muscle,

(b) a population of elastic fibers and fenestrated membranes, less than observed in larger elastic arteries.

(c) an *external elastic membrane* separating the tunica media and the tunica externa. This membrane is not as well defined as that of the internal elastic membrane.

(3) Tunica externa [adventitia] of **arteria myotypica** contains a few longitudinally oriented nonstriated (smooth) myocytes, a few fibroblasts, adipocytes, and collagen fiber types I, III, and IV.

(a) In *aging*, there is excessive production of types I and III, known for their affinity for platelets (Trelstad, 1974).

(b) Vasa vasorum, nervi vasorum, and **vas lymphaticum vasorum** accompany one another in the tunica externa to supply subjacent layers.

d. *Arterioles*, the smallest arteries, measuring 400 nm or less in diameter, form a network, the **rete arteriolare**, prior to connecting with capillaries (Rhodin, 1967). Arterioles

(1) have a small tunica media (one to three layers of myocytes) and almost no elastic fibers.

(2) have a pronounced refractile *internal elastic membrane* but no *external elastic membrane*.

(3) mark the connection with capillaries by the disappearance of nonstriated (smooth) myocytes.

(4) terminate (with a lumen reducing from 30 μm down to 8 μm) as *precapillary arterioles* (or *metarteriole*).

(5) regulate blood flow into the capillary plexus via a *precapillary sphincter* of myocytes. Sympathetic motor nerves stimulate contraction and relaxation of the myocytes in this region.

(6) possess gap junctions between myocytes and endothelial cell processes to mediate communications between them.

(7) are surrounded by a thin tunica externa, with connective tissue elements common to loose connective tissue.

E. Venae (*veins*) have a larger lumen and thinner walls than corresponding arteries. Though they possess the same named layers, they are difficult to delineate because of the paucity of nonstriated (smooth) myocytes and the minimal elastic connective tissue.

1. Venulae (*venules*) are the smallest veins draining the capillary plexuses (Rhodin, 1968). A **rete venosum** (venous network) unites several venules to form successively larger venules ᴜ̩til a few veins are formed.

a. *Postcapillary venules*, formed by the union of several capillaries, have diameters ranging from 10 to 20 μm and are up to 700 μm long. Postcapillary venules are characterized by

(1) a continuous layer of *pericytes* surrounding the venule.

(2) a **tunica interna** that has

(a) an **endothelium** with occasional fenestrations. Junctional attachments of endothelial cells are the loosest in the entire vascular system and there are no gap junctions (Simionescu et al, 1978). Leaks between cells are common.

(b) a *basement membrane* interrupted by pericytes and adhering to a poorly developed *subendothelial stratum*.

(3) a negligible **tunica media** with neighboring pericytes so plentiful that they are mistaken for myocytes,

(4) a **tunica externa [adventitia]** consisting of scattered elements of loose connective tissue.

(5) thin venule walls with a special permeability to facilitate important blood-connective tissue fluid exchange.

(6) reactions to temperature extremes, allergic conditions, and tissue inflammation causing blood to leak between the loose endothelial cell junctions.

b. **Venula colligens**, characterized by an increased amount of collagen fibers in the tunica externa, is slightly larger (20 to 50 μm in diameter) than the postcapillary venule.

c. **Venula muscularis** resembles other venules (50 μm in diameter) but has *partially differentiated* nonstriated (smooth) myocytes scattered between the endothelium and the tunica externa. *Differentiated* myocytes proliferate and aggregate to increase the diameters up to 200 μm, after which venules are classified as small veins. Venulae musculares accompany arterioles.

2. **Venae** (*veins*) accompany named arteries that supply the same area that they drain.

a. **Tunica interna [intima]** possesses an irregularly arranged layer of endothelial cells supported by a loosely organized layer of connective tissue, the *subendothelial stratum*. Elastic fibers form a poorly definable network of elastic fibers, the **rete elasticum**, to separate the next tunica (if present).

b. **Tunica media** varies considerably, depending on the function and size of the vessel.

(1) In *large veins*, inconspicuous *nonstriated (smooth) myoctes* intermingle with collagen fibers.

(2) A conspicuous layer of *nonstriated (smooth) myocytes* is best observed in pulmonary veins, deep veins of the penis, and the uterine veins during pregnancy. These veins are classified as **vena myotypica** (muscular-type veins).

(3) In contrast, veins of the central nervous system and those of the bone marrow lack *nonstriated (smooth) myocytes* in the tunica media.

(4) In veins without a tunica media, there are considerably

more connective tissue fibers, classifying these veins as **vena fibrotypica** (fibrous-type veins).

    c. Tunica externa [adventitia] of all veins is the thickest layer. In large veins (*vena cava*), it is distinguished by longitudinal bundles of smooth muscle (entwined with collagen fibers and elastic networks) to facilitate changes in length brought about by excursions of the diaphragm.

    d. *Valves* are confined to the limbs.

    (1) The thinness of venous walls would seriously impair the flow of blood against gravity were it not for the presence of *valves* arranged along the course of the veins.

    (2) An outpouching of endothelium on opposite walls, filled with a thin layer of elastic and collagen fibers for added strength, forms two cup-shaped *valves*.

    (3) The free edges of the valves face the direction of blood flow. Between cardiac pulsations, a back flow of blood fills the valve depressions, **sinus valvulae**, forcing the free edges to slap shut, thus preventing pooling of blood. Loss of valvular integrity results in pooling, recognized as varicose veins.

    e. A *portal system* of *veins* develops when a small vein branches into a capillary plexus instead of flowing into a larger vein.

    (1) A *portal system* collects blood from one or more sites and diverts it to another organ, for additional processing, prior to delivery to the heart. Example:

    (a) The *hepatic portal system* collects blood from the gastrointestinal tract, pancreas, and spleen and transports it to the liver via a single large vessel, the *hepatic portal vein*.

    (b) The hepatic portal vein divides repeatedly into a plexus of *sinusoids* (modified capillaries) within small liver lobules. Digested foods, enzymes, and hemoglobin are transferred to the hepatocytes (liver cells) and products of the hepatocytes are deposited into the blood.

    (c) From the sinusoids, blood is routed to successively larger veins and to the inferior vena cava leading to the right atrium of the heart.

IV. *Heart*

  A. *Histogenesis*

    1. Prior to the appearance of the somites (20 days), scattered masses of mesodermal *cardiogenic cells* appear at the anterior margin of the three-layered embryonic disc at about 18 days. The *cardiogenic masses* react like the blood islands of the yolk sac, forming *endothelial* *cells* around developing blood cells. The masses fuse to form short right and left *endocardial primordia* in the form of tubes.

2. The *endocardial tubes* unite superiorly to form the first aortic arch and a venous tube inferiorly. The intraembryonic developing vessels join the primitive vascular network of the yolk sac and umbilical veins developing in the placenta.

3. Mesenchymal cells surrounding the endocardial tubes differentiate into a layer of primitive cardiac myoblast cells, the *epimyocardial primordium.*

    a. The interval between the **endothelium** of the endocardial tubes and the *epimyocardium* is occupied by a wide layer of embryonic (mucous) connective tissue, which eventually disappears except for a few regions.

    b. Processes from the *endothelial cells* reach through the mucous connective tissue to contact the *epimyocardial cells.*

4. The simple tubular embryonic heart develops three layers, corresponding to the three layers of the blood vessels.

    a. **Endocardium**, from endocardial primordium.

    b. **Epicardium**, composed of squamous **mesothelium** and **tela subepicardiaca [subserosa]**, develops from outer layers of the epimyocardial primordium.

    c. **myocardium**, the intermediate muscular layer, develops from the major part of the epimyocardial primordium.

  B. *General anatomy* of the *heart*

1. The heart, the contractile organ of the cardiovascular system, is responsible for pumping blood to the lungs and to the body tissues.

2. Though the four-chambered heart lies almost on its right side in the pericardial sac, it is still described as having an *atrium* and a *ventricle* in the right half and an *atrium* and *ventricle* in the left half.

3. Deoxygenated blood is returned from the body tissues and organs via the *superior vena cava* and the *inferior vena cava* to the *right atrium.*

4. When the heart relaxes, blood drains out of the right atrium through the *tricuspid valve* (with three leaves) and into the *right ventricle.*

5. Muscular contractions of the right ventricle force deoxygenated blood into the lungs via the *pulmonary artery.* Oxygenated blood returns to the *left atrium* of the *heart* via the *pulmonary veins.*

6. During relaxation of the heart, blood drains out of the left atrium and enters the *left ventricle* through the *bicuspid valve*.

7. Blood exiting the left ventricle during contraction is pumped to the body tissues and organs via the *aorta*.

C. *Microscopic anatomy* of the *heart*

1. Endocardium lining the lumen of all four chambers is composed of

(a) an **endothelium** resting on a basement membrane,

(b) a thin *subendothelial stratum* consisting of a loose arrangement of connective tissue cells, collagen fibers, and some branching refractile elastic fibers,

(c) a thicker **stratum myoelasticum** of dense connective tissue with many elastic and isolated nonstriated smooth muocytes.

2. A **tela** (the term *tela* always signifies connective tissue) **subendocardialis**, a looser connective tissue layer, unites the **endocardium** to the **myocardium**. Traveling in this layer are the

a. stimulatory and inhibitory nerves of the ANS,

b. intramural branches of blood vessels,

c. myofibra conducens cardiaca (cardiac conduction fibers), composed of specialized **myocytus cardiacus conducens** (cardiac conduction myocytes) that do not contract, but convey the inherent beat from the point of origin, the SA node, and the AV node [The eponym Purkinje has been deleted from the current *Nomina Histologica*.] (Anderson et al, 1984).

[**Author's note:** A myofibra is a series of cardiac myocytes juxtaposed end-to-end; it is not a synonym for myocytus.]

3. Myocardium: During development, reticular fiber networks bind the loosely arranged cardiac muscle myocytes into a unified compact mass.

a. On the luminal surface of the adult heart, protruding bundles of remnant embryonic muscle (covered by endocardium) give the appearance of a spongy network. Some of these muscle fascicles are the **trabeculae carneae.**

b. Elastic fibers, prevalent in the myocardium of the atria, are scarcer in the ventricles.

4. Tela subepicardiaca [subserosa] is the layer of connective tissue separating the epicardium from the myocardium. The major coronary vessels and nerves travel in this layer prior to sending branches through the myocardium.

5. The outermost **epicardium** consists of

    a. a layer of connective tissue, with all its cellular and fibrillar elements,

    b. covered by a *visceral mesothelium* that faces the pericardial cavity surrounding the heart.

6. The *pericardial sac* in which the heart is suspended by its base, consists of

    a. pericardium fibrosum, a dense fibrous connective tissue covered by the looser connective tissue **tela subpericardialis [subserosa].** The connective tissue from this layer forms a strong connection, the **ligamenta sternopericardiaca,** to the sternum.

    b. pericardium serosum consisting of two layers enclosing a space, the **cavitas pericardialis:**

        (1) lamina parietalis, with mesothelium facing the cavity, and

        (2) lamina visceralis, with mesothelium continuing over the epicardium and facing the cavity.

    c. Approximately one cup of a watery fluid, the *serous fluid*, in the *pericardial cavity* keeps the heart lubricated during its excursions. Should the serous fluid escape or dry up, the two layers of facing mesothelium might adhere to one another ("adhesions").

        (1) New fluid, produced continually from **vas capillare arteriale** in the connective tissue under the mesothelium, passes through the mesothelial cells via micropinocytotic vesicles.

        (2) Old fluid is resorbed through the mesothelium by reverse micropinocytosis and picked up by the **vas capillare venosum.**

D. The *cardiac skeleton*: A ring of connective tissue of the epicardium separates the contiguous atria and ventricles and provides origin and insertion sites for cardiac myofibers. Connective tissue fibers from this ring form the *cardiac skeleton*. The connective tissue gives origin to a series of dense collagenous fiber bundles arranged into fibrous rings:

    1. annulus fibrosus of the *tricuspid orifice* between the right atrium and the right ventricle,

    2. annulus fibrosus of the *bicuspid orifice* between the left atrium and the left ventricle,

    3. annulus fibrosus of the *pulmonary trunk* surrounds the exit point of the main pulmonary artery.

    4. The **annulus fibrosus** surrounding the *aorta* resides in a triangular area situated between the adjacent atrioventricular rings (1 and 2

above) and that of the pulmonary trunk. This **annulus fibrosus** consists of three recognizable segments:

    a. *left fibrous trigone*: on the left side between the bicuspid orifice and the aorta,

    b. *right fibrous trigone*: anteriorly, between the two atrioventricular rings (annuli) and the aorta,

    c. *conus ligament*: posteriorly, between the pulmonary trunk and the aorta.

    5. Septum interventriculare, interventricular septum, separating the right and left ventricles, consists of two parts:

    a. the **pars membranacea**, dense connective tissue originating from the right fibrous trigone, extending into the myocardium of the pars muscularis,

    b. the **pars muscularis**, consisting of myocardium covered on the luminal surfaces by endocardium. The right and left bundle branches of the cardiac conduction system travel beneath the endocardium.

    E. *Valves of the heart* have a core of connective tissue that is chondroid (cartilage like). In some species (ie, ungulates) the valve tissue may have extensions of cartilage from the cartilaginous rings.

    1. The *bicuspid* and *tricuspid valves* are extensions of the atrioventricular fibrous rings.

    a. Endocardium of the atria and ventricles covers the valves and fuses at the free edges.

    b. *Nonstriated (smooth)* myocytes may migrate into the subendocardial tissue of the valves proper.

    c. Chordae tendineae, tendinous cords, extend from *papillary muscles* (composed of cardiac myocyte myofibers) of the ventricles to insert into the connective tissue of the valves. Endothelium covers the papillary muscles and the cords. Chordae tendineae prevent the valves from everting during contraction, not unlike the cords of a parachute.

    2. The *valves* of the *pulmonary artery* and the *aorta* are composed of connective tissue covered with endothelium.

    a. Each set of valves has three cusps with a little node of thickened tissue at the midpoint of the free edges.

    b. Valves prevent blood from reentering the heart.

    F. *Coronary arteries*, the major vessels of the heart, deserve particular attention because they are susceptible to atherosclerosis. The primary feature of this disease is *atheroma*, a localized plaque in the tunica interna, characterized by increased lipid content and fibrosis of loose connective tissue.

1. *Coronary arteries* arise immediately from the aorta to bring the *first oxygenated blood* to the heart walls.

2. In situ, coronary arteries resemble any other muscular artery. However, some authors maintain that the tunica media is separated into two layers by an intermediate elastic membrane. This "characteristic" occurs primarily in newborn infants. Jaffe et al (1971) demonstrated that the tunica media is not divided. In reality, a thickened musculoelastic cushion occurs in the tunica interna at sites where the coronary arteries branch. The cushion causes a thickening of the tunica interna between the endothelium and internal elastic membrane. Undifferentiated nonstriated (smooth) myocytes migrate from the tunica media into the tunica interna through fenestrations of the internal elastic membrane. These cells give rise to longitudinally oriented nonstriated (smooth) muscle bands, elastic fibers, and collagen fibers.

3. Lipid droplets accumulate in the extracellular matrix, the cytoplasm of monocytes, nonstriated (smooth) myocytes, and endothelial cells. This thickening of the tunica interna should be appreciated because it is characteristic in adults with focal deposits in atherosclerosis.

4. Coronary arteries traveling within the epicardial connective tissue divide into branches that penetrate the myocardium and then break up into capillary plexuses. *Arterial-arterial anastomoses* (A-A) are situated between the main branches of the coronary arteries in the epicardium and between the myocardial penetrating branches (Fig. 11-4).

5. Blood returns from the capillary plexuses via veins with no valves, which in turn join larger cardiac veins situated in the epicardium. *Venous-venous anastomoses* (V-V) occur between the main cardiac veins and the penetrating veins. The A-A and V-V anastomoses are complicated by direct *arterio-venous anastomoses* (A-V). Anastomoses are significant in providing collateral (alternate) channels of blood flow in certain cases of coronary artery obstruction (Fig. 11-4).

6. The significant difference in this pattern from other tissues is the presence of *arterioluminal* vessels bringing blood from the penetrating arteries directly into the lumen of the atria or the ventricles. Likewise, the **venae cordis minimae** (minute veins) begin at the luminal surface and drain either into the penetrating veins or into the capillary plexuses (Fig. 11-4).

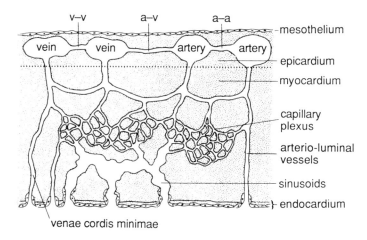

Figure 11-4 Intramural vasculature of the heart.

7. Another significant variation is the presence of capillary-like *sinusoids* with thinner and more flaccid walls for holding large quantities of blood under lower pressure for maximal metabolic exchange. The *sinusoids* drain blood from the capillary plexuses and pass it into the heart chambers (Fig. 11-4).

Questions

DIRECTIONS: Each group of questions below consists of five lettered headings followed by a list of numbered words or statements. For each numbered word or statement, select the one lettered heading that is most closely associated with it. Each lettered heading may be selected once, more than once, or not at all.

Questions 1–3
A. Pericytes
B. Zonulae occludentes
C. Fenestrae
D. Micropinocytotic vesicles
E. Diaphragms

1. Capillaries of blood–tissue barriers
2. Capillaries of renal glomeruli
3. Capillaries surrounding skeletal myocytes

Questions 4–6
A. Vasa vasorum
B. Sinus venularis
C. Aorta
D. Pulmonary artery
E. Muscular-type artery

4. A specialized postcapillary venule
5. Possesses some cardiac muscle in tunica media
6. An undulating prominent internal elastic membrane

Questions 7–9
A. Vena cordis minimae
B. Postcapillary venules
C. Sinus valvula
D. Portal vein
E. Uterine veins in pregnancy

7. Conspicuous tunica media with nonstriated myocytes
8. Surrounded by a conspicuous layer of pericytes
9. Prevents blood from pooling

Questions 10–12
A. Endocardial tubes
B. Mesothelium
C. Endothelium
D. Annulus fibrosus
E. Musculoelastic cushion

10. Lines the pericardial sac
11. Occurs in the tunica interna of coronary arteries
12. Form the first aortic arch

Explanatory Answers

1. B. Capillaries of blood–tissue barriers are best characterized by the necessity of zonulae occludentes or tight junctions to prevent leakage of substances between cells. A second feature of these capillaries is the lack of micropinocytotic vesicles.

2. C. The capillaries of the renal glomeruli are characterized by the presence of fenestrae without diaphragms. Although there have been reports of diaphragms, consensus agreement exists that these are diaphragmless.

3. D. Capillaries surrounding skeletal and other myocytes are thick continuous capillaries, necessitating an abundance of micropinocytotic vesicles for efficient transendothelial transport.

4. B. The sinus venularis is a specialized capillary of the spleen, with longitudinally arranged endothelial cells. These vessels were formerly incorrectly called venous sinuses.

5. D. The pulmonary artery is distinguished by the presence of some cardiac myocytes within the tunica media for only a short distance.

6. E. In contrast to the aorta and pulmonary artery, muscular-type arteries display a prominent, birefringent, wavy internal elastic membrane.

7. E. In addition to the uterine veins during pregnancy, the pulmonary veins and deep veins of the penis have a pronounced tunica media with nonstriated (smooth) myocytes.

8. B. Postcapillary venules are surrounded by a continuous layer of pericytes, resembling nonstriated (smooth) myocytes. Pericytes encountered along some capillaries do not form the continuous layer as in postcapillary venules.

9. C. The sinus valvula formed by the valves of veins catches blood between pulsations (causing the valves to slap shut), thereby preventing pooling of blood in the lower extremities.

10. B. Mesothelium lines the visceral and parietal laminae of the pericardial sac. Endothelium lines lumina of the heart and blood vessels.

11. E. Musculoelastic cushions occur in the tunica interna of coronary vessels where the coronary vessels branch. Myocytes from the tunica media migrate into the tunica interna, giving rise to longitudinally oriented muscle bands along with elastic fibers and collagen fibers.

12. A. The union of embryonic tubes anteriorly form the first aortic arch. Posteriorly they form the vena cava.

12 The Lymphopoetic Organs

I. *Introduction*

  A. Higher vertebrates and man possess *lymphopoetic organs* to

    1. assist *hemopoetic organs* in blood cell production,

    2. participate with the blood vascular system in returning excess tissue fluids to the general circulation,

    3. develop and maintain the body's immune responses.

  B. The lymphopoetic organs considered in this chapter are *lymph nodes, spleen,* and *thymus.* Other lymphatic tissues will be discussed as they occur in other tissues and organs.

II. The unidirectional *lymphatic system* consists of *lymph nodes* united by lymphatic vessels. *Lymph* flow through the lymphatic vessels is directed by valves. The significance of lymphatic vessels can be appreciated by their association with the blood vascular system.

  A. *Arterioles* deliver blood to capillary plexuses in connective tissues. *Venules* drain the capillary plexuses to redirect blood to the heart. Interposed lymphatic vessels play the following role:

    1. An ultrafiltrate of *blood plasma* exiting arterial capillary vessels permeates the connective tissues as *tissue fluid.* Some of this tissue fluid is recovered by the venous capillary vessels.

    2. The remaining *tissue fluid*, containing particulate and colloidal material, is recovered from the connective tissue by blind (unidirectional) *lymphatic capillaries.*

    3. *Lymphatic capillaries* unite to form progressively larger vessels which ultimately empty into veins.

4. *Lymphatic nodes,* positioned at advantageous sites along the path of the lymphatic vessels, filter *tissue fluid* and add *lymphocytes.* Tissue fluid thus becomes *lymphatic fluid.*

B. Histogenesis of *lymphatic vessels* and *lymph nodes*

1. Lymphatic vessels develop similarly but independently from blood vessels.

2. Interposed at designated anatomical sites along the path of the lymphatic vessels are aggregates of mesenchymal cells that will develop into bean-shaped *lymphatic nodes.* These densities are vascularized by vessels entering and exiting at the concave surface or **hilum.**

[**Please note**: The term lymphatic "follicle" should not be used, for it was a misnomer based on the misconception that the nodules had cavities.]

3. Several developing blind-ended lymphatic vessels approach the convex surface of mesenchymal cell aggregates and are flattened on contact.

4. Reticular and collagen fibers, around the flattened lymphatic ends, form a connective tissue *capsule* around the developing lymphatic node.

5. The flattened lymphatic vessel ends fuse to form a *subcapsular sinus* under the connective tissue *capsule.*

6. Commencing at the **hilum,** connective tissue elements accompany and surround the entering and exiting blood vessels.

a. The hilar mass of connective tissue separates and follows the blood vessels as they branch in the mesenchymal mass.

b. Each connective tissue branch is a *trabecula,* and the protected blood vessels within are the *trabecular vessels.*

c. The *trabeculae* subdivide the developing mesenchymal cells into

(1) a peripheral *cortex,* containing the *lymphatic nodules,* and

(2) a central *medulla* extending to the hilum. Later the central region differentiates into a subnodular *paracortex* and the juxtahilar *medulla.*

7. At the hilum entrance, a bulbous expansion of the *subcapsular sinus* invades the node to form a network of *medullary sinuses* and *trabecular sinuses* around the trabeculae.

8. The radiating trabecular *sinuses* eventually contact and re-unite with the subcapsular sinus. Continuity thus forms between the subcapsular sinus, trabecular sinuses, and medullary sinuses.

9. Thus, the basic flow pattern of the mature lymphatic node is established:

    a. several *afferent lymphatic vessels* (with valves) enter the *subcapsular sinus* of the lymphatic node.

    b. *tissue fluid* (entering the first set of lymphatic nodes) is filtered in the lymphatic node and lymphocytes are added. The combination of *tissue fluid + lymphocytes = lymphatic fluid.*

    c. lymphatic fluid exits the lymphatic node via one or two valved *efferent lymphatic vessels*, which convey it to the next set of lymphatic nodes and so on, until the lymphatic fluid is delivered to the cardiovascular system.

C. *Microscopic structure* of *lymphatic vessels*

1. *Lymphocapillaries*, slightly larger and more irregular in cross section than blood capillaries, have *nonfenestrated* thin *endothelial cells*:

    a. that *overlap* at their *junctional edges*. Closely adherent edges may have some tight adherence spots and some seepage spaces,

    b. with scattered *microvilli* on the luminal surface,

    c. covered by a *poorly developed basement membrane*, with *no* associated *pericytes*.

2. *Lymphatic anchoring filaments* from the surrounding connective tissue insert on fragmented patched of basement membrane and directly onto the external (abluminal) plasmalemma of the endothelial cells. Anchoring filaments maintain vessel patency during inflammation, when the pressure of excess tissue fluid in contiguous connective tissue would collapse them.

3. *Local dilatations* at branching sites distinguish a *lymphocapillary* from a blood capillary.

4. Superficial and deep *lymphocapillary plexuses* accompany blood capillary plexuses, but usually *reside deeper* in the connective tissue layers of

    a. skin,

    b. digestive system,

    c. respiratory system,

    d. urinary system,

    e. male and female reproductive systems,

    f. under mesothelium (serous membranes).

5. *Lymphocapillary* plexuses are *absent* in
  a. the central nervous system,
  b. bone marrow,
  c. the eye.

6. Blind-ended *lymphocapillary* terminals range from simple tubes (ie, intestinal *central lymphatic vessels* [lacteals]) to branched ends, and from flattened to circular in cross section.

D. *Lymphatic vessels*

1. *Medium-sized lymphatic vessels* have the three layers common to blood vessels, but are extremely difficult to distinguish. These collecting vessels, *provided with valves* aimed in the direction of flow, have a structure and function similar to those of veins.

  a. The **tunica interna [intima]** has *longitudinally oriented connective tissue fibers.*

  b. The **tunica media** has *circularly* disposed connective tissue fibers and nonstriated (smooth) myocytes.

  c. The **tunica externa [adventitia]**, the thickest coat, resembles that of veins, with scattered *longitudinally* coursing nonstriated (smooth) myocytes.

2. *Large lymphatic vessels* ultimately terminate in the *thoracic duct* and *right lymphatic duct*, both of which are *provided with valves.*

  a. The *right lymphatic duct*, at the site of entrance in the right subclavian vein, is guarded by bicuspid valves to prevent reflux of venous blood into the duct (Clemente, 1985).

    (1) The *right lymphatic duct* is formed by the union of the
      (a) *right jugular trunk*, which receives lymphatic fluid from right side of the head and neck,
      (b) *right subclavian trunk*, which drains the right upper extremity,
      (c) *right bronchomediastinal trunk*, which drains the right side of the thorax, right lung, right side of the heart, and part of the convex surface of the liver.

    (2) *Variations*: The right lymphatic duct is formed by the union of these three trunks, but in keeping with the variability of the lymphatic system, the three trunks may enter separately or in any combination, near the angle of junction of the right internal jugular and right subclavian veins.

  b. The *thoracic duct*, the largest lymphatic channel in the body, receives lymphatic fluid from the rest of the body and delivers it to the blood vascular system at the junction of the *left internal jugular vein* and the *subclavian vein.*

(1) The thoracic duct, originating as a dilated sac, the **cisterna chyli,** is an evolutionary consolidation of a series of lymphatic sacs.

(2) Its structure resembles that of a comparable sized vein, but differs in three characteristics:

(a) the tunica media and externa are difficult to distinguish,

(b) an internal elastic membrane helps to distinguish the tunica interna from the tunica media,

(c) there is more muscle than a vein.

(3) At the termination, bicuspid valves directed toward the vein prevent reflux of venous blood into the duct (Clemente, 1985).

E. *Microscopic structure* of *lymphatic nodes* (Fig. 12-1)

1. The **stroma** consists of an external *capsule,* internal *trabeculae,* and meshes of *reticular fibers.*

a. The external *capsule* covering the *subcapsular sinus* of the flattened bean-shaped *lymphatic node* consists of

(1) dense bundles of collagen fibers and reticular fibers intermingled with a finer network of elastic fibers,

(2) scattered nonstriated (smooth) myocytes, which play a negligible role in accelerating lymphatic flow. In lower vertebrates, capsular muscle assists fluid flow.

b. *Trabeculae* divide the *lymphatic node* into compartments.

Figure 12-1 Structure of a lymphatic node.

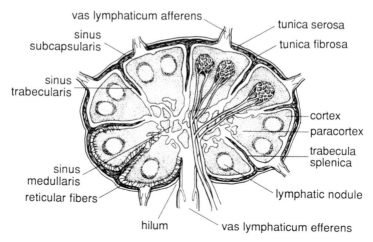

From the trabeculae, fine branching *reticular fibers* permeate the parenchyma of the lymphatic node and the lumena of the sinuses (subcapsular, trabecular, and medullary sinuses).

   c. *Reticulocytes* (old name: reticular cells) and fixed macrophages attach to and invest the reticular fibers to complete the stroma. *Reticulocytes* resemble those of bone marrow stroma and possess similar developmental potencies, especially as progenitors of hemocytoblasts.

   2. *Lymphatic nodes* produce *lymphocytes* for distribution to the body. *Macrophages* ingest pathogenic bacteria, dust (in the pulmonary lymphatic nodes), and aged erythrocytes. The lymphatic node is divided into a peripheral *cortex*, an inner *medulla*, and an intermediate *paracortex*.

   a. The *cortex* houses *lymphatic nodules*:

   (1) consisting of aggregations of *lymphocytes* supported in reticular fiber networks,

   (2) with *small lymphocytes* forming a dense *corona* (ring) around a *germinal center* of less compacted *large lymphocytes*.

   b. The *paracortex* consists of a less dense distribution of lymphocytes (Greaves et al, 1974).

   c. The *medulla* lymphocyte population is arranged into *medullary cords* by the network of medullary sinuses.

   F. *Topography* of *T lymphocytes* and *B lymphocytes*. Within mature lymphatic nodes it is possible to recognize T and B compartments (Parrott and DeSousa, 1971).

   1. *Thymus-dependent areas.* Originally in neonatally thymectomized rats and mice (Waksmann et al, 1962) and in congenitally hypothymic mice (DeSousa et al, 1969), selective areas of lymphocyte depletion were seen in the *paracortex* of *lymphatic nodes* (also in periarteriolar sheaths of the spleen and internodular areas of gastrointestinal lymphoid tissues).

   2. *Thymus-independent areas* are the germinal centers of *lymphatic nodules* and *medulla* of lymphatic nodes (also lymphatic nodules and plasma cells in the gastrointestinal tract, lymphatic nodules and peripheral regions of splenic white pulp) (Parrott et al, 1966).

   G. *Aging*

   1. During inactivity, the *germinal center* may be replaced by a dense migration of small lymphocytes.

   2. From the embryo through the first few postnatal months, and in aged adults, lymphatic nodules are rather inconspicuous.

3. With advancing age, lymphatic nodules *involute*; that is, lymphocytic activity decreases and the nodules are invaded by *adipocytes*.

III. The *spleen*

A. *Introduction*: The *spleen*, a lymphatic organ about the size of a fist (4 × 8 × 12 cm) and weighing between 150 to 200 g, possesses the largest amount of lymphatic tissue in the body. While the spleen is unnecessary for life, its loss increases chances for succumbing to massive infections.

1. Unlike lymphatic nodes, which are interposed along chains of lymphatic vessels, the spleen is inserted directly in the course of the blood vascular system.

2. The spleen is located in the upper left quadrant of the abdomen, posterior to the stomach, closely related to the diaphragm at the level of the 9th, 10th, and 11th ribs.

3. The spleen is perhaps the least understood abdominal organ, especially with regard to knowledge of the microcirculatory patterns.

4. Clinically, it is involved in many generalized systemic disease processes, necessitating competent hematologic evaluation of the patient.

B. *Histogenesis of the spleen*: One of the first lymphatic tissues to appear in the embryo, the spleen is hemopoetically active until the fifth or sixth month of intrauterine life.

1. About the 32nd day of development, the anlage of the spleen appears as a mass of rapidly dividing mesenchymal cells between the two mesothelial layers of the *dorsal mesentery*. The mesothelium thus provides the outer **tunica serosa**.

2. The cell mass, probably receiving cellular contributions from the adjacent mesothelium, increases in mass until it bulges into the peritoneal cavity.

3. The highly vascularized mass of mesenchymal cells differentiates into *parenchymal* and *stromal* cells.

   a. The **stroma** consists of

     (1) a connective tissue **tunica fibrosa [capsula]**,

     (2) anastomosing *splenic trabeculae* (from the tunica fibrosa) penetrating the parenchyma,

     (3) networks of *reticular fibers* (from the trabeculae) forming a spongy stroma. *Reticulocytes* and fixed macrophages coat the reticular fibers.

b. The **parenchyma** consists of
(1) free basophilic cells (lymphocytes?) in the "compartments" between stomal fibers,
(2) macrophages and scattered transient cells.

4. The spleen initiates activity after it achieves its adult form,
with
a. the *external surface*, impressed by adjacent organs,
b. a **hilum**, where vessels and nerves exit and enter.

C. *Microscopic structure of the spleen* [Lien]

1. The *spleen* is covered by a **mesothelium** (with a basement
membrane) anchored to a thin *loose* connective tissue layer. The outer
surface of the mesothelium faces the peritoneal cavity.
Mesothelium + basement membrane + connective tissue = **tunica serosa.**

2. Deep to the **tunica serosa** is a *denser* connective tissue layer,
the **tunica fibrosa [capsule]** composed of collagen fibers, elastic fibers,
and a few nonstriated (smooth) myocytes.

3. *Splenic trabeculae*, penetrating from the tunica fibrosa, give
origin to collagen fibers that branch repeatedly as *reticular fibers* of a
spongy stroma. (These fibers were called "argyrophilic" because they
attract silver stains. A good silver preparation is valuable in demon-
strating the reticular stroma.) Reticulocytes (formerly: reticular cells)
and fixed macrophages associate with stromal fibers.

4. In freshly cut sections, the spleen presents
a. a *red pulp*, appearing like tomato paste,
b. a *white pulp* of irregularly shaped, whitish gray areas speckled in the red pulp.

5. The *white pulp* consists of densely packed *lymphocytes* and
diffuse *lymphocytes.*
a. Densely packed lymphocytes form the **lymphonodulus
splenicus** (splenic lymphonodules) with *germinal centers* that may
appear and disappear.
b. Both dense and diffuse lymphocytes are supported by a
stroma of reticular fibers (macrophages). Elastic fibers intermingle
with reticular fibers, especially around *arteries of the white pulp.*

6. The *red pulp* is characterized by specialized postcapillary venules, each of which is termed a **sinus venularis**. (The previous term,
venous sinus, is preempted by the *Nomina Histologica* for certain
large venous channels.)

a. Parenchymal tissue fills the interstices around the sinuses.

b. The term *red pulp* is attributed to the abundance of erythrocytes surrounding and within the **sinus venulares** (pl.).

c. Free and fixed macrophages are observed digesting erythrocytes in TEMs. Thus one of the most important functions of the spleen is revealed, the breakdown of aged erythrocytes to recover iron from hemoglobin.

d. The adult spleen retains its potentiality for hemocytopoesis, and in certain emergency conditions requiring *extramedullar hemocytopoesis* resumes its fetal capability to produce erythrocytes, granulocytes, and megacaryocytes.

D. *Circulatory patterns of the spleen*

1. Although blood circulation through the spleen is the least understood of all body organs, it may be comprehended by examining what is known and what is speculative (Fig. 12-2).

2. The *splenic artery* enters at the **hilum** and immediately branches into several *trabecular arteries*, protected and supported within the *splenic trabeculae*.

3. Upon reaching the smallest *splenic trabeculae* (after which the

Figure 12-2 Circulatory patterns of the spleen. *1.* Closed system. *2.* Open system. *3.* Combination open/closed.

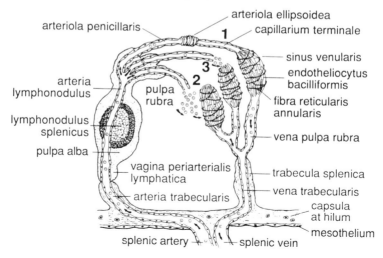

trabeculae become indistinguishable from reticular networks), the smallest arteries exit and enter the *white pulp* as the **arteria pulpae albae** (artery of the white pulp).

a. *Lymphocytes* coating the *artery of the white pulp* form a **vagina periarterialis lymphatica** (periarterial lymphatic sheath) (Weiss, 1974).

b. *Splenic lymphonodules* with germinal centers may appear, disappear, and reappear anywhere along the periarterial lymphatic sheath.

c. The *artery* within a splenic lymphonodule was referred to as the "central" artery. However, because it rarely traverses the center of a lymph nodule, "central artery" has been replaced by the more precise term, **arteria lymphonoduli** (artery of the lymphonodule).

d. The **arteria lymphonoduli** distributes capillaries to the white pulp to provide nutrients and oxygen to the energetically dividing lymphocytes.

4. Prior to entering the red pulp, the arteria lymphonoduli branches into several thin *penicillar arterioles*.

a. After the penicillar arterioles acquire sheaths of concentrically arranged cells (possibly reticulocytes), they are termed **arteriola ellipsoidea** (Blue and Weiss, 1981). *Ellipsoid arterioles*, large enough to resolve (via LM) in the cat, dog, or pig, are rare in humans.

b. The **arteriola ellipsoidea** conducts blood into the **vas capillarium terminale** (terminal capillary vessel).

5. From this point on, the mechanism of distribution is unclear, but three plausible explanations based on experimentation and observation have been offered. Before considering these, it is advantageous to examine the *venous* drainage pathways.

a. *Venous drainage* commences in the **sinus venularis**, a modified postcapillary venule connecting the *terminal capillary vessel* and the *vein of the red pulp*.

b. The walls of the **sinus venulares** (pl.) are lined, not by interdigitating diamond-shaped endothelial cells, but by elongated endothelial cells, the **endotheliocytus fusiformis**, arranged along the longitudinal axis of the sinus venularis.

(1) The sinus venularis features *large spaces* between occasional *tight junctions* of the *fusiform endothelial cells*.

(2) Fibra reticularis annularis wrap around the exterior of the fusiform endothelial cells to provide structural support. The branching *annular reticular fibers* blend with those of the surrounding stroma.

(3) The sinus venularis may be compared to a *barrel*, composed of staves and hoops:

    (a) *staves* = fusiform endothelial cells,

    (b) *hoops* = reticular fibers.

    c. The *fusiform endothelial cells* stand as "sentries" along the sinus venularis to permit passage of erythrocytes through the spaces between them (Chen and Weiss, 1973).

    d. In the surrounding red pulp, *phagocytic macrophages*, with a unique ability to recognize aged or damaged erythrocytes, inspect erythrocytes. Failure to pass inspection subjects the erythrocytes to phagocytosis. Old erythrocytes with depleted sialic acid on their surfaces expose galactose residues, which are recognized by macrophages.

    (1) *Phagocytosis*, following engulfment of a whole erythrocyte, is recognized in TEMs by the following phenomena:

    (a) erosion of the erythrocyte periphery,

    (b) electron density increase of the cell.

    (2) The remaining *hemosiderin* (an iron-containing pigment) condenses into small electron-dense masses within the macrophage.

    (3) *Bilirubin*, derived from the breakdown of hemoglobin, is returned to the bloodstream and delivered to the liver for further processing and elimination in bile.

    6. Blood released from the sinus venularis flows through the *trabecular veins*, which unite at the hilum of the spleen to form the *splenic vein*.

    7. The *splenic vein* joins the *portal vein*, which brings blood to the liver prior to returning blood to the heart, via the inferior vena cava.

    E. *Theories of splenic circulation* (Chen, 1978): From the *terminal capillary vessels*, blood reaches the **sinus venularis** by three postulated routes (Fig. 12-2):

    1. *Closed system* (Kinsely, 1936): The *terminal capillary vessel* empties directly into the closed end of the sinus venularis. Erythrocytes pass into the red pulp through the spaces between the fusiform endothelial cells and return the same way.

    2. *Open system* (McCuskey and McCuskey, 1977, 1985): The *terminal capillary vessel* ends in the red pulp and pours its contents into the spongy reticular stroma. From the red pulp, blood cells find their way into the sinus venularis through gaps between fusiform endothelial cells.

3. *Combination theory* (Groom and Song, 1962; Groom et al, 1971): Terminal capillary vessels empty into the sinus venularis at one particular time, but may withdraw at other times to empty into the red pulp. In a contracted spleen the circulation is said to be closed; while in a relaxed one, the circulation is open. Entering and reentering blood cells pass through the gaps between the *fusiform endotheliocytes.*

F. *Functions of the spleen*

1. *Blood filtration* occurs by phagocytic removal of
   a. lipid droplets from the bloodstream,
   b. old, abnormal, or damaged erythrocytes, leucocytes, and thrombocytes,
   c. particulate material.

2. *Hemoglobin degradation*
   a. *Iron* stored as ferritin or hemosiderin in macrophage lysosomes is transported to the liver by blood *plasma transferrin* and then to bone marrow for reuse in erythroblasts.
   b. *Heme*, a pigment degraded by macrophages to bilirubin, binds to *albumin* in the blood plasma for delivery to the liver, where it is secreted as a component of bile.

3. *Removal* of pathogens, via phagocytosis or immune responses, to control infectious diseases.

4. *Removal* of partially differentiated cells (reticulated erythrocytes, T and B lymphocytes, thrombocytes, etc) from the circulation to provide a proper environment for completion of differentiation. Monocytes removed from circulation are transformed to splenic macrophages.

5. *Production* of immunologically functioning lymphocytes.

6. *Resumption* of hemocytopoesis in some pathological conditions (extramedullary hemopoesis).

7. *Storage* of blood via *blood–spleen barriers* in the red pulp. Barriers, closing down the entire spleen, may also be erected as protective mechanisms. Blood is sequestered for varying periods of time in red pulp compartments by reticulocyte (old name: reticular cells) activity, which closes down selected areas:
   a. *Fast flow compartment (1)* (Groom and Song, 1962): lets 90% of blood pass through in about 30 seconds.
   b. *Intermediate flow compartment (2)* (Groom et al 1971): 9% of the blood flow passes through in about 8 minutes. Thus blood is stored and expelled by contraction of the spleen.

    c. *Slow flow compartment (3)* (Weiss et al, 1986): 1% of the blood is held in storage for 1 hour. Reticulated erythrocytes and some granulocytes achieve final maturation prior to reentering the circulation.

    8. Possible *synthesis* of *splenin*, a hormone that regulates
    a. hemocytopoesis in bone marrow,
    b. destruction of erythrocytes.

    9. *Production* of antibodies (Mitchel and Abbott, 1971)

IV. The **thymus** (Kendall, 1981) (Fig. 12-3)

    A. *Introduction*: The **thymus** is described as a lymphoepithelial organ, with endodermal stromal cells derived from endoderm and mesodermally derived lymphocyte stem cells from the blood. The thymus functions for a short time as an embryonic hemopoetic organ, before assuming its role in producing

    1. *T lymphocytes* (*thymocytes*), involved in cell-mediated responses (immunological reactions transferable by cells and not by serum). The T lymphocytes produced in the thymus originate in the bone marrow and reach full maturity in the spleen or lymph nodes. Although structurally difficult to distinguish on their journey, they can be differentiated by monoclonal antibody methods.

    2. *Humoral factors* (*thymopoetin, thymosin*), presumably polypeptide hormones produced by *thymic epithelioreticulocytes*, which promote the differentiation and maturation of stem cell lymphocytes by inducing formation of T-lymphocyte surface markers (Goldstein, 1984; Bach and Papiernik, 1981).

    B. *Histogenesis of the thymus* (The pharyngeal pouches are considered in the next chapter.)

    1. The embryonic pharynx, lined by endoderm, forms the segment of the digestive tract following the oral cavity.

    a. The developing pharynx pushes bilateral pouches of pharyngeal endoderm into the surrounding mesoderm.

    b. The set of bilateral pouches closest to the oral cavity are the *first pharyngeal pouches*; the next more posterior, the *second pharyngeal pouches*; the next, the *third pharyngeal pouches*; and finally those closest to the origin of the esophagus are the *fourth pharyngeal pouches*. Sometimes there are *fifth pharyngeal pouches*.

    2. Toward the end of the *sixth week* of prenatal life, the *thymus*

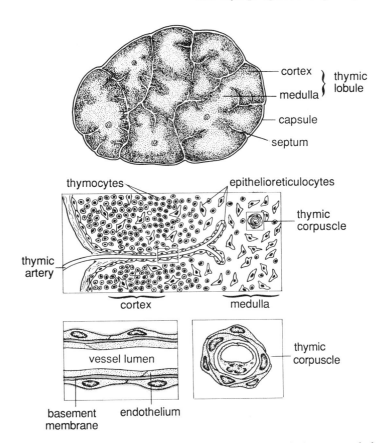

Figure 12-3 The thymus. Note T lymphocytes and the stromal thymic epithelioreticulocytes. Capillaries are sheathed by thymic epithelioreticulocytes, which contribute to the blood–thymus barrier.

develops as bilateral sacculations of the *third pharyngeal pouches* and sometimes contributions from the *fourth pharyngeal pouches*.

a. The hollow *endodermal thymic primordia* descend ventrally and caudally until they reach their site of permanent residence, the superior mediastinum.

b. Cellular endodermal growth into the lumen forms solid cords, which sever ties with their pharyngeal origins.

c. The leading right and left ends enlarge and unite. Finger-like lobular extensions, from the anlage, protrude into the surrounding mesoderm forming the general configuration of the organ.

3. *Thymic corpuscles* (formerly: Hassall's corpuscles) may be composed of one cell or many cells in the aging thymus. Their formation results from the arrangement of

a. free *endodermal cells* rolled into tight balls.

b. free *thymic epthelioreticulocytes* surrounding
   (1) cysts formed by aberrant embryonic pharyngeal epithelium,
   (2) kerato-hyaline granules,
   (3) cytoplasmic filaments, or
   (4) degenerated calcified cells.

4. During the 12th week of development, the organ develops an outer **cortex** and an inner **medulla**.

a. *Thymocytes* (lymphocytes), tightly packed at the periphery of the finger-like lobules, form the **cortex**.

b. **Epithelioreticulocytus thymi** (derived from endoderm) are stellate-shaped cells forming the major portion of the lightly stained medulla.

c. Mesenchymal cells, through which the thymic anlage penetrated, form a delicate connective tissue *capsule* and *cortical septae* between the cortical lobules.

5. During development, the trailing ends of the migrating lobes usually atrophy or break away to be incorporated into the thymus proper. In some instances, the ends fail to descend and may persist as solid *accessory thymic nodules* or *cysts* at the level of the thyroid gland in the neck or anywhere along the pathway to the mediastinum.

6. From the sixth prenatal month to puberty, the thymus continues *proliferative growth* until it reaches a maximum weight of 40 g in its residence site, the superior mediastinum.

7. *Involution* (Clarke and MacLennan, 1986)

a. *Age involution* begins shortly after puberty, during which regression occurs with a concomitant infiltration of adipocytes and connective tissue fibers. During involution, the thymus remains functional. With advancing age, the following components undergo sequential involution:
   (1) **medulla** first,
   (2) **cortex** second,

(3) *thymic corpuscles* decrease in number during involution, but those remaining grow to 100 μm in diameter.

(4) *lobular* atrophy causes the *septae* to widen, making lobulation more apparent.

    b. *Accidental involution* prior to puberty results from

      (1) disease or infection,

      (2) unmanageable stress,

      (3) poor diet,

      (4) various endotoxins and steroids.

C. *Microscopic structure of the thymus*

    1. The sponge-like **stroma** is composed of stellate-shaped, endodermally derived *thymic epithelioreticulocytes.*

    a. Reticular fibers are not associated with stromal cells, except those accompanying blood vessels.

    b. Blood vessels and nerves penetrating the organ through the septae carry their own connective tissue fibers and cells.

    c. Adipocytes of involution are thought to be derived from connective tissue cells and not *thymic epithelioreticulocytes.*

    d. *Thymic epithelioreticulocytes* have

      (1) an oval nucleus (7 to 10 μm) with one or two nucleoli and thinly distributed euchromatin,

      (2) occasional profiles of rER and sER that are inadequate to distinguish the cytoplasm. Occasional membrane-bound vesicles, resembling lysosomes, appear in the cytoplasm.

      (3) cell processes attached to adjacent cell processes via desmosomes. Cytoplasmic intermediate processes appear to insert into the desmosomal plaques.

    2. Parenchymal *thymocytes (T lymphocytes)*

    a. *Small thymocytes* have heterochromatic nuclei, enveloped by a thin coating of basophilic cytoplasm.

    b. *Larger thymocytes* occur only at the periphery of the cortex. Mitotic thymocytes at the periphery indicate that newly generated cells migrate toward the medulla, where they are inserted into the circulation.

    c. *Degenerating thymocytes* occur at the interface between cortex and medulla.

    d. *Thymocytes* are far fewer in number in the medulla than in the cortex.

    3. *Other cells in the parenchyma*

    a. *Macrophages*, while few in number, are present to destroy aging lymphocytes, ineffective lymphocytes, or foreign substances.

b. *Plasma cells* occur rarely, but their presence has not been clarified.

c. *Acidophils* (eosinophils) occasionally occur.

d. *Tissue basophils* (mast cells) when present appear in the peripheral connective tissue (Ginsburg and Sachs, 1963).

4. *Efferent lymphatic vessels*, starting from blind-ended lymphatic vessels, exit the medulla via the septae to the capsular vessels, carrying T lymphocytes. The T lymphocytes must be able to cross the blood–thymus barrier in the medulla. Afferent lymphatic vessels have not been reported.

D. *Functions of the thymus*: The fetal thymus is populated by lymphocyte stem cells from the liver, until bone marrow assumes the role of the hemopoesis. Thereafter, bone marrow functions as the major source of lymphocyte stem cells. Developmental activity within the thymus produces more cells than necessary, necessitating massive destruction of lymphocytes. Enough T lymphocytes are produced to colonize the lymph nodes, spleen, and other tissues (see below).

1. *Neonatal thymectomy* in mice results in the following sequelae of events (Miller, 1962):
   a. failure of immunological competence,
   b. descreased capacity to produce antibodies,
   c. failure to reject transplants of foreign tissue,
   d. death.

2. *Neonatal thymectomy* in mice results in selective depletion of T lymphocytes from these *thymus-dependent areas* (Parrott et al, 1966):
   a. *periarteriolar lymphatic sheath* of the spleen,
   b. *paracortex* of lymphatic nodes,
   c. *internodular areas* of lymphatic nodes, *gut-associated lymphatic tissue* (GALT), and *bronchiolar-associated lymphatic tissue* (BALT).

3. *Thymus-independent areas* or B lymphocyte areas:
   a. all *lymphatic nodules*, ie,
      (1) lymphatic nodes,
      (2) splenic white pulp.
      (3) GALT and BALT,
      (4) tonsils.
   b. *medulla* of lymphatic nodes.

4. Production of thymopoetin and thymosin.

5. T lymphocytes are involved in cell-mediated responses.

6. The thymus monitors T-lymphocyte production by destroying T lymphocytes that attack body tissues rather than foreign invaders.

    E. The *blood–thymus barrier* is a tight barrier between the blood vessesls and the parenchyma of the cortex. The blood–thymus barrier is impermeable to many substances. The barrier in the medulla is not as tight. The barrier consists of

    1. In capillaries:

    a. blood vascular nonfenestrated (continuous) endothelium lining the lumen covered by its

    b. continuous basement membrane,

    c. perivascular connective tissue,

    d. basement membrane of the epithelioreticulocytes,

    e. tightly apposed thymic epithelioreticulocytes.

    2. In arteries and veins, there are nonstriated myocytes around the perivascular connective tissue.

Questions

DIRECTIONS: Each of the questions or incomplete statements below is followed by suggested answers or completions. Select the *one* that is the *best* answer.

---

    1. The endothelial cells of lymphocapillaries
       1. are elongated, fusiform cells
       2. overlap at their junctional edges
       3. have a well-developed basement membrane
       4. are nonfenestrated

    2. Lymphatic nodes are divided into
       1. cortex
       2. paracortex
       3. medulla
       4. white pulp

    3. Thymus-independent areas of lymphatic nodes are the
       1. germinal centers of lymphatic nodules
       2. cortex
       3. medulla
       4. paracortex

4. The red pulp of the spleen is characterized by the presence of
   1. trabecular sinuses
   2. endodermally derived stromal cells
   3. efferent lymphatic vessels
   4. sinus venularis

5. Annular reticular fibers
   1. maintain the patency of lymphocapillaries
   2. can be stained with silver stains
   3. form the major part of the splenic capsule
   4. wrap around fusiform endothelial cells

6. Erythrocytes in the spleen may be
   1. inspected for depletion of membrane sialic acid
   2. removed if not fully differentiated
   3. subjected to phagocytosis by macrophages
   4. sequestered in a blood–spleen barrier to mature

7. The thymus
   1. originates from the third and sometimes fourth pharyngeal pouches
   2. produces T lymphocytes
   3. is recognized in the aged by the presence of thymic corpuscles
   4. may leave bilateral trails of accessory thymic nodules

8. Thymic corpuscles (Hassall's) form from free thymic epithelioreticulocytes surrounding
   1. kerato-hyaline granules
   2. degenerated calcified cells
   3. cytoplasmic filaments
   4. aberrant pharyngeal cysts

9. Thymic epithelioreticulocytes have
   1. a basophilic cytoplasm
   2. an endodermal ancestry
   3. an oval nucleus with clumped heterochromatin
   4. desmosomes connecting cell processes

10. The arteria elliposoidea is
    1. surrounded by a sheath of concentrically arranged cells of possible reticulocyte (old name, reticular cells) origin
    2. coated with a sheath of lymphocytes
    3. rare in humans
    4. found within a splenic lymphonodule

Explanatory Answers

1. **C.** 2 and 4 are correct. Elongated fusiform endothelial cells are unique to the sinus venulares of the spleen. The endothelial cells of lymphocapillaries resemble those of blood capillaries, except that they overlap at their edges, providing some open spaces. Additionally, the endothelium is characterized by scattered microvilli on the luminal surface. The basement membrane on the abluminal surface is poorly developed.

2. **A.** 1, 2, and 3 are correct. White pulp is descriptive of the whitish speckled areas in the red pulp of the spleen.

3. **B.** 1 and 3 are correct. Thymus-independent areas are sites where B lymphocytes reside, thus they occur in the germinal centers of lymphatic nodules and the medulla. T lymphocytes can occur in the internodular areas of the cortex as well as the paracortex.

4. **D.** 4 is correct. The sinus venularis, of which there are many, is a specialized postcapillary venule that is interposed between the terminal capillary and the vein of the red pulp. These sinuses possess the elongated fusiform endotheliocytes. Trabecular sinuses and efferent lymphatic vessels are found in lymphatic nodes. The endodermally derived stromal cells are peculiar to the thymus.

5. **C.** 2 and 4 are correct. Annular reticular fibers describe those fibers that support the fusiform endotheliocytes of the spleen. These can be stained with silver stains as can all reticular fibers. Lymphatic anchoring filaments are those that insert on the lymphocapillary endothelial cells to prevent them from collapsing. While the capsule has reticular fibers, only those associated with the sinus venularis are called annular reticular fibers.

6. E. All are correct. The spleen is specialized to deal with many situations. In particular, all the listed items involve the erythrocytes. Iron and the pigment heme are recovered by the spleen. Only 1% of the blood, retained in the spleen for maximum periods, provides the proper environment for reticulated erythrocytes and some granulocytes to achieve final maturation.

7. E. All are correct. The thymus originates bilaterally from the third and sometimes the fourth pharyngeal pouches. As it descends to its final position in the superior mediastinum, bilateral "rests" (left behind) of cysts or accessory thymic nodules may occur along the path. While thymic corpuscles decrease in number with age, those that remain get larger and persist into old age. Lymphocytes seeded to the thymus are transformed into T lymphocytes.

8. E. All are correct. The thymic corpuscles form from all of the numbered items. It appears that all that is needed is a seed of substance and free thymic epithelioreticulocytes will spiral around the "seed" to begin a thymic corpuscle.

9. C. 2 and 4 are correct. The cytoplasm of thymic epithelioreticulocytes is distinguished by cytoplasmic structures, and the oval nucelus has thinly distributed euchromatin and one or two nucleoli. These endodermally derived cells have a number of cell processes that connect to their partners by desmosomes.

10. B. 1 and 3 are correct. The arteriola ellipsoidea in the splenic red pulp conducts blood from the pencillar arteriole to the terminal capillary vessel. A sheath of concentrically arranged cells, possibly derived from reticulocytes, surrounds the arteriole, which occurs only rarely in humans. The vessel in a splenic lymphonodule is the arteria lymphonoduli, derived from the artery of the white pulp. This was called the central artery, but because it almost never occurs in the center of a lymphonodule, the name was changed to *artery of the lymphonodule.*

13 The Branchial Region

I. The branchial region is outlined prior to the major systems of the body because references will be made to development of this region in subsequent chapters. The reader should review this outline not only during anatomical courses, but also in subsequent courses.

II. The adult musculomembranous **pharynx** extends for 12.5 cm from the inferior surface of the skull to the sixth cervical vertebra.

    A. The **pharynx** is

        1. *widest* at the inferior surface of the skull,

        2. *narrowest* at the esophageal junction.

    B. Seven openings communicate with its cavity:

        1. *two* from the nasal cavity,

        2. *one* from the mouth,

        3. *one* from the esophagus,

        4. *one* from the larynx,

        5. *two* from the tympanic cavities.

    C. The **pharynx** receives

        1. *air* filtered through the nasal cavity and conducts it to the *larynx* and to the lungs.

        2. *solids* and *liquids*, prepared in the oral cavity, and conducts them to the esophagus.

    D. *Development:* As the head of the embryo flexes and grows larger than the body, the pharynx follows suit. It has a wide cephalic end opening from the oral cavity and a narrow caudal end leading into the enteron (foregut). The pharynx is a flattened, flexed triangular tube with developing bilateral sacs (Fig. 13-1).

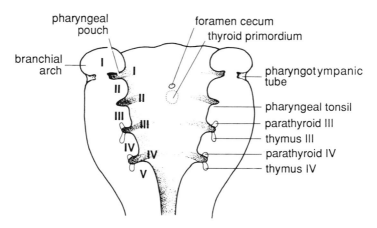

Figure 13-1 The embryonic pharynx.

1. The pharynx serves as the developmental site of important organs that detach and migrate to nearby areas.

2. In the embryo

a. *mesoderm* occupies the interval between the *endoderm* lining the pharynx and the *ectoderm* covering its exterior,

b. *ectodermal* invaginations, the *branchial sulci* (grooves), penetrate the mesoderm and move toward simultaneously developing *pharyngeal sacs.*

(1) In fishes and some amphibians, the *pharyngeal sacs* and *bronchial sulci* meet, fuse, and perforate to become *gill slits* (most obvious in sharks).

(2) In humans, perforations may develop as embryological anomalies called *fistulae.*

c. corresponding *endodermal* evaginations, the *pharyngeal sacs*, invade the mesoderm and migrate toward the invaginating *branchial sulci.* The *first branchial sulcus* gives origin to the concha of the ear and external acoustic meatus. No traces of the second, third, and fourth branchial sulci persist.

(1) The first sac to develop, closest to the oral cavity is *pharyngeal sac I.*

(2) In rapid succession, other pharyngeal sacs develop until by the end of the first month of development, *pharyngeal sac IV*, located more caudally, completes the sacculations.

(3) The rudimentary *pharyngeal sac V* is associated with *pharyngeal sac IV*.

E. Below are listed some of the important derivatives of

1. *pharyngeal sac I*
   a. *auditory tube,*
   b. *tympanic cavity* of the middle ear.

2. *pharyngeal sac II*: forms the sinus tonsillaris where the *palatine tonsils* develop.

3. *pharyngeal sac III*
   a. ventral part: major portion of the **thymus,**
   b. dorsal part: *inferior parathyroids.*

4. *pharyngeal sac IV*
   a. ventral part: a small portion of the **thymus,**
   b. dorsal part: *superior parathyroids.*

5. *pharyngeal sac V*
   a. *Ultimobranchial (UB) bodies* become incorporated and converted into thyroid tissue or degenerate. Some experimental data indicate that these bodies may become cystic and lead to pathology.
   b. Though their function is poorly understood, some evidence implicates these bodies as the source of *parafollicular endocrine cells,* which produce the hormone calcitonin (lowers blood calcium levels). Transplantation experiments indicate that *neural crest cells* migrate to the *UB* bodies to differentiate into parafollicular endocrine cells. From this site, they are incorporated into the developing thyroid gland (Taylor, 1968).

III. The *branchial arches*

A. *Mesoderm* confined between the *pharyngeal sacs* and the *branchial sulci* forms cores of cartilage or bone around the *aortic arches* (arteries) that loop through the arches of mesodermal tissue. These are the *branchial arches,* of which six appear but only four are visible externally. The fifth and sixth arches are somewhat rudimentary, less defined, and visualized only on the internal surface of the developing pharynx. Below are listed some of the more important derivatives of these arches.

1. *Branchial arch I* (mandibular arch): appears at the 14-somite stage as right and left arms of the **pars ventralis** of the *first branchial cartilage* (Meckel's cartilage). This arch is associated with the development of the face. Since the nerve of the first arch is the *mandibular*

division of the trigeminal nerve, all derivatives retain innervation from this source.

    a. *bone*
- **(1)** mandible,
- **(2)** incus,
- **(3)** malleus,
- **(4)** maxillary process.

    b. *muscles*
- **(1)** of mastication,
- **(2)** mylohyoid,
- **(3)** anterior belly of the digastric,
- **(4)** tensors tympani and palati.

    c. *tongue*: anterior part.

    d. *ligament*: sphenomandibular.

    e. *lip*: lower, and lateral part of upper lip.

2. *Branchial arch II* (hyoid arch): assists in forming the lateral and anterior (front) sides of the neck. The nerve of this second arch, cranial VII (facial nerve), innervates all its derivatives.

    a. *bone*
- **(1)** stapes bone of the middle ear,
- **(2)** styloid process,
- **(3)** hyoid bone, the lesser horn.

    b. *ligament*: stylohyoid

    c. *muscles*
- **(1)** of expression,
- **(2)** stapedius,
- **(3)** stylohyoid,
- **(4)** digastric, posterior belly.

3. *Branchial arch III:* Cranial nerve IX or glossopharyngeal nerve innervates the third branchial arch and its derivatives.

    a. *bone*
- **(1)** hyoid, greater horn,
- **(2)** hyoid, body.

    b. *muscles*
- **(1)** pharynx, upper musculature,
- **(2)** stylopharyngeus.

    c. *tongue*: posterior part.

4. *Branchial arch IV:* The recurrent laryngeal branches of cranial nerve X or vagus nerve innervates arches IV, V, and VI.

    a. *cartilage*: thyroid cartilage, part of,

    b. *muscles*: pharynx, lower musculature.

5. *Branchial arch V and VI*
  a. *cartilage*
    (1) thyroid cartilage, remainder of,
    (2) laryngeal cartilages
      (a) arytenoid,
      (b) corniculate,
      (c) cuneiform,
      (d) cricoid.
  b. *muscles*: of the larynx

IV. Other important derivatives

  A. *Tongue*: develops partly from the floor of the oral cavity and partly from the floor of the pharynx. The tongue will be considered in the chapter on the digestive system.

  B. *Thyroid gland:* develops from the floor of the pharynx. The thyroid will be considered in the chapter on endocrine organs.

Questions

DIRECTIONS: Each group of questions below consists of five lettered headings followed by a list of numbered words of statements. For each numbered word or statement, select the one lettered heading or lettered component that is most closely associated with it.
    A if only *1, 2, and 3* are correct
    B if only *1 and 3* are correct
    C if only *2 and 4* are correct
    D if only *4* is correct
    E if *all* are correct

Questions 1–5
A. Pharyngeal sac I
B. Pharyngeal sac II
C. Pharyngeal sac III
D. Pharyngeal sac IV
E. Pharyngeal sac V

  1. Palatine tonsil
  2. Major portion of the thymus
  3. Inferior parathyroid gland
  4. Ultimobranchial body
  5. Auditory tube

		Directions Summarized		
A	**B**	**C**	**D**	**E**
1,2,3	1,3	2,4	4	All are
only	only	only	only	correct

Questions 6–10
A. Branchial arch I
B. Branchial arch II
C. Branchial arch III
D. Branchial arch IV
E. Branchial arch V

6. Mandible
7. Muscles of expression
8. Stapes bone of the middle ear
9. Muscles of mastication
10. Muscles of the larynx

Explanatory Answers

1. B. The pharyngeal sac II gives rise to the palatine tonsil.

2. C. The pharyngeal sac III gives rise to the major portion of the thymus *and* the inferior parathyroid gland. (Since these are bilateral sacs, there are two inferior parathyroids developed, as there are two arms to the thymus.)

3. C. See question 2.

4. E. If indeed a fifth pharyngeal sac develops, it will be resorbed into the fourth. Strong evidence supports the ultimobranchial body as a derivative of this sac.

5. A. The auditory tube, opening into the pharynx via the pharyngeal ostium, is derived from pharyngeal sac I. The auditory tube opens into the cavity of the middle ear.

6. A. The mandible and all bony derivatives (incus, malleus, and the maxillary process) from branchial (mandibular) arch I are innervated by the mandibular division of cranial nerve V (trigeminal).

7. B. The facial muscles of expression (too numerous to list here) derive from branchial (hyoid) arch I, and as such are innervated by cranial nerve VII (facial).

8. B. The stapes (shaped like a stirrup) bone of the middle ear develops from branchial arch II. Attention is directed to this tiny bone since it is important in surgical restoration of some hearing problems. This bone is innervated by cranial nerve VII (facial).

9. A. The muscles of mastication (the temporalis, masseter, medial pterygoid [mandibular sling], and lateral pterygoid), which move the mandible during chewing and speech, are innervated by the nerve of branchial arch I, the mandibular division of cranial nerve V (trigeminal).

10. E. The laryngeal musculature derives from the lower arches, primarily branchial arch V (since VI is more rudimentary). Like branchial arch IV, this area is innervated by recurrent laryngeal nerve branches of cranial nerve X (vagus).

14 The Endocrine System

I. *Introduction to the Endocrine Glands*

 A. The *endocrine system* is comprised of widely separate, seemingly unrelated glands, which differentiate from epithelial cells derived from any one of the three primary germ layers.

 1. In contrast to exocrine glands, which secrete products onto related epithelial surfaces via ducts, endocrine secrtions (*hormones*) are transported to nearby or distant sites of activity via the blood vascular system. They are frequently called "ductless glands," or glands of "internal secretion."

 2. The specialized, chemically complex *hormones* are cellular products of highly vascularized glands that exert discernible influences on *targets* as diverse as specific
  a. cells,
  b. tissues,
  c. organs,
  d. the body as a whole.

 3. Patterns of secretion affect the microscopic ultrastructure of the parenchymal gland cells. *Hormones* may be secreted
  a. as rapidly as they are formed in some glands,
  b. when necessary in others, or
  c. stored until required.

 B. The *endocrine glands* complement the nervous system in integrating total behavioral patterns of the body.

 1. Nerve impulses account for the rapid motor responses, which may be either coarse or extremely precise.

 2. The endocrine glands coordinate sustained intricate responses of their targets after a latent period associated with the delivery time of hormones via the bloodstream.

C. *Endocrine* glands may be subject to control by

1. the nervous system,

2. other endocrine glands,

3. both.

D. The cooperative activity of *hormones* is responsible for the maintenance of cells, tissues, or organs. In general, the endocrine glands secrete substanes that influence reproduction, growth, development, and general maintenance of the individual.

II. *The suprarenal glands* (adrenal) [Nomenclature: ad-renal means "toward the kidney." *Suprarenal*, meaning "on top of the kidney," is the correct internationally accepted term used in this text.]

A. *Introduction*: The human suprarenal glands, capping the cranial poles of the kidneys, are roughly triangular flattened glands

1. each weighing 5 g and measuring approximately
a. 5 cm in the lateral dimension,
b. 3 cm in the anteroposterior plane,
c. 1 cm in thickness.

2. with a yellow cortex (attributed to the high content of lipid droplets in the parenchymal cells of the cortex) and a reddish brown medulla (attributed to the numerous vascular plexuses).

B. *Development*: The suprarenal glands are composed of two distinct endocrine glands of different developmental origin. In higher vertebrates, *mesodermal* and *ectodermal* derivatives proliferate cells that form two intimately related glands, the **cortex** and the **medulla**, respectively (Gardner, 1975).

1. The **cortex** (Johannison, 1968) develops from the *mesothelium* of the abdominal peritoneal lining, adjacent to the root of the mesentery.

a. In 9-mm embryos, the mesothelium thickens into columnar epithelial cells that undergo mitoses. Cell division produces two cells: one that remains behind as part of the mesothelium to generate other cells and another that migrates retroperitoneally into the mesenchyme lateral to the mesenteric root to differentiate as a stem cell for suprarenal cortical cells.

b. Continued proliferation forms a mass of large differentiating spherical acidophilic cells, the *fetal cortex*. The relatively large fetal suprarenal gland (equal in size to the kidney in an 8-week fetus) is accounted for by the *fetal cortex*, which slowly regresses and completely involutes after birth.

c. In 12-mm embryos, the *fetal cortex* is capped by a further proliferation of smaller, less acidophilic cells, similarly derived from peritoneal mesothelium. These smaller cells constitute the *definitive cortex*, which is organized by midterm into two recognizable regions in juxtaposition to the fetal cortex:

(1) an outer **zona glomerulosa**,

(2) an inner **zona fasciculata**.

d. At term (birth) a third zone, the **zona reticularis** develops between the **zona fasciculata** and the involuting fetal cortex.

2. The **medulla**, wrapped by the cortex, makes up only 10% of the suprarenal gland.

a. The **medulla** develops from neuroectodermal *chromaffin cells* migrating from the anlage (mass of primitive cells) of the sympathetic ganglia lateral to the primitive neural tube.

b. It stains *red-brown* following treatment of the *chromaffin cells* with chromic acid or its salts. This chemical reation is attributed to the catecholamines *epinephrine* and *norepinephrine* within these cells. Electron microscopic studies distinguish two cell types, the *clear* and *dense endocrine cells*.

3. The association of **cortex** and **medulla** forms a dual gland of the following sizes related to the kidney:

a. at *birth*: one third the size,

b. *adult*: one thirtieth the size.

C. *Structure* of the suprarenal gland

1. The **cortex** (Neville and O'Hare, 1982), with its *lipid-loaded parenchymal cells*,

a. is protected by a connective tissue *capsule* consisting of

(1) a *thick* **lamina fibrosa** on the inner surface contacting the kidney and

(2) a *loose* **lamina fibrosa** on the outer surface, blending with the surrounding connective tissue. Blood vessels, nerves, and lymphatics snake through this looser capsular lamina. Finer collagenous and reticular fibers from this layer penetrate the three reegions of the cortex and the medulla to form the stroma and provide pathways for blood vessels to follow.

b. *Light microscopy* reveals three definitive zones:

(1) an outer **zona glomerulosa**, under the *capsule*, is so named because the *cortical endocrine cells* are arranged into balls of large and small *columnar cells* (glomerulus: Latin for "a ball of thread"). The **zona glomerulosa** constitutes *15% of the cortex.*

(a) *Capillaries* following the penetrating connective tissue fibers from the capsule invade the center of the balls of cells and form plexuses around their periphery, contacting every *cortical endocrine gland cell* on at least two surfaces.

(b) The *basement membranes* of the *cortical endocrine gland cells* are fused with those of the typical *capillary* endothelium. Thus, *hormone* products to be delivered to the lumen of the capillaries must pass through the following six barriers:

[1] cell membrane of the gland cell,

[2] lamina lucida of the bland cell,

[3] lamina densa of the gland cell, *fused to the*

[4] lamina densa of the capillary,

[5] lamina lucida of the capillary,

[6] endothelial wall.

(2) a middle **zona fasciculata**, continuous with the **zona glomerulosa** *endocrine gland cells*, can be compard to "balls of thread" unwinding to send long, parallel, wavy "fascicles" of cells cascading toward the medulla. The **zona fasciculata** constitutes the largest portion (*78%*) *of the cortex.*

(a) Each *fascicle* of the *cortical endocrine gland cells* is surrounded by *sinusoidal capillary vessels*, which descend from the zona glomerulosa.

[1] Thin fused basement membranes form between the *endothelial cells* and *cortical endocrine gland cells*. The basement membrane surrounding the endothelium is continuous.

[2] Like other *sinusoidal capillaries*, they sequester relatively large quantities of blood under lower pressures. Thus, blood is retained longer, to permit the *endocrine gland cells* a greater opportunity to secrete products into the bloodstream and to extract nutritional substances.

(b) Small *interstital cells* migrating in the perivascular space between the sinusoidal endothelium and the endocrine gland cells may

[1] become actively phagocytic, to engulf and destroy bacteria or foreign substances.

[2] produce reticular fibers to form a gossamer network around the *cortical endocrine cell* columns.

(c) *Microvilli* of the *endocrine cells* protuding into the perivascular space provide greater surface area.

(d) Processing tissues preparatory to histological staining extracts lipid droplets from the polyhedral cells and imparts a more distinctive foamy appearance to the **zona fasciculata** than the zona glomerulosa.

(3) an inner **zona reticularis** consisting of more closely packed gland cells continuous with the fasciculi of the zona fasiculata. The **zona reticularis** constitutes the smallest portion (*7%*) *of the cortex.* Compare the fasciculata vs the reticularis:

    (a) The **zona fasciculata** has relatively large polyhedral cells aligned in columns, surrounded by straight sinusoidal capillaries.

    (b) The **zona reticularis** has cell cords arranged in a network (hence the name *reti*cularis) surrounded by a network of larger sinusoids.

    c. *Ultrastructure* (electron microscopy) resembles that of other steroid-secreting cells such as the endocrine cells of the ovary and endocrine cells of the testes (Mota, 1984).

    (1) Mitochondria in the

    (a) zona glomerulosa are round to oval and occasionally elongated, with lamellated cristae.

    (b) zona fasciculata are characterized by the vesicular cristae common to steroid-secreting cells.

    (c) zona reticularis have both the lamellated and vescicular cristae.

    (2) Cytoplasmic *lipid droplets* serve as storage depots for *cholesterol,* which is the precursor of *steroid hormones.* The lipid droplets in the

    (a) zona glomerulosa are small in size and number.

    (b) zona fasciculata are larger and more numerous.

    (c) zona reticularis have the least amount of lipid droplets. Instead, *lipofuscin pigment granules* occupy considerable space. Their increase in number with age is the reason they are called the "wear and tear pigment" and "aging pigment."

    (3) The *endoplasmic reticulum* is tubular.

    (a) Any one section through a cell shows crowded circular profiles of tubular smooth endoplasmic reticulum.

    (b) Occasionally, a confined juxtanuclear array of parallel *rER* membranes are encountered.

    (4) *Polyribosomes* lie free in the cytoplasm, except for those associated with the ER.

    d. *Hormone synthesis* and secretory mechanisms are still poorly understood. Some 100 steroid hormones are synthesized from cholesterol, but only a few are released and active. The endocrine cells of the following zones have been implicated (by experimental evidence) as sites of synthesis:

    (1) Zona glomerulosa

(a) *mineralocorticoids* are the hormones participating in mineral metabolism.

(b) *aldosterone* is a hormone that promotes retention of sodium by kidney tubules.

(2) **Zona fasciculata**

(a) *glucocorticoids* are hormones that participate in metabolism of lipids, proteins, and carbohydrates:

[1] *cortisol*, the most important, also provides resistance to infections, resistance to stress (Axelrod and Reisine, 1984), and inhibits allergic reactions.

[2] *dehydroepiandrosterone* is also a weak androgen sex steroid hormone.

(3) **Zona reticularis** also produces *glucocorticoids*. This zone may be more active in producing androgens.

e. *Hormone production* and *maintenance* of suprarenal cortical morphology is governed by *adrenocorticotrophic hormone* (ACTH) secreted by the *corticotrop(h)ic endocrine cells* of **pars distalis** of the adenohypophysis.

(1) Failure of ACTH production results in atrophy and nonproductivity of the **zona fasciculata** and **zona reticularis**.

(2) The **zona glomerulosa** is affected only slightly by experimental removal of the **hypophysis cerebri**, for it continues producing aldosterone (Nickerson and Brownie, 1975).

f. The **cortex** is indispensable for life. Its loss or pathological destruction results in *Addison's disease* and ultimately death. Administration of exogenous cortical hormones will avoid death.

2. The **medulla** of the suprarenal gland (Carmichael, 1983), a separate endocrine component, is quite unnecessary for maintenance of life. In vertebrates lower than mammals (fishes), the medulla does not relate morphologically to the cortex.

a. Some cords of cortical endocrine cells may extend into the **medulla**, causing some problems in identification of the medulla. However, careful histological examination of the **medulla** and the **cortex** distinguishes the

(1) *acidophilia* of *cortical endocrine cells*,

(2) *basophilia* of *medullary endocrine cells*. Also, fixatives containing potassium dichromate produce the *chromaffin reaction*, imparting a brownish color to the cytoplasm.

b. Two *medullary endocrine cell* types, derived from neural crest ectoderm, are present:

(1) *clear endocrine cells* (epinephrine cells, adrenalin cells)

in the human are more numerous than the dense endocrine cells, and hence 10 times more epinephrine than norepinephrine is produced. Two chromaffin granular forms are recognized (Winkler and Westhead, 1980):

(a) electron-dense membrane-bound cytoplasmic granules, with no prominent space between the granule and the membrane.

(b) nongranular sER membranes are short and scattered, but on occasion stacks of rER are seen.

(c) prominent glycogen accumulations in the cytoplasm.

(2) *dense endocrine cells* (norepinephrine cells)

(a) extremely electron-dense granules about 100 to 300 nm in diameter and located eccentrically in dilated sacs (large space or halo between the membrane and the granule).

(b) nongranular sER membranes similar to clear endocrine cells.

c. The two cell types are arranged in small groups of cords separated by very wide flaccid *medullary venous plexuses*, which empty into the *central vein* of the medulla.

d. Scattered among the medullary endocrine cells are ganglia of autonomic *multipolar neurons* characterized by vesicular nuclei with single nucleoli. Postganglionic neuronal fibers emanate from these ganglia.

e. Careful examination reveals a large population of lymphocytes in the medulla, particularly in the loose connective tissue surrounding the venous plexuses.

f. Storage of preformed hormones in the suprarenal cortical endocrine cells is minimal, but in the **medulla** catecholamine hormones stored in high concentrations are

(1) *epinephrine*, forming 80% of catecholamines:

(a) increases cardiac rate,

(b) increases output of blood (per minute),

(c) increases *only* systolic blood pressure because arterioles in muscle become dilated (vascular congestion in muscle),

(d) dilates bronchi (causesd by relaxing muscles),

(e) stimulates glycogenolysis in the liver and subsequent release of glucose.

(2) *norepinephrine*, which may be considered to be an intermediary precursor to epinephrine, has

(a) little effect on heart rate,

(b) little effect on cardiac output, and

(c) functions as a neurotransmitter in certain CNS synapses.

g. The medulla appears to be under the control of the nervous system, although there is a suggestion that the sinusoids of the cortex passing into the medulla carry substances that may influence the secretory activity of the medulla.

D. *Blood supply of the suprarenal gland* (Hamaj and Harrison, 1984)

    1. The *arterial supply* is derived from three sources:

      a. *superior suprarenal artery*, from the inferior phrenic artery,

      b. *middle suprarenal artery*, from the aorta,

      c. *inferior suprarenal artery*, from the renal artery.

    2. Branches of these arteries ramify through the loose connective tissue of the capsule and then dip into the cortex and medulla along with accompanying connective tissue (Fig. 14-1).

      a. In the **zona glomerulosa**, arterioles become capillaries leading into the straight sinusoidal capillary vessels of the **zona fasciculata**. Glomerulosa sinusoids are characterized by small fenestrations up to 100 nm in diameter. Larger fenestrae up to 400 nm are found in the inner part of the zona fasciculata and zona glomerulosa (Ryan et al, 1975).

      b. The *sinusoidal capillaries* gradually diminish in size and ultimately exit via the following sequence:

        (1) *venous capillary plexuses* in the **medulla** also have large fenestrations to permit better exchange with the medullary parenchymal cells. Medullary capillary endothelium is typical.

        (2) large *central vein*,

        (3) *suprarenal vein* (exits via furrow, the *hilus*, on the anterior surface of each gland).

      c. Other arterial branches pass through the cortex directly to the venous plexuses of the medulla that empty into the venous system. The **medulla** therefore possesses a *dual blood supply*:

        (1) sinusoidal capillaries from the cortex,

        (2) arteries directly from the capsular artery.

III. *The* **paraganglia** (Mascarro and Yates, 1970)

    A. The **paraganglia** are groups of cells capable of reacting with chromic acid or its salts. These *paraganglion sympathetic glomerocytes* are scattered widely in close association with major blood vessels and organs such as the kidney, testes, ovaries, liver, and the heart.

    2. These *glomerocytes* resemble those of the suprarenal medulla and are *derived from neural crest cells* that failed to differentiate into neurons. Two types are recognized:

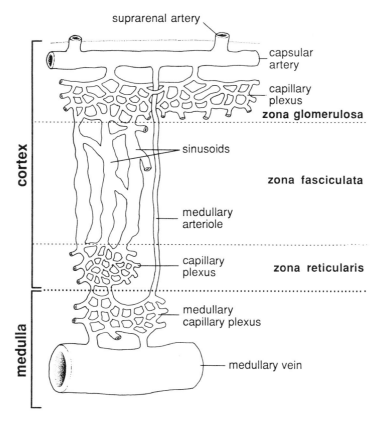

Figure 14-1 Blood supply of the suprarenal gland.

    a. *Granular endocrine cells,* similar to those of the suprarenal medulla, also respond to potassium dichromate with the chromaffin reaction.

    b. Epithelioidocytus sustentans (supporting epithelial cells)

  B. Generally, *paraganglionic sympathetic glomerocytes* reside in or near the autonomic ganglia. The most easily recognized cell clusters are the *lumbar aortic paraganglia* (formerly: the organs of Zuckerkandl) located at the junction of the inferior mesenteric artery with the aorta.

  C. Neuroectodermal cells of the neural crest, streaming toward the suprarenal medulla, may be delivered to nearby structures such as the testes, ovaries, and kidneys. In descent of these organs to their adult position, the *chromaffin cells* follow the course of the arteries that supply them and take up residence within these organs.

D. The paraganglia possess the **vas capillare sinusoideum** or sinusoidal capillary vessels similar to those of the pars distalis of the adenohypophysis and the zona fasciculata of the suprarenal gland.

E. The significance of these accessory structures is primarily clinical, for they become involved in the production of *chromaffin tumors*, the *pheochromocytomas*, similar to those of the suprarenal medulla. Tumors of this nature cause increased blood pressure and hypertension. The patient complains of severe headaches and appears pale and sweaty. Removal of the tumor removes the problems.

IV. *The* **hypophysis cerebri** (pituitary gland)

A. *Introduction*: Probably the single most important endocrine gland, the **hypophysis cerebri** is also one of the smallest organs in the human body.

1. *Size*: Its far-reaching generalized and specific effects do not seem to be those of a structure as small as a green pea and weighing about a half-gram.

2. *Location*: It occupies a small depression, the **sella turcica**, in the *sphenoid bone* and is roofed by a dense connective tissue membrane, the **diaphragma sella**.

3. *Connection*: A central aperture in the diaphragma sella offers a passageway to the infundibular stalk connecting the gland to the floor of the diencephalon (third ventricle of the brain).

B. *Development* (Fig. 14-2) (Moore, 1988)

1. Like the suprarenal gland, the hypophysis cerebri is derived from two embryonic sources:

    a. the *ectoderm* of the roof of the *stromatodeum* [stomodeum] forming the *hypophyseal sac* (Rathke's pouch),

    b. the *ectoderm* of the neural **hypothalamus**.

2. The embryonic *stomatodeum*, the primitive oral cavity, is sealed off from the pharynx by the *oropharyngeal membrane* (buccopharyngeal membrane).

    a. The anterior surface of this membrane is a continuation of the ectoderm of the stomatodeum.

    b. The posterior surface is endoderm of the pharynx.

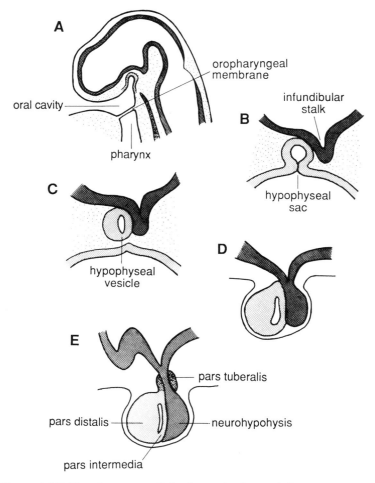

Figure 14-2 Development of the hypophysis cerebri.

3. Directly in front of the oropharyngeal membrane, on the roof of the stomatodeum (base of cranial cavity),

    a. the ectoderm pushes upward as if pushed by a finger, forming the *hypophyseal sac*, into the mesenchymal tissue plate separating the brain from the stomatodeum. (This mesenchyme gives rise to the bones and connective tissue of the cranial cavity floor.)

b. While the *hypophyseal sac* grows upward, another sac, the *infundibular stalk*, descends from the floor of the *hypothalamus* of the diencephalon (third ventricle) toward the same area.

4. As these two sacs approach one another, active mitotic growth of the surrounding *mesenchyme* produces waves of cells that concentrate around the base of the *hypophyseal sac* and gradually constrict it.

    a. As a result, the *hypophyseal sac* separates from the stomodeal ectoderm, yielding a cyst-like vesicle, the *hypophyseal vesicle*.

    b. The anterior wall of the *hypophyseal vesicle* increases in thickness by cellular proliferation.

    c. The posterior wall, only a few cells thick, is compressed against the *infundibular stalk*.

5. The *infundibular stalk*

    a. retains attachment with the floor of the **hypothalamus**, but

    b. its lumen is gradually obliterated by neuroectodermal cells and axons growing in from groups (nuclei) in the hypothalamus.

6. Thus the gland is formed. *Compare* the formed *fetal* hypophysis vs the *adult* hypophysis cerebri (Table 14-1).

7. The upper portion of the adenohypophysis, known as the **pars tuberalis**, sends out lateral extensions to embrace the neurohypophysis.

8. The entire gland is surrounded by a connective tissue *capsule* carrying branches of the major vessels. From this capsule, delicate connective tissue septae and blood vessels pervade the gland.

C. *Microscopy of the* **pars distalis** (Tixier-Vidal and Farquhar, 1975)

1. This portion of the adenohypophysis is channeled by thin-

Table 14-1 Comparison of the Fetal and Adult Hypophysis Cerebri

Fetal	Adult
Hypophyseal vesicle	Adenohypophysis (anterior lobe)
Thick anterior portion	Pars distalis and
	Pars tuberalis
Residual lumen	Potential lumen
Thin posterior portion	Pars intermedia
Posterior infundibular stalk	Neurohypophysis (posterior lobe)

walled sinusoidal vessels supported by delicate reticular fiber networks. Grossly, the vasculature imparts a striking redness to the gland.

2. The endocrine parenchymal cells (which developed from ectodermal epithelium of the stomatodeum) are forced into cord like arrangements that rest on the reticular fiber networks surrounding the sinusoidal capillary vessels.

3. *Association of cell types and hormones* (Fig. 14-3): The historical perspective must be understood in light of available technology. Basically, the existence of at least six (perhaps nine) hormones had to be reconciled with only three recognized cell types.

    a. With *hematoxylin* and *eosin* stains, *two groups* of cells are distinguished, one of which has two subtypes:

        (1) *chromophils*, those attracting stain
        (a) *acidophil endocrine cells*,
        (b) *basophil endocrine cells*.
        (2) *chromophobes*, which do not stain.

    b. With newer techniques (combining histochemistry, immunocytochemistry, and electron microscopy on normal and pathological tissues), the *chromophil* subtypes have been identified (Pelletier et al, 1978).

        (1) *Acidophilic endocrine cells*
        (a) *Somatotro(h)ic endocrine cells*
        [1] selectively stained with orange G.
        [2] Electron microscopy shows
        [a] electron-dense, membrane-bound granules, 300 to 350 nm in diameter.
        [b] golgi complex is relatively large, with immature, less electron-dense granules in formation.
        [c] profiles of rought ER.
        [d] mitochondria.
        [e] granules are expelled at the plasmalemma surface by exocytosis.
        [3] Hormone produced = *somatotrop(h)in (STH)*. *Human growth hormone (HGH)* stimulates the epiphyseal plate in growing long bones.
        [a] *Hypofunction* (underproduction) of this hormone prior to closure of the epiphyseal plate leads to *dwarfism*.
        [b] *Hyperfunction* (overproduction) prior to closure of the epiphyseal plate leads to *gigantism*.
        [c] *Hyperfunction* after closure of the epiphyseal plate results in excessive deposition of bone substance of mature bones, a condition known as *acromegaly*.

251

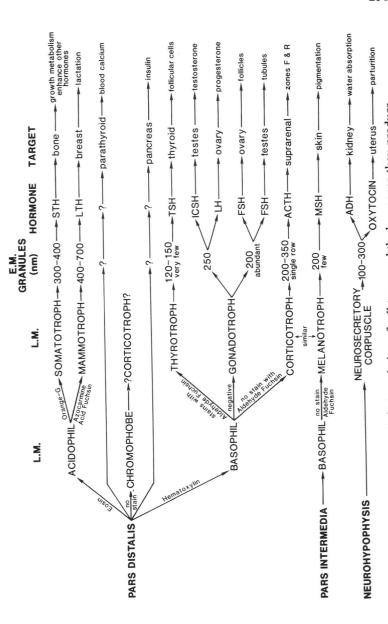

Figure 14-3 The hypophysis cerebri. Association of cell types and the hormones they produce.

[4] *Somatotrop(h)in* also regulates protein, lipid, and carbohydrate metabolism

[5] The action of other hormones is enhanced by *somatotrop(h)in.*

(b) *Mammotrop(h)ic endocrine cells* are the second type of acidophil endocrine cells selectively stained with azocarmine, erythrosin, or acid fuchsin.

[1] Secretory membrane-bound *granules* are larger (600 to 900 nm) and vary in shape.

[2] The large *golgi complex* contains smaller, smooth-surfaced membranes packaging dense secretory immature granules.

[3] The endoplasmic reticulum of flattened, rough-surfaced membranes fills a large portion of the cytoplasm.

[4] The mammotrop(h)s produce the hormone *mammatrop(h)in* (other names in the literature: prolactin, lactogenic hormone [*LTH*]), which stimulate lactation in the breast.

(2) *Basophilic endocrine cells* are subdivided into three subtypes by stains:

(a) *Thyrotrop(h)ic endocrine cells*, stained specifically by aldehyde fuchsin, are the smallest endocrine cells in the pars distalis and often appear somewhat elongated (Phifer and Spicer, 1973).

[1] Membrane-bound *granules*, measuring only 120 to 150 nm, line up in a single row under the plasmalemma.

[2] The hormone produced is *thyroid-stimulating hormone (TSH)* or *thyrotrop(h)in*, which stimulates secretory activity of the thyroid follicular cells.

(b) *Gonadotrop(h)ic endocrine cells* are distinguished by electron microscopy into two types on the basis of their *granule size*:

[1] *Granules 250 nm in diameter* are rather uniform in size and tend to polarize to one side of the cell. Mitochondria and free ribosomes are scattered evenly between sparse flattened rER membranes.

[a] In the *female* these cells produce *luteinizing hormone*, which stimulates conversion of the ruptured ovarian follicle (after explusion of the egg) into a **corpus luteum**, which produces *progesterone.*

[b] In the *male* these cells secrete *interstitial cell-stimulating hormone (ICSH)*, which stimulates the testicular interstitial endocrine cells to produce the male sex hormone *testosterone.*

[2] *Granules 200 nm in diameter* are abundant in the cytoplasm. Irregularly dilated cisternae of rER contain medium electron-dense material.

[a] In the *female* these cells produce *follicle-stimulating hormone* (*FSH*), which stimulates *growth of ovarian follicles*.

[b] In the *male*, this *FSH* stimulates the seminiferous epithelium to *produce* **spermatozoa**.

(c) *Corticotrop(h)ic endocrine cells* are large basophilic cells responsible for producing the *adrenocorticotrop(h)ic hormone* (*ACTH*), which stimulates the zona fasciculata and zona reticularis to produce glucocorticoids. These cells are readily distinguished in electron micrographs by the following criteria (Phifer et al, 1970):

[1] a few scattered membrane-bound *granules* about 200 nm in diameter,

[2] an eccentric indented nucleus,

[3] rER membranes isolated among smooth surfaced vesicles,

[4] an extensive golgi complex occupying a large portion of the cell.

(3) *Chromophobic endocrine cells*, claimed to be a reserve or degranulated *chromophil endocrine cell*, are easily distinguished from *chromophilic endocrine cells* because they

(a) do not contain a significant population of granules,

(b) do not stain with any of the differential stains,

(c) do not secrete a hormone, although some investigators now report that *ACTH* is produced and secreted.

D. The **pars tuberalis**, the small superior portion of the pars distalis embracing the **infundibulum**, is separated from it only by a thin connective tissue layer.

1. The extensive vascular supply (to be described) is concentrated in the pars tuberalis, making it the most vascularized region of the hypophysis.

2. The parenchyma consists of a few

a. acidophil endocrine cells,

b. basophil endocrine cells, and some

c. cells that are difficult to classify either as chromophobes or chromophils. They appear to be stem cells for the chromophils and hence are designated *undifferentiated adenocytes*.

3. Other cell types, squamous in nature, form *islands of squamous epithelium*. No function has been attributed to these cells. They may be *epithelial rests* derived from the embryonic *stomatodeal epithelium*.

E. The **pars intermedia**, the thinnest portion of the pars distalis, is compressed against the neurohypophysis (infundibulum) (Stoeckel et al, 1981).

1. A space present in the embryo, between the thick pars distalis and the thin pars intermedia

    a. is recognizable in the young.

    b. With increasing age, the cleft decreases and may appear as a discontinuous series of vesicles or cysts filled with an acidophilic colloidal substance. These colloid-filled cysts may be confused with thyroid follicles, possibly the prostrate and perhaps even the active mammary gland.

2. The parenchymal cells of the **pars intermedia** are the *basophilic melanotrop(h)ic endocrine cells*. The cytoplasmic granules are the source of *melanocyte-stimulating hormone (MSH)*, which initiates the production of melanin responsible for darkening of skin (Lerner and McGuire, 1961; Hadley et al, 1981).

    a. These cells possess a faintly basophilic cytoplasm and an eccentric nucleus, *resembling* the *corticotrop(h)ic endocrine cells*.

    b. Via TEM, it is possible to differentiate the corticotrop(h)s from melanotrophs as follows:

        (1) melanotrophs are polygonal and smaller,

        (2) the nucleus of the melanothroph is smooth, whereas that of the corticotroph is much indented,

        (3) the granules are very similar and impart the cytoplasmic basophilia. The granules measure between 200 and 300 nm.

F. The **neurohypophysis** (posterior lobe of the hypophysis)

1. The neurohypophysis is derived from the floor of the hypothalamus of the brain. The important elements of this neural structure are considered.

    a. The **gliocytus centralis** (pituicytes). Under the electron microscope, the relationship of *axon fibers* (of the neurosecretory cells below) to the *gliocytes* is quite intimate.

        (1) The *gliocyte* plasmalemma is indented in several areas from the partially embedded axons which ar supported and protected.

        (2) Cellular organelles and extracellular matrix are not remarkable. The ER is sparse and the indented nucleus has uniformly dispersed chromatin.

        (3) The gliocyte does not secrete a hormone, but provides support similar to the neuroglia of the CNS.

    b. The *hypothalamohypophysial tract* is an axon fiber tract originating from cell bodies in the lateral walls of the hypothalamus. These are *neurosecretory cells*, responsible for producing the hormones stored in the axon terminals in the infundibulum (Scharrer, 1969).

(1) The *axons* of the *neurosecretory cells* originate from cell bodies located in *nuclei* (groups of cell bodies) in the lateral walls of the hypothalamus.

c. The *supraoptic nucleus*, located over the *optic chiasma*, provides axons of the *supraopticohypophyseal tract.*

d. The *paraventricular nuclei* (in the medial portion of the hypothalamic walls) provide axons of the *paraventriculohypophyseal tract.*

e. Other minor tracts contribute to the mass of axon fibers terminating in the **neurohypophysis.**

2. Occasional swellings along the axon fiber tracts are resolved by the TEM. Extremely large swellings were called Herring bodies, but the new nomenclature emphasizes their primary function:

a. The name is *stored neurosecretory corpuscles* with *accumulations* of *neurosecretory substance.*

b. These corpuscles contain granules of varying electron density which are said to contain the hormones *oxytocin* and *vasopressin.*

3. Elegant studies have demonstrated that these granules migrate within the axon to be stored in their localized swellings in the neurohypophysis.

4. In addition to electron-dense granules, TEM reveals large clear vesicles that are interpreted as

a. *synaptic vesicles* (of nerve fibers) containing acetylcholine for nerve transmission,

b. *residual vesicles* from which hormones were extracted.

5. *Hormones of the neurohypophysis*

a. *Oxytocin* is a hormone manufactured in the cells of the hypothalamic nuclei and stored in the axon-forming tracts in the neurohypophysis. Two essential functions are attributed to this hormone (Dierickx and Vandesande, 1977):

(1) Contraction of uterine nonstriated (smooth) myocytes during coitus and parturition.

(2) Contraction of *myoepithelial cells*, which clasp the terminal ends (alveoli) of the mammary glands, resulting in ejection of milk, in response to tactile suckling by the infant.

(a) *Mammotrophin* (from the pars distalis) stimulates lactation.

(b) *Oxytocin* causes the ejection of milk.

(c) *Milk* is withdrawn by mechanical suckling.

b. *Vasopressin (antidiuretic hormone, ADH)* is manufactured by cells of the hypothalamic nuclei and stored in the neurosecretory corpuscles. The following functions have been reported (Bonner and Brownstein, 1984):

(1) Contraction of the nonstriated myocytes of the tunica media of small blood vessels, resulting in an increase of blood pressure.

(2) Conservation of water via the direct influence of *ADH* upon the cells of the distal convoluted tubules of the kidney. This results in the reabsorption of water.

(a) The disease *diabetes insipidus* results when nuclei of the hypothalamus are involved in tumor growth or injury.

(b) Failure to produce *ADH* causes excess loss of water by the kidney, and the patient is driven to drink large volumes of water.

(c) Sections of the neurohypophysis show little or no vesicles containing the electron-dense granules believed to be the source of ADH.

(d) Sections of the hypothalamic nuclei reveal hypertrophy of the cells and no neurosecretory granules.

G. *Vascular supply of the hypophysis* (Fig. 14-4)

1. The blood supply of the **hypophysis** introduces the *portal system* (Wislocki, 1938; Farquhar, 1961).

a. In most tissues of the body, the conventional pattern is sequential: artery – arteriole – capillary plexus – venule – vein.

Figure 14-4 Vascular supply of the hypophysis.

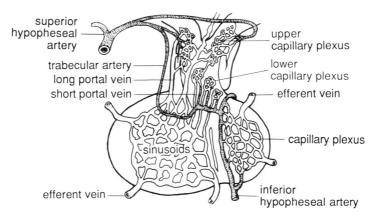

superior hypopheseal artery

trabecular artery
long portal vein
short portal vein

upper capillary plexus

lower capillary plexus

efferent vein

sinusoids

capillary plexus

efferent vein

inferior hypopheseal artery

b. In a *portal system*: artery – arteriole – capillary plexus – *portal veins – sinusoidal capillaries* – efferent veins.

2. The hypophysis is supplied by two sets of arteries:

a. two *superior hypophyseal arteries* (right and left)

(1) encircle and anastomose around the upper portion of the neurohypophyseal stalk,

(2) branch into short arterioles leading to *upper capillary plexuses* in the pars tuberalis and hypothalamic stalk,

(3) send trabecular artery branches down along the hypophyseal stalk which loop back to supply the *lower capillary plexuses* of the hypophyseal stalk.

(4) *Long portal veins* from the upper capillary plexuses descend into the pars distalis to feed the sinusoidal capillary plexuses. *Efferent veins* drain the sinusoids.

(5) *Short portal veins* drain the lower capillary plexuses and descend into the sinusoids of the pars distalis, drained by efferent veins.

(6) The *sinusoidal capillary network* retains blood in the vessels for relative long periods of time to permit

(a) transfer of *hormones* to the blood, and

(b) interchange of chemical information between the blood and endocrine cells of the pars distalis.

b. two *inferior hypophyseal arteries* (right and left) send branches to anastomose with the trabecular artery, and smaller branches to supply the

(1) *lower capillary plexus* of the hypophyseal stalk and

(2) *capillary plexus* of the **neurohypophysis**. This plexus is drained by its own efferent veins.

3. Barring massive vascular occlusions, the hypophysis is probably one of the best supplied organs in the body and is assured of an adequate blood supply via extensive collateral circulation.

IV. *The thyroid gland* (Werner and Ingbar, 1971)

A. Introduction: The *thyroid gland* (Greek: "like a shield"), weighing between 20 and 30 g, shields the lower anterior part of the neck and may be palpated as a soft mass at the anterior border of the sternocleidomastoid muscle.

1. A connective tissue capsule continuous with the pretracheal fascia assists in fixing the thyroid across the trachea and larynx.

2. Generally, two *lobes*, a right and a left, are united by a thin

band of glandular tissue, the *isthmus*, giving it an *H* or *U* shape. In rare conditions the *isthmus* is missing.

3. In about four out of ten cases, a *pyramidal lobe* extending upward from the *isthmus* represents residual tissue of the *thyroglossal duct* marking the midline developmental pathway.

B. *Development of the thyroid* (Shepard, 1975). The *thyroid gland*, the very first endocrine gland, appears at 24 days of gestation.

1. At a stage when the *stomatodeum* is separated from the primitive pharynx by the *oropharyngeal membrane*, a ventral sac grows downward from the floor of the pharynx into the underlying mesenchyme of the pharynx.

a. This is the *median thyroid diverticulum*, which develops at the level of the first pharyngeal pouch, where the tongue anlage originates. This site is marked in the adult tongue by a pit, the *foramen cecum*.

b. The *median thyroid diverticulum* elongates into the recognizable *thyroglossal duct* (the tube connecting the foramen cecum to the thyroid gland).

2. The advancing flash-like blind end bifurcates into two lobes and continues migration toward its permanent position in the neck.

3. Proliferation of endodermal cells within the duct results in a solid cord of cells that will atrophy and disappear after the sixth week of development. Should atrophy fail to occur, residual thyroid tissue (epithelial rests) cysts (Marshall and Becker, 1949) or even a patent duct might remain in the path of the descending gland.

4. Failure to commence migration results in thyroid tissue remaining in the tongue beneath the foramen cecum.

C. *Histology of the thyroid gland*

1. The most conspicuous feature of the thyroid is the appearance of about *three million* spheres of colloid-filled follicles varying in size from 50 to 900 μm. The *size* reflects the activity. Generally, bound hormone is stored in follicles surrounded by cuboidal epithelium.

a. When the follicles are *inactive*, they accumulate colloid (containing bound hormones of the thyroid) causing the epithelium to flatten.

(1) *Colloid* in the *inactive* state is a dense *gel*.

(2) *Dense* colloid usually stains intensely acidophilic.

(3) Fixation hardens the colloid to the point of brittleness. The microtome knife leaves repetitive "chatter marks" as it cuts through.

b. In smaller *active* follicles, in which hormone is being released,

(1) colloid is depleted,

(2) *active colloid* is a *semifluid* that loses its acidophilia,

(3) the epithelium increases in size to columnar,

(4) tissue fixation may create vacuoles at the periphery of the colloid, which becomes more pronounced during increased *activity.*

c. Follicles are separated from one another by loose connective tissue continuous with the *septae,* which separate the *lobes* into *lobules.* The septae proliferate fropm the capsule. A *capillary* plexus surrounds each follicle.

d. Sections through the upper and lower poles of each lateral lobe may include portions of the *parathyroid glands*

e. The *ultimobranchial bodies* may be incorporated into the thyroid.

(1) They appear as cysts enclosed by stratified squamous epithelium.

(2) The lumen contains desquamated cells, pyknotic nuclei, and other debris.

2. The *parenchymal cells of the thyroid* surrounding the colloid follicle are distinguished by a variety of techniques (histological, immunocytochemical, electron microscopy). They are *follicular endocrine cells, parafollicular endocrine cells,* and *colloid cells.*

a. *Follicular endocrine cells* produce the hormones *thyroxine* and *triiodothyronine.*

(1) *Cellular characteristics*

(a) They surround the colloid material and may vary from simple squamous to simple cuboidal to simple columnar epithelium, to reflect the state of activity of the follicle.

(b) The *apical ends* of the follicular cells are covered with microvilli that extend into the colloid, providing enormous surface area for absorption.

(c) The *basal surfaces,* anchored to the basement membrane, are fairly smooth and *not invaginated* at any point.

(d) A central oval *nucleus* is surrounded by *rER* distinguished by cisternae dilated with flocculent material.

(e) A rather large *golgi complex* of stacked, smooth-surfaced membranes occupies the side of the nucleus facing the colloid.

(f) Free *polyribosomes* and *mitochondria* are dispersed randomly throughout the cytoplasm.

(2) The *secretory process* (Taurog, 1978) introduces varia-

tions not encountered in other secretory cells. The sequences of secretion are controlled by *TSH* (*thyroid-stimulating hormone*) secreted in the adenohypophysis (pars distalis). *Follicular endocrine cells*

    (a) *produce* the hormone components,

    (b) *transfer* the components out of the cell bodies into the colloid (for storage),

    (c) *extract* the components from the colloid and process them for subsequent introduction into the circulation. (Fig. 14-5).

    (3) *Protein synthesis* occurs in the rER and most probably is formed continuously in homeostatic conditions, as evidenced by the dilated cisternae.

    (4) *Polysaccharide components* are produced in the *golgi complex*. *Protein* and *polysaccharides* are released together at the apical end of the cells for storage in the colloid.

    (5) The *follicular endocrine cells* also concentrate *iodine*, which is oxidized prior to iodination of *tyrosine* into the *mono-* and

Figure 14-5 The secretory process of thyroid follicular and parafollicular cells.

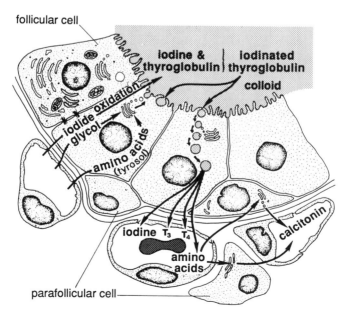

diiodotyrosine forms. Following coupling of these forms, they yield the principal *hormones*

(a) *thyroxine (T4)*

(b) *triiodothyronine (T3)*

(6) The hormones T3 and T4 are bound to a protein polysaccharide-thyroglobulin complex for subsequent storage as *colloid.*

(7) *Hormonal extraction from the colloid*

(a) Colloid droplets are returned to the cell at the base of the microvilli via *micropinocytosis* or *endocytosis* (Seljelid et al, 1970).

(b) Within the cell, the following events may occur:

[1] Captured colloid droplets fuse with electron-dense, membrane-bound granules formed in the golgi complex. These migrate through the cell to be released at the base, which is in contact with the basement membrane.

[2] Large colloid droplets, less dense than the electron-dense granules, may migrate unaltered all the way through the cell.

[3] Some dense membrane-bound granules may also migrate unaltered through the cell until released. It is suggested that the dense granules contain *acid phosphatase* which assists in the degradation of thyroglobulin for the release of the hormone.

(8) *Functional considerations*: The thyroid hormones control metabolic rate by controlling the metabolism of carbohydrates, lipids, and proteins affecting growth of the whole body.

(a) *Hypofunction* of the thyroid results in decreased hormone production.

[1] In the *infant*, the resulting fall in metabolic rates is reflected by *cretinism*, exemplified by inadequate physical and mental growth.

[2] In the *adult*, hypofunction results in the condition known as *myxedema*, in which the face is puffy and sallow. Cerebration and physical efforts are difficult.

(b) *Hyperfunction* leads to an increase in metabolic rate, a condition referred to as *exophthalmic goiter*. The patient presents with protruding eyes and an obvious enlargement of the thyroid gland in the neck. Biopsies show the *follicular endocrine cell* epithelium as tall cuboidal or columnar.

(c) The thyroid is functionally more *active* in *puberty*, during *pregnancy*, and under physiologic *stress*.

b. *Parafollicular endocrine cells*, associated with the thyroid follicular endocrine cells, are responsible for secreting the hormone *thyrocalcitonin* or, as frequently known, *calcitonin*. They have been referred to in the literature as *C-cells* (from calcitonin cells). *Thyrocal-*

citonin lowers serum calcium levels by suppressing bone resorption. The *parafollicular endocrine cells* (Fig. 14-5)

(1) *develop* in the *neural crest* and migrate to the *ultimobranchial body* or directly to the developing *thyroid* for maturation.

(2) are *located*

(a) within the follicular cell basement membrane, but do not reach the colloid substance in the lumen of the follicle.

(b) in greater numbers in the interfollicular loose connective tissue, either singly or in small groups. In this location they are more elongated.

(3) are *characterized* by

(a) a central oval *nucleus,*

(b) an extensive *golgi complex*, with small vesicles, apparently pinched off from the golgi complex gathered in the vicinity.

(c) a *granular* (rough) *ER*, interspersed with free polyribosomes.

(4) have electron-dense, membrane-bound *granules* (Ekholm and Erickson, 1968):

(a) 100 to 200 nm in diameter, in spaces between the sparse endoplasmic reticulum,

(b) often concentrated on the side facing the interfollicular space, when they are enclosed by the basement membrane,

(c) dispersed evenly in the cytoplasm, indicating that the granules may be secreted at any surface close to capillaries surrounding the parafollicular endocrine cells in the interfollicular spaces (Bussolati and Pearse, 1967).

c. *Colloid cells* found next to the follicular endocrine cells contain small droplets of colloid-like material. The current interpretation maintains that these cells are degenerating follicular cells. Formerly they were referred to as Langendorf cells.

D. *Vascular patterns in the thyroid gland* (Fujita and Murakami, 1974)

1. The *thyroid gland* receives blood via the superior and inferior thyroid arteries, which form an extensive *perifollicular capillary network* (plexus). The capillaries are surrounded by basement membranes in contact with the basement membranes of the follicular cells.

2. The *capillaries* drain into progressively larger veins, finally emptying into the superior, middle, and inferior thyroid veins.

E. *Lymphatic drainage in the thyroid gland* is very extensive. Surrounding each follicle is a *perifollicular lymphocapillary network* as extensive as the *perifollicular capillary network*.

1. Drainage of lymphatic fluid passes to a larger *perivascular plexus* and subsequently to a still larger *superficial lymphatic plexus*.

2. The larger lymphatic vessels pass to the deep cervical lymph nodes and to the pretracheal nodes prior to final drainage into the venous system.

V. The *parathyroid glands* are essential to life and to maintaining the serum calcium levels in the body (Roth, 1971).

A. *Introduction*

1. *Location*: The parathyroid glands are located

a. on the posterior surfaces of the superior and inferior poles of the right and left lobes of the thyroid gland (in 50% of the cases). They are usually enclosed by the thyroid gland capsule.

b. within the substance of the thyroid gland,

c. within the thymus,

d. within the tunica adventitia of the esophagus,

e. in a variety of places in the lateral neck, reflecting developmental epithelial "rests."

2. *Hormone produced*: *parathyroid hormone*, a protein that regulates calcium levels in blood serum.

3. The *parathyroid gland* has colorations throughout life reflecting the abundant vasculature (characteristic of endocrine glands in general) and an increasing content of adipocytes with advancing age. The fresh parathyroid appears

a. bright pink in young individuals,

b. red to red-brown in older patients,

c. yellow in aged individuals.

4. The *gross parathyroid gland* may be mistaken for a lymph node or a fat body. *Histological sections* may be confused with other tissues as well. If a particular tissue is confused with the parathyroid, then it is imperative that the tissues be studied side by side for specific characteristics.

B. *Development* of the *parathyroid glands*

1. The parathyroid glands are derived primarily from the pharyngeal endoderm of pouch III and from pouch IV.

a. A local thickening on the cranial aspect of pouch III appears opposite the caudal evagination of the developing thymus.

b. Descent of the thymus III drags the parathyroid to the inferior poles of the lateral thyroid lobes.

c. Thymus IV does not travel as far as pouch III and subsequently the parathyroid anlage on pouch IV settles on the superior poles of the lateral thyroid lobes.

2. It should not be surprising then, to encounter aberrant thymus tissue and parathyroid tissue embedded anywhere in the thyroid. Recall, thyroid tissue descends in the midline and spreads laterally, while the thymus and accompanying parathyroids descend laterally and encounter the thyroid. The descent patterns, especially of parathyroid III (pouch III), account for most of the aberrations.

C. *Microscopic structure* (Davis and Enders, 1961)

1. Stroma: A delicate connective tissue capsule surrounds the parathyroids in all locations. From the capsule, fine connective tissue septae subdivide the gland into vague lobules.

2. *Vasculature*: Blood vessels captured from any nearby vessel, together with nerves and lymphatics, accompany the connective tissue septae into the substance of the gland. A rich capillary plexus pervades the gland and drains into two networks of small veins at the periphery, one inside the capsule and one outside the capsule.

3. Parenchyma: Two cell types predominate: *principal endocrine cells* and *oxyphil endocrine cells.*

a. *Principal endocrine cells*, the most numerous, are characterized by their polygonal shape and central vesicular nuclei. Two subtypes have been distinguished: *clear* and *dense.*

(1) *Clear principal endocrine cells* outnumber the smaller dense cells. Electron micrographs reveal a small golgi complex, increased glycogen granule content, and practically *no* electron-dense secretory granules, suggesting inactivity.

(2) *Dense principal endocrine cells* possess fine membrane-bound granules that apparently are the same as the argyophilic granules of the principal cells revealed by the light microscopists. An *rER* and a large golgi complex indicate that this cell is functionally active (Munger and Roth, 1963).

b. *Oxyphil endocrine cells* usually appear between 5 to 10 years of age and increase in number throughout life. However, the exact function of these cells has not been established. In histology slide collections that do not have human, monkey, or cow parathyroids, the student will have difficulty locating these cells.

(1) The excessive content of **mitochondria** crowding out other cytoplasmic structures is responsible for the *granular appearance* and *acidophilia* of these cells under the microscope. The **cristae** of the mitochondria are closely packed.

(2) Free *polyribosomes* and *glycogen particles* may be found scattered between the mitochondria.

(3) The golgi complex, if present, is hidden, and the endoplasmic reticulum is negligible.

D. *Functional considerations*: The parathyroids are indispensable for life. Following their destruction, death can be avoided by the administration of calcium, animal parathyroid extract, and diet.

1. Parathyroid hormone produced by the *principal endocrine cells* regulates calcium ion levels in the body.

a. If calcium levels fall, *parathyroid hormone* stimulates the osteoclasts to commence resorption of bone.

b. Parathyroid hormone decreases the concentration of phosphatase ion in the blood.

(1) Cessation of activity by the parathryoids results in an increase in the concentration of phosphatase ion in the blood.

(2) Diagnosis is facilitated by proper understanding of phosphate levels in the blood.

2. *Hyperparathyroidism* (Roth, 1962) causes extensive bone resorption and possibly deposition of calcium in soft tissues, leading to their calcification.

3. *Hypoparathyroidism*, resulting in a decrease of blood calcium, is recognized by *tetany*, a disorder marked by intermittent tonic muscular contractions, tremors, and severe muscular pains.

E. *Aging*: The parathyroid reflects the following changes with advancing age:

1. invasion of connective tissue and adipocytes, similar to the changes observed in the involuting lymph nodes and thymus and remarkably similar to the increase of adipocytes in the aging parotid gland.

2. increase in the number of oxyphil cells after puberty and throughout life.

3. from the one-year infant and on, cords of parenchymal cells and some colloid material continue to increase with age.

VI. The **epiphysis cerebri** (pineal gland) (Wolstenholme and Knight, 1971)

A. *Introduction*: This derivative of the diencephalon is considered an endocrine organ which develops like the neurohypophysis. It grows as a flat outgrowth to a size averaging 7 mm long by 4 mm wide at the caudal end of the third ventricle, attached by a hollow stalk. Its location is useful as a major landmark of the brain in the diagnostic procedure employing computerized axial tomography.

    1. A *capsule* of loose connective tissue, **pia mater**, invests the organ and from it delicate trabeculae divide the parenchymal cells into vague lobules.

    2. Blood vessels and nerves enter via the capsule and the *trabeculae.*

    3. Postganglionic sympathetic nerve fibers originating from the superior cervical ganglion innervate the organ. This is *one of the rare parts of the CNS that receives a sympathetic supply.*

    4. Once described as a vestigial "third eye" of the evolutionary process, convincing new evidence attributes a significant role in regulating rhythmicity of the entire endocrine system.

    B. *Microscopic structure* (Ariens-Kappers and Schade, 1965): The cell responsible for elaborating the suspected hormone is the stellate-shaped, lightly basophilic *pineal endocrine cell.* Lateral swellings terminate in bulbous swellings.

    C. *Electron microscopy* (Arstila, 1967) reveals that some of these *pineal endocrine cells* are *clear* and some are *dense.* Perhaps these reflect stages in the synthesis process. The following appear:

    1. an extensive smooth-surfaced tubular ER with vesicular cisternae (resembling that of steroid-secreting cells),

    2. clumps of polyribosomes occur in the cytoplasm,

    3. a large golgi complex with many neighboring clear vesicles and some membrane-bound granules,

    4. microtubular filaments randomly dispersed throughout the cytoplasm. In the process, the microtubules are oriented parallel to the fiber axis.

    5. lipid droplets and lysosomes.

    D. The **stroma**: The structural cells comprising some of the stroma are *central gliocytes*, resembling the astrocytes of the CNS.

    1. They are more basophilic than the pineal endocrine cells, and like the astrocytes contain numerous cytoplasmic filaments.

    2. The stellate processes of the pineal endocrine cells embed into the walls of the central gliocytes, somewhat like the supportive cells of the CNS.

3. A helpful identifying characteristic is found in the pattern of chromatin distribution:

    a. *Central gliocytes* have a high concentration of heterochromatin.

    b. *Pineal endocrine cells* have less heterochromatin.

E. *Aging changes*: The gland reaches maximal development between 5 and 10 years of age.

    1. Usually at age 14, regression sets in.

    2. With increasing age, small mulberry-shaped concretions, the **corpora arenacea** accumulate (Latin: arena = sand, hence the common name brain sand). These occur not only in the substance of the gland but in the capsule. Computerized axial tomography depends on the density of the corpora arenacea to show the position of the cerebral epiphysis. Any deviation from its position would alert the diagnostic radiologist to seek greater detail.

F. *Functional considerations*

    1. Two substances secreted by the corpora arenacea have been identified:

    a. the hormone *melatonin* (Reiter, 1980), which causes blanching of the skin in lower animals (especially salamanders). In this respect *melatonin* may be the antagonist of *MSH* (from the adenohypophsis).

    b. the *HIOMT* (5-hydroxyindole-O-methyltransferase), an enzyme that mediates the synthesis of melatonin.

    2. Exposure to *light* (photons) (Wurtman, 1966) may influence the activity of the cerebral epiphysis by causing a decrease in the activity of *HIOMT*, which results in the failure of *melatonin* synthesis.

    3. *Melatonin* may have an inhibitory effect on the development and maturation of the gonads. *Pinealectomy* in animals causes early maturation and enlargement of the gonads.

    4. From the two reported findings (effect of light and effect of melatonin on gonadal development), it may postulated that *light* stimulates ovarian and testicular maturation by inhibiting production of *melatonin*.

    5. *Tumors* of the supportive *central gliocytes* crowd out the pineal endocrine cells with subsequent supression of *melatonin* production. In young boys with tumors of this type, precocious sexual growth occurs.

Questions

DIRECTIONS: Each group of questions below consists of five lettered headings with five lettered components, followed by a list of numbered words or statements. For each numbered word or statement, select the one lettered heading or lettered component that is most closely associated with it. Each lettered heading may be selected once, more than once, or not at all.

Questions 1–5 (cell types)
A. Central gliocytes [gliocytus centralis]
B. Parafollicular endocrine cells
C. Oxyphil endocrine cells
D. Chromophobe endocrine cells
E. Dense endocrine medullary cells

1. Suprarenal medulla
2. Neurohypophysis
3. Thyroid gland
4. Parathyroid
5. Cerebral epiphysis

Questions 6–10 (development)
A. Mesoderm
B. Stomatodeal ectoderm
C. Pharyngeal endoderm
D. Neural crest
E. Hypothalamic ectoderm

6. Parafollicular endocrine cells
7. Somatotrop(h)ic endocrine cells
8. Clear medullary endocrine cells
9. Cortical endocrine cells
10. Parathyroid endocrine cells

Questions 11–15 (cellular components)
A. Lipofuscin pigment granules
B. Corpora arenacea
C. 600 to 900 nm cytoplasmic granules
D. Mitochondria loaded cytoplasm
E. Microvilli extending into colloid

11. Mammotrop(h)ic endocrine cells
12. Oxyphil endocrine cells
13. Cerebral epiphysis
14. Follicular endocrine cells
15. Zona reticularis

Questions 16–20 (hormones)
A. Epinephrine
B. Melatonin
C. Mineralocorticoids
D. Thyrocalcitonin
E. Thyroid-stimulating hormone

16. Zona glomerulosa
17. Medullary clear endocrine cells
18. Basophilic endocrine cells (pars distalis)
19. Pineal endocrine cells
20. Parafollicular cells

Questions 21–25 (functions)
A. Provides resistance to infections and stress
B. Promotes retention of sodium by kidney tubules
C. Increases cardiac rate and output of blood
D. Stimulates the epiphyseal plate
E. Stimulates the seminiferous epithelium

21. Epinephrine
22. Somatotrop(h)in
23. Cortisol
24. Follicle-stimulating hormone
25. Aldosterone

Questions 26–30 (vasculature)
A. Sinusoidal capillary vessels
B. Venous capillary plexuses
C. Perifollicular capillary networks
D. Venous sinuses
E. Arterial venous anastomoses

26. Zona fasciculata
27. Suprarenal medulla
28. Pars distalis
29. Thyroid gland
30. Paraganglia

Questions 31–35 (aging)
A. Parathyroid
B. Thyroid
C. Cerebral epiphysis
D. Suprarenal
E. Hypophysis

31. Accumulation of corpora arenacea
32. Increase in oxyphil cells
33. Colloid vesicles or cysts appear
34. May retain attachment to foramen cecum
35. Reaches maximal development between 5 and 10 years of age

Explanatory Answers

1. E. The *suprarenal medulla* consists of two types of cells: clear (secrete epinephrine) and dense endocrine cells (secrete norepinephrine). Likewise, the *parathyroid* has two types of principal cells, light and dark. A third endocrine gland, the epiphysis, also has light and dark endocrine cells. Light (lucida) and dense (densus) refers to electron density.

2. A. Gliocytus centralis, or *central gliocytes*, are supporting cells. Glial cells are peculiar to the central nervous system and its derivatives, such as the **neurohypophysis** and the *cerebral epiphysis*.

3. B. The *parafollicular cells*, though derived from neural crest ectoderm and which probably mature in the ultimobranchial body, are found most commonly in the thyroid gland, either in the interfollicular connective tissue or enclosed within a follicle by the follicular basement membrane (though they never reach the colloid).

4. C. The *parathyroid* is distinguished by the presence of the acidophilic oxyphil cells. The acidophilia is attributed to the great numbers of mitochondria packing the cytoplasm.

5. A. Same answer as question 2. Central gliocytes are the supporting cells of the neurohypophysis and the cerebral epiphysis.

6. D. Parafollicular cells are neuroectodermal cells, derived from the neural crest.

7. B. The somatotrop(h)ic endocrine cells, which produce human growth hormone (HGH), are derived from the ectoderm of the stomatodeum. In fact, all parenchymal endocrine cells of the adenohypophysis (acidophilic endocrine cells, basophilic endocrine cells, and chromophobic endocrine cells) are derived from stomatodeal ectoderm.

8. D. Both the clear and dense endocrine cells of the suprarenal medulla are derived from neuroectoderm of the neural crest.

9. A. The cortical endocrine cells develop from mesodermally derived mesothelium of the abdominal peritoneal lining, adjacent to the root of the mesentery.

10. C. The principal parathyroid endocrine cells are derived from the endodermal lining of pharyngeal sacs III and IV. They migrate initially with their thymic partners.

11. C. The acidophilic and basophilic endocrine cells of the adenohypophysis all possess cytoplasmic granules. Those of the mammotrop(h)s are the largest (600–900 nm dark).

12. D. As noted above, the oxyphil endocrine cells, of which we really know little, are recognized by the presence of large quantities of mitochondria crowding all other cytoplasmic structures.

13. B. The cerebral epiphysis is characterized by the presence of sand granules, corpora arenacea, which increase with age. These are mulberry shaped and serve as an important landmark in CAT scans.

14. E. The thyroid follicular endocrine cells range from low cuboidal to columnar in shape. The apical surfaces facing the colloid lumen are studded with microvilli, which serve to increase the surface area. In contrast, the basal surface attached to the basement membrane is rather smooth.

15. A. The zona reticularis endocrine cells of the suprarenal cortex have the least amount of lipid in the cytoplasm. Instead, one finds lipofuscin pigment granules that accumulate with age.

16. C. The zona glomerulosa of the suprarenal cortex produces mineralocorticoids and aldosterone, while the zona fasciculata and the reticularis produce the glucocorticoids and some androgens.

17. A. The clear (lucida) endocrine cells of the suprarenal medulla are associated with the secretion of epinephrine, while the dense cells are associated with norepinephrine secretion.

18. E. The thyrotrop(h)ic endocrine cells of the adenohypophysis are classed as basophilic endocrine cells, and they secrete TSH or thyroid-stimulating hormone.

19. B. The pineal endocrine cells (lucida and densus) are associated with the secretion of melatonin, a hormone involved with skin pigmentation.

20. D. The parafollicular secrete the hormone thyrocalcitonin, which lowers serum calcium levels by suppressing bone resorption.

21. C. Epinephrine, in addition to increasing the cardiac rate and output of blood, dilates bronchi and stimulates liver glyconeogenesis.

22. D. Somatotrop(h)in acts directly on the epiphyseal plate of growing long bones, to promote growth in length.

23. A. Cortisol, as a glucocorticoid, participates in metabolism of lipids, proteins, and carbohydrates. As the most important glucocorticoid, cortisol provides resistance to infections, stress, and allergies.

24. E. Follicle-stimulating hormone in the female stimulates the ovarian follicles into development. However, in the male it stimulates the seminiferous epithelium to produce spermatozoa.

25. B. Aldosterone, a mineralocorticoid produced by the zona glomerulosa of the suprarenal cortex, promotes retention of sodium by kidney tubules.

26. A. Sinusoidal capillary vessels are found in the zona fasciculata of the suprarenal cortex, as well as the pars distalis of the adenohypophysis (28) and the paraganglia (30).

27. B. The suprarenal medulla is characterized by venous capillary plexuses that have large fenestrations to permit better interchange with the light and dark medullary endocrine cells.

28. A. See 26.

29. C. The follicles of the thyroid gland are encased in a perifollicular capillary network, not unlike a basketball hung up in a basketball net.

30. A. See 26.

31. C. With aging, the corpora arenacea increase in the cerebral epiphysis.

32. A. That oxyphil cells of the parathyroid increase with age is a mystery. One should ask why does a cell increase the major cellular structure associated with respiratory enzymes in an aging tissue? An answer has not come forth.

33. E. Although colloid vesicles may appear in any of the pharyngeal derivatives, because of their intimate developmental association, the developmental cleft between the pars distalis and the pars intermedia shows an increase in colloid vesicles or cysts with increasing age.

34. B. The thyroid gland develops from the floor of the pharynx at the junction of the anterior two thirds and posterior one third of the tongue. The site is marked by the foramen cecum. Usually the thyroglossal duct trailing behind the descending gland atrophies. However, it may remain attached to the foramen cecum and be attached to the thyroid by a patent thyroglossal duct. More serious is the situation in which the gland remains in the tongue.

35. C. The cerebral epiphysis reaches maximal development between the ages of 5 and 10. Usually at age 14 regression sets in, with the accumulation of corpora arenacea.

15 The Integument

I. *Introduction:* The *skin* (Montagna and Parakkal, 1974) encloses the tissues and organs of the body and acts not only as a protective shield, but at junctions with the various body apertures facilitates exchange between the external environment and the internal systems: digestive, respiratory, urinary, and reproductive. The *skin* also provides the following biological functions:

A. *Control:* The quantity of water that may *enter* (*absorption*) and *exit* (*excretion*) is controlled by a physiological barrier between the environment and the underlying structures it protects. Its control over water is significant in preventing osmotic injuries and maintaining fluid balance.

B. *Protection:* Dangerous *radiation*, such as ultraviolet light, penetrates skin only a short distance, and consequently the epidermal thickness provides remarkable protection. Ultraviolet light also acts on 7-dehydrocholesterol in the squamous epitheliocytes to form vitamin D. Protection is afforded against invasion by a variety of microorganisms.

C. *Selection:* While many physical and chemical agents are prevented from entering the body through the skin, certain chemical poisons and drugs are readily admitted.

D. *Thermal regulation:* Sweat glands and the unique vascular supply of skin serve admirably to regulate temperature.

E. *Sensory reception:* The variety of sensory receptors (cf chapter on nerve tissue) in the skin register pain, temperature, touch, pressure, and two-point discrimination. The value of skin in conveying emotional or pathological states via vascular reflexes and facial expressions is significant in clinical diagnoses.

1. Sensory information relayed to the brain stimulates appropriate motor responses.

274

2. In physical examinations, this information assists in diagnoses.

F. *Statistics:* Skin

1. comprises 16% of the total body weight,

2. presents a surface area of 1.5 m² to 2.0 m², which equals the filtration area of both kidneys.

3. epidermis about 0.1 mm in thickness is thin skin.

4. epidermis 1 mm thick (palms, soles) is thick skin.

II. *Composition of the skin* (Latin: *cutis*): The *skin* consists of three intimately related layers: an outer **epidermis**, a middle **dermis [corium]**, and a deep **tela subcutanea**. (*Tela* always specifies a connective tissue layer.)

A. The **epidermis** is a stratified squamous epithelium that is pliant, supple, resists ordinary wear and tear, and has a capacity for self-renewal every 28 days. The epidermal surface presents geometrical patterns composed of grooves and "friction" ridges on every part of the body. The sweat glands open onto the surface of the "friction" ridges. On fingertips, the ridges form fingerprints that differentiated during the 13th to 20th week of fetal life. Other than enlargement of the patterns, they remain identifiable throughout life.

1. *Development* (Moore, 1988)

a. In the early embryo, the external protective covering is a monolayer of simple cuboidal *ectoderm*, resting on a layer of *mesoderm*.

(1) *Ectoderm* gives rise to the **epidermis**.

(2) *Mesoderm* gives rise to the **dermis** and **tela subcutanea**. Interactions between ectoderm and mesoderm (and their derivatives) provide a proper milieu for growth and differentiation. In the adult, dermal–epidermal interactions are necessary for regeneration and repair (Billingham and Silvers, 1968).

b. During the fifth week of development (5-mm embryo), ectoderm multiplies (by mitosis) into two layers:

(1) an *external protective layer* and

(2) an *internal layer* that proliferates the strata recognized in the adult epidermis.

2. *Layers of the* **epidermis** are described below, starting at the basal layer and working out to the exterior (Montagna and Lobitz, 1964).

a. Stratum basale, or *basal layer*, in all areas of the body consists of a *single layer* of *columnar cells* resting on the dermis, with only a thin *basement membrane* intervening. Each *basal epithelial cell* retains the embryonic ability to undergo mitosis throughout life. From the time a cell is "born" until it reaches the surface as a keratinized dead cell, 28 days or one month elapses. Important structural features of these cells, as revealed by electron microscopy, are described below.

(1) The *basilar surfaces* of the basal epithelial cells project irregular folds, to

(a) *increase* the absorptive surface area facing the underlying capillary plexuses,

(b) *provide* more anchoring surface.

(2) *Hemidesmosomes* are small intracellular thickenings of the basal plasmalemma that anchor the basal cells to the basement membrane. (*Desmosomes* are localized thickenings of the plasmalemma of two opposing cells.) Since epithelial cells do not exist in the dermis, only *half* a desmosome, a *hemidesmosome*, forms.

(3) *Desmosomes* occur along the lateral and upper surfaces of the cells, with opposing cells providing a half desmosome.

(4) *Nuclei*, with one or two nucleoli, are indented and outlined by a thin peripheral rim of heterochromatin.

(5) *Mitotic index* (frequency of mitoses) of the **stratum basale** is 0.002, or 2 cells in mitosis for every 1000 counted. The mitotic index, normally, is far greater in the **stratum spinosum.**

(a) Should the mitotic index of the stratum basale exceed 0.002, then the pathologist might be facing a case of *hyperplasia* (rapid increase in cell number by mitosis) which may precede *basal cell carcinoma*.

(b) The old name "stratum germinativum" for the stratum basale suggested that this layer expressed the highest mitotic index. This concept was proved incorrect and the terminology was abandoned.

(6) The *endoplasmic reticulum* consists of a few short profile membranes studded with polyribosomes. Clusters of polyribosomes, scattered freely throughout the cytoplasm, contribute to producing two important cellular components: *tonofilaments* and *keratohyalin granules*.

(a) *Tonofilaments* aggregate into fascicles of *tonofibrils*, some of which loop against the desmosomes, while others form the *cytoskeleton*.

(b) *Keratohyalin granules* formed in these cells are extruded and assimilated by the cells in the upper layers.

b. Stratum spinosum, the *spiny layer* [Historical note: The stratum spinosum together with the stratum basale was called the stratum Malpighii. This eponym is no longer used.]

(1) The **stratum spinosum** consists of newly differentiated polyhedral cells (each cell = **epitheliocytus spinosus**) in a varying number of layers. The number of cells diminishes close to the dermal papillae and increases between them.

(2) *Mitotic figures* are found in this layer to a greater extent than any other layer of the epidermis.

(3) The name *spinosum* derives from the cellular appearance in normal and pathological tissues prepared for light microscopy.

(a) That *tonofibrils do not cross* from one cell to the other (at sites now recognized as desmosomes) has been established by electron microscopy. Artifact of fixation caused shrinkage of the plasmalemma except at the desmosomes, giving a spiny appearance.

(b) The intercellular spaces between desmosomes provide adequate channels for nutrients, for dendritic processes of melanocytes, and for free nerve endings (cf chapter on nerve tissue).

(c) Nutrients (from dermal capillary loops) reach the avascular epithelial cells via diffusion through the intercellular spaces.

c. Stratum granulosum, the *granular layer*, varies from *one* to *five* cells in thickness. Each cell is an **epitheliocytus squamosus** (*squamous epithelial cell*).

(1) The squamous epithelial cells are filled with irregular angular aggregates of *keratohyalin granules* intimately associated with the tonofibrils. (Keratohyalin should not be confused with melanin pigment, which is colored even in its untreated state.)

(2) *Keratin* formation in the outer layers (**stratum corneum**) depends on keratohyalin as a chemical precursor. *Keratin*, confined to the outer protective layers, is an insoluble protein produced by the epidermal cells.

(3) Although "spiny" projections are fewer in this layer, typical desmosomes are still present.

(4) A vesicular nucleus lacking nucleoli offers morphological evidence of waning productivity.

d. Stratum lucidum (*clear layer*) is a thin homogeneous layer of flattened squamous epithelial cells (each cell = **epitheliocytus squamosus**).

(1) This layer, interposed between the stratum granulosum and the outermost **stratum corneum**, is most pronounced in *thickened epidermis*, particularly from the sole of the foot and the palm of the hand.

(2) Absent nuclei and nucleoli indicate nonfunction.

(3) The inactive cytoplasm lacks mitochondria, endoplasmic reticulum, polyribosomes, and golgi complex.

(4) *Tonofilaments* align along the longitudinal axis of the cells, parallel to the skin surface.

e. **Stratum corneum**, the *horny layer*, is a composite of structureless, dehydrated, dead squamous epithelial cells. These are flattened into horny plates or squames that are continuously sloughed off or desquamated. The cytoplasm is replaced by *keratin granules* produced in the stratum granulosum. Desmosomes may be recognized in electron micrographs, attesting to their (the squames) derivation from the deeper cell layers.

3. *Additional cells of the epidermis*

a. *Melanocytes* (Fitzpatrick et al, 1979), pigment-producing cells of the stratum basale, appear about the 13th week of development in proportions of 4 to every 12 epidermal cells.

(1) The *melanocyte*, resting directly on the basement membrane, sends dendritic processes into the stratum spinosum. The melanocyte produces *melanin*, which is distributed to the other cells and hair via the dendritic processes (Quevedo, 1972). Melanin granules determine the degree of skin pigmentation.

(2) *Melanin* pigment, a polymer of tyrosine (an amino acid), forms within melanocytes via the action of the enzyme *tyrosinase*. *Melanin* production is stimulated by

(a) hormone influences (*melanocyte-stimulating hormone, MSH*) from the pars intermedia of the hypophysis,

(b) ultraviolet (UV) light, by (1) darkening resident melanin, (2) distributing of melanosomes to the squamous epitheliocytes, and (3) increasing tyrosinase activity, thus producing more melanin. Excessive UV causes carcinomas (basal cell or squamous cell) and malignant melanomas (involving melanocytes). UV has proved beneficial in treating psoriasis, a disease characterized by scaly patches (usually on extensor surfaces) by inhibiting mitotic activity of basal and squamous epitheliocytes.

(c) irritations involving excessive blood supply for long periods of time.

(3) Typically, the cell body lacks tonofibrils and desmosomes. A rounded nucleus, mitochondria, rER, and a well-developed golgi complex are found.

(4) The *melanosome* is a football-shaped structure about 0.7 μm long and 0.3 μm at its widest diameter. The melanosome encloses

a series of concentrically arranged sheets in the longitudinal axis, surrounding an electron-dense *melanin pigment granule.*

(5) Following maturation, *melanin pigment granules* are expelled and incorporated into the squamous epitheliocytes. Two types of melanin pigments are produced:

(a) brown/black *eumelanin*

(b) red/yellow *pheomelanins.* Redheads and blondes carry the gene for pheomelanin.

b. *Melanophorocytes* are phagocytes of epithelial and connective tissues that ingest only melanin.

c. *Intraepidermal macrophages* (formerly the Langerhans' cells) have been interpreted as effete melanocytes. However, most of the current literature recognizes these to be cells with well-developed cytoplasmic structures (Wolff and Stingl, 1983). The best available evidence depicts this cell as distinctly different and unrelated to the melanocytes.

(1) A most conspicuous feature revealed by TEM are rod-shaped granules, related to the golgi complex. Some granules possess a dilated vesicle, usually at the end of the rod.

(2) While the morphology is well described, the functions and origins are unknown. It has been suggested that they are probably dermal macrophages that migrated into the epidermis.

d. *Tactile epithelioid cells* (Merkel cell) (Gould et al, 1985) (Fig. 10-6B) were presented in the chapter on nerve tissue. This cell has been compared to a neurosecretory cell or an amine precursor uptake and decarbosylation cell (Winklemann, 1977).

B. The **dermis** (Montagna et al, 1970), a mesodermal derivative, provides epidermal support and a rich vascular bed for metabolic exchange processes. Good histologic preparations show nerves and their various free endings, lymphatic vessels, and epidermal derivatives (glands, hair).

1. The *thickness* of the **dermis** generally averages about 1.5 mm. In thin skin of the eyelids and penile prepuce, the thickness is reduced to about 0.5 mm. In regions subjected to contraction and relaxation (eg, the penis, scrotum, areola of the nipple, and the perineum), nonstriated (smooth) myocytes occur. The dermis tends to be somewhat thinner in the anterior than the posterior body surface. Males usually have thicker dermis than females.

2. Two inseparable strata comprise the dermis:

a. An external **stratum papillare**: a narrow band of loose connective tissue in contact with the basement membrane of the epidermal **stratum basale**.

(1) Enzymatic digestion of skin fragments permits the ready separation of epidermis from the dermis.

(a) Examination of the superficial surface of the exposed **dermis** reveals finger-like projections, the dermal **papillae**, studding the surface.

(b) Correspondingly, the basilar surface of the **epidermis** shows invaginations from where **papillae** were withdrawn.

(2) The papillary stratum is a typical loose connective tissue composed of

(a) *fibers:* randomly arranged reticular, collagen, and elastic fibers.

(b) *cells:* fibroblasts, lymphocytes (which may migrate into the epidermis), neutrophils, fixed and free macrophages, plasma cells, and tissue basophil granulocytes (mast cells). The tissue basophil granulocytes are particularly abundant along capillaries.

(3) The rich capillary bed of the **stratum papillare** is significantly extensive to nourish the epidermis and serve as a thermoregulator.

(4) Dermal papillae usually reach their highest peak opposite the site where the epidermal grooves are deepest. This location brings the dermal capillary loops close to nourish the upper cells of the **stratum spinosum**.

b. **Stratum reticulare**, composed of dense, irregularly arranged bundles of collagen fibers, extends from the **stratum papillare** down to the less dense **tela subcutanea**.

(1) As with most dense connective tissues, the cell population consists primarily of fibroblasts. Aggregates of adipocytes appear in scattered sites.

(2) Capillary plexuses are not as rich as in the stratum papillare.

(3) The visible "stretch marks" following pregnancy are caused by the stretching of the skin by the enlarged uterus, resulting in ruptured collagen fibers in this layer. The marks (striae gravidarum) remain permanently.

C. **Tela subcutanea** (old name: *hypodermis*) extends from (and is continuous with) the dermis, down to the *deep fascia* covering muscle or bone. This layer functions as a thermal insulator of the body.

1. The *character* of the connective tissue components in this layer determines whether the skin moves freely or is bound down.

a. When the *skin moves freely*, the connective tissue is extremely loose and contains little or no adipose tissue.

b. When the *skin* is *bound tightly*, considerably more adipose tissue is present in lobules separated by thick, dense connective tissue septae.

(1) Adipose tissue is absent from thin skin of the eyelids, penis, and scrotum.

(2) Adipose tissue of abdominal skin forms a fat pad, the **panniculus adiposus**, which may exceed 3 cm in thickness.

2. Large vessels, nerves, and lymphatics penetrate the **tela subcutanea** to reach the dermis.

3. In the **tela subcutanea** next to the dermis, there may be parts of sudoriferous glands and hair follicles.

4. Subcutaneous injections should be administered into the **tela subcutanea**, particularly where the dermis is freely movable.

D. *Appendages* of the skin: The epidermis may be modified in a variety of ways to produce hair, nails, and glands. (The *mammary gland*, a special appendage of the skin, is considered with the female reproductive system.)

1. *Hair* (Montagna and Dodson, 1969), a familiar epidermal specialization, varies in amounts on the body surface.

a. The following sites are *glabrous* (hairless):

(1) *Appendages*

(a) palms of hands and soles of feet.

(b) palmar and plantar surfaces of the fingers and toes.

(c) sides of the hands and the feet.

(2) *The lips*

(3) *Genitalia*

(a) *male:* glans penis and prepuce.

(b) *female:* clitoris, labia minora, and inner surface of the labia majora.

(4) *Mammary glands:* the nipples.

b. *Lanugo* in the newborn is the very smooth, almost woolly *hair* that covers a good part of the body. *Lanugo* disappears for the most part, but remains on the forehead in the adult.

c. Coarse hairs occur on the face (beard), eyebrows, pubis, and axilla.

d. Hair is a keratinized filament composed of a **scapus** (shaft), an **apex** (exterior end), and a **radix** (root) anchored deep in the dermis.

(1) The external surface of the hair shaft is surrounded by a

cuticle of cylindrical *cuticular epitheliocytes*, which become extremely flattened toward the **apex**. The *cuticle* covers a cortex of horny squames containing melanin granules.

(2) The **medulla**, or center of the shaft, is composed of *polyhedral epitheliocytes* at the root and horny squames toward the apex. Tonofibrils, melanin granules, and *trichohyalin* granules occupy the cytoplasm of the polyhedral epitheliocytes.

(3) The **folliculus** of the hair is a long pit lined by cells that are continuous with the surface epithelium. The *follicle* in which the hair shaft resides is surrounded by connective tissue of the dermis. Thus, two sheaths surround the hair:

(a) **vagina epithelialis radicularis** (epithelial root sheath) derived from the epithelium, and a

(b) **vagina dermalis radicularis** (connective tissue root sheath) derived from the dermis.

(4) Deep in the dermis, the follicle expands into a **bulbus** (bulb-shaped base) with a **cervix** (neck) and a **cavitas** (cavity). The dermis invaginates upward into the root of the future hair shaft.

(a) The epithelial cells making up the invaginated cervix are undifferentiated epidermal cells that generate the keratinized cells of the hair shaft.

(b) The **cavitas** (invagination) is filled with connective tissue dermal papilla cells that provide the nutritional elements necessary for hair growth.

e. Mitosis of the undifferentiated cells at the root yields an accumulation of cells that form the hair shaft.

f. SEM reveals that the outer cuticle of human hair is covered with fine scale-like plates, each called **epitheliocytus cuticularis**.

(1) These are the same as the dehydrated, dead **stratum corneum** squames, but are an extremely flattened version.

(2) *SEM* further reveals distinctive differences in the arrangement of *cuticular epitheliocytes* in hair from different sites:

(a) *scalp hair*
   [1] *borders:* smooth,
   [2] *cells:* run transversely at regular intervals,

(b) *eyebrows*
   [1] *borders:* smooth,
   [2] *cells:* irregularly arranged,

(c) *pubic hair*
   [1] *borders:* less smooth
   [2] *cells:* extremely irregular in arrangement,

(d) *axillary hair*

    [1] *borders:* serrated,

    [2] *cells:* randomly oriented around the shaft.

    g. The epidermal surface cells surrounding the folliculus entrance may become extremely dried by improper shampoos or bacteriocidal action and flake off as dandruff. To prevent excessive drying, *sebaceous glands* empty their secretions into the surface provided by the hair follicle:

    (1) From within the follicle, an oily secretion ascends the hair shaft.

    (2) One duct provides access for the lobules of the sebaceous gland located at an angle to the hair shaft and usually on the same side of the hair follicle as the *arrector pili muscle.*

    h. The *arrector pili muscle* consists of bundles of nonstriated (smooth) muscle strands, which pull the hair follicle so that the hair appears to stand up. Contraction of the *arrector pili* causes the "goose bumps" frequently seen on skin when one shivers from cold or an emotional stimulus.

    2. Unguis = *nails* (Zaias and Baden, 1979): The nails are flattened, slightly convex horny plates with the following components.

    a. The **corpus** (body) of the nail corresponds to the outer cornified layers of skin and has

    (1) an *external face* (surface).

    (2) an *internal face* (surface) attaches to a nail bed made up of the **stratum basale** and the **stratum spinosum.**

    (3) a free *distal edge* projects over the **hyponychium**, which is the stratum corneum of the skin under the distal edge.

    (4) a nail *root* under the *proximal skin fold.* The **eponychium** (cuticle) is the extension of stratum corneum of the proximal skin fold onto the nail.

    (5) a *lateral nail fold*, the skin at the lateral edge of the nail.

    (6) The **lunula** is a whitish half-moon of the nail surface projecting out from the proximal nail fold. The thicker epidermis, proximally, prevents the pink color from appearing through the lucent nail body.

    b. The **dermis penetrates the epidermal strata under the nail as longitudinal ridges of** *dermal papillae*, rather than finger-like papillae.

    c. *Nail growth:* nails, unlike hair, grow continuously and have no resting cycle.

    (1) The fastest rate of growth occurs during childhood and following any trauma. Nail biting increases the rate of growth.

(2) Aging slows down nail growth, as does illness, disease, and poor nutrition.

3. *Exocrine glands of the skin* are derivatives of the ectoderm and retain connections via ducts. Their products are liberated freely onto the skin surface.

a. *Sebaceous glands* (Strauss et al, 1976) exist in body skin that possesses hair follicles. The **glandula sebacea pili** have *ducts* that empty into the troughs surrounding *hair*, and the arrector pili muscles on contraction help to empty the gland. The **glandula sebacea libera** are free and have ducts emptying directly onto the surface of the epidermis. Both types are not controlled by nerves, but by androgenic hormones.

(1) The large polyhedral *sebaceous exocrine cells* contain a spherical vesicular nucleus.

(2) TEM resolves numerous lipid droplets in the cytoplasm, with moderately dense material at the periphery of each droplet surrounding a clearer central substance.

(3) Cisternae and vesicles of agranular (smooth) endoplasmic reticulum are layered around the lipid droplets.

(4) Lipid droplets and portions of the surrounding cytoplasm contribute to the product called *sebum*, which contains bacteriocidal agents.

(5) *Sebum* lubricates hairs, prevents skin from drying and cracking, and deposits a waxy waterproof coat.

b. *Sudoriferous glands* form two types based on whether they are connected to hair follicles: *sudoriferous merocrine glands* (not connected) and *sudoriferous apocrine glands* (connected).

(1) The *sudoriferous merocrine glands* (Sato, 1983), or sweat glands, are simple branched tubular glands of epidermal origin located everywhere *except* the margins of the lips, glans penis, and nail bed. These gland forms are not connected with hair follicles. Secretion is controlled by postganglionic *cholinergic* sympathetic nerve fibers.

(a) The secretory **portico terminalis** begins in the **dermis** close to (and often in) the **tela subcutanea**. The secretory portion appears as a coiled ball of yarn, from which ascends a wavy duct directly to the epidermis. In the **stratum corneum**, a spiraled lumen confined by the squames of dehydrated dead cells exits at a **porus glandularis** (glandular pore) on an epithelial ridge.

(b) The cells of the **ductus glandularis** in the dermis are called **exocrinocytus densus** or dense exocrine cells, in contrast to the **exocrinocytus lucidus** or light exocrine cells of the coiled secretory portion.

[1] The *dense exocrine cells* possess

[a] large electron-dense granules rich in protein polysaccharides in the apical portion of the columnar-shaped *duct cells.*

[b] less electron-dense granules around the golgi complex, which resides on the side of the nucleus facing the duct lumen.

[c] a few short microvilli on the luminal surface, while the basilar surface invaginates to increase the surface area.

[2] The *light exocrine cells,* of the secretory portion, expel their aqueous contents into the small intercellular canaliculi that lead into the duct. The aqueous product probably plays an important role in salt secretion and probably contains bacteriocidal agents.

[a] The apical surface facing the intercellular canaliculi is covered with small microvilli.

[b] The lateral surfaces possess deep invaginations, similar to those of the *dense cells,* which serve to interdigitate with cells next to them.

[c] Most characteristic is the high content of polyribosomes, which confer a cytoplasmic basophilia.

(2) The *sudoriferous apocrine glands* (Hurley and Shelly, 1960), *connected with hair follicles*, possess granules probably containing some keratin. These glands, controlled by sex hormones and postganglionic *adrenergic* sympathetic nerves, are represented by

(a) *apocrine sweat glands* of the axilla, pubis, and circumanal glands, which produce a viscous secretion. The characteristic odor is attributed to bacterial action on secretion, because in the absence of bacteria the secretion is odorless.

(b) *ceruminal glands* of the external acoustic meatus, which produce a waxy secretion (cf ear),

(c) *ciliary glands* (spiraled sweat glands) between the eyelash follicles (old name: glands of Moll) (cf eye).

c. *Classification* of the three basic types of secretory patterns, based on electron microscopy:

(1) *Holocrine secretion* is the loss of an entire cell as a result of lipid accumulation in the cytoplasm and nuclear pyknosis. The flattened cell ghost is discharged along with the secretory products. Undifferentiated cells at the periphery of the gland replace the lost cells. *Example:* sebaceous glands next to hair follicles.

(2) *Merocrine secretion* (eccrine): Exocrine cells of this category elaborate secretory products without any substantial loss of any part of the cell. *Example: sudoriferous merocrine gland* of the skin (not associated with hair).

(a) The originating secretory granule is packaged intracellularly in smooth-surfaced membranes of the golgi complex.

(b) The membrane-bound granule moves to the luminal surface of the cell where it fuses to the plasmalemma.

(c) At the site of fusion of membranes, an opening appears and the granule is discharged in toto or in smaller particles.

(d) The empty membranous sac (which surrounded the granule) evaginates to form a microvillus, thus conserving the membrane.

(3) *Apocrine secretion:* A non-membrane-bound secretory product exits the cell with a fragment of the plasmalemma. *Example: sudoriferous apocrine glands* associated with the hair in the axillary, pubic, and circumanal regions; also the ceruminal and ciliary glands.

(a) In apocrine exocrine cells, globular secretory products, like lipid droplets, migrate to the cell surface at the lumen.

(b) At the cell surface, the lipid droplet forces the plasmalemma upward.

(c) The lipid droplet protrudes sufficiently to be enclosed by a portion of the plasmalemma.

(d) At this point, the cell membrane seals tight around the droplet as it moves into the lumen.

(e) At the exit site, the plasmalemma seals itself to prevent any loss of cytoplasm.

III. *Vasculature of the skin*

A. *Blood vessels* (Winkelmann et al, 1961): In addition to ordinary metabolic needs of the skin, the vasculature controls body temperature and provides for storage of blood. In some tissues and organs, blood storage is accommodated by thin-walled sinusoidal vessels. Within the skin, veins approaching the nature of sinusoids also store great quantities of blood under low pressure.

1. The vascular patterns are

a. *plexus I:* large vessel network under the tela subcutanea. This plexus is fed and drained by major vessels.

b. *plexus II:* a smaller plexus, **rete arteriosum dermidis**, situated between the dermis and the tela subcutanea.

c. *plexus III:* the smallest plexus, **rete arteriosum subpapillare**, immediately under the epidermis.

2. The largest arterial vessels in *plexus I* send perpendicular branches directly to *plexus II*.

a. Smaller arteries, emanating from *plexus II*, ascend to *plexus III* under the epidermis.

b. From *plexus III, intrapapillary capillary loops* ascend into the *dermal papillae*. Since the epidermis is avascular, nutritional elements and waste products must be exchanged via these capillary loops. Cells of the stratum basale obviously have a better exchange rate than cells of the more superficial layers.

c. Blood from the capillary loops returns to venules in *plexus III*, the **plexus venosus subpapillaris superficialis**. Larger venules drain this plexus into *plexus II* and larger venules and veins back to *plexus III* and thereafter to the general circulation.

d. Islands of adipocytes in the **tela subcutanea** are supplied by ascending arteries from the *plexus I*. Capillary plexuses in the adipose lobules are drained by small veins leading directly to those veins in *plexus I*. Similarly, adipose lobules in the dermis are supplied and drained by neighboring vessels of *plexus II*.

e. the **papillae** of the *hair follicles* in the dermis are supplied and drained by vessels from *plexus II*. The terminal secretory portions of the *sudoriferous merocrine glands* are likewise fed and drained from the vessels of *plexus II*.

3. The vasculature provides exceptional storage for blood. Venous plexuses, with large-diameter lumina surrounded by thin endothelial walls, resemble sinusoids of other tissues. Those of the areola and nipple of the breast are good examples of this tendency to resemble sinusoids.

4. *Arterio-venous anastomses (AVA)*, previously noted in the vasculature of the heart walls, are represented in the dermis of the palmar surface of the hand and plantar surface of the feet and in the nail beds.

a. Under relatively normal conditions, the *AVA* permit little or no blood to pass from the artery to the vein. Blood travels from the ordinary route of artery to arteriole to capillary bed to venule to vein.

b. Increase of blood flow with the *AVA open* causes the skin to become warmer, with a concomitant loss of heat. This may be recognized on examination by simply feeling the skin and observing the flushed reddish color imparted by the increased blood flow. Many situations bring this condition about, especially emotional states in which the entire face and neck or patches are reddened by *"blushing."*

B. *Lymphatic vessels:* The dermis possesses a rich supply of lymphatic vessels, but no lymph nodes.

1. In contrast to the blood vasculature of the skin, which has three plexuses of arteries and veins, only one lymphatic plexus is certain, the **rete lymphocapillare cutis profundum** or deep plexus.

2. Blind lymphocapillaries commence in the dermal papillae and join the deep plexus. From the deep plexus, lymph fluid exits the skin in the company of large arteries.

IV. *Aging of skin*

A. *General changes*

1. Skin achieves its optimal appearance between the ages of 20 and 30. Thereafter, signs of aging begin to appear, vis-à-vis "crows-feet" wrinkles at the lateral corners of the eyes.

2. Other signs presenting evidence of skin aging are
a. gradual increases of pigment spots on the dorsum of the hand and face,
b. graying (loss of pigmentation) of hair,
c. drying of skin,
d. loss of elasticity, at the same time that elastic fibers increase in number and thickness,
e. loss of subcutaneous adipose deposits.

3. Redheads and blonds, with less protective brown-black pigmentation, age more rapidly than those with brown or black hair, and those with brown hair age more rapidly than those with black hair.

4. the degree of pigmentation expresses itself in skin color: Caucasians age most rapidly at one end of the spectrum, while blacks age the least at the opposite end of the spectrum.

B. Changes in the **epidermis**

1. The number of cell layers is reduced. In senile skin, particularly of the buttocks, only two to three living cell layers may be present above the stratum basale.

2. The stratum corneum may have only one or two dead cells to protect the underlying living cells. Frequent cracks in this layer expose the underlying living cells to bacteria, dessication, trauma, and a host of problems of concern to the physician.

3. Patients allowed to lie in bed for prolonged periods are subjected to decubitis ulcers (bed sores) brought about by prolonged pressure on the thinning epidermis.

C. Changes in the **dermis**

1. Loss of elasticity is due to the fragmentation of the thicker elastic fibers, while collagen fibers loose flexibility. Females possess less collagen in the dermis than males, and thus aging changes occur more rapidly.

2. The irregularity of the dermal–epidermal junction straightens out, as evidenced by

    a. the basal surface of the stratum basale cells becomes smooth,

    b. the dermal papillae decrease in size and number, and eventually most disappear.

3. The loss of vibrant skin color gradually disappears as the capillary loops and plexuses recede. The dermis vascularity, in fact, is markedly reduced. In histological sections, capillaries are difficult to find, and the blood vessels that are present are sclerosed.

  D. *Glands*

    1. Most *sebaceous* glands are unchanged.

    2. *Sudoriferous merocrine glands* (sweat glands) are reduced in number (by atrophy and disappearance).

    3. *Sudoriferous apocrine glands* (in the axilla, acoustic auditory meatus, and ciliary glands) atrophy and gradually disappear.

Questions

DIRECTIONS: Select the best answer to the question or incomplete statement. There may be other options that are partially correct, but there is only one best answer.

  1. A patient presents with contact dermatitis. The dermatologist prescribes a steroid cream to improve the condition and explains that visible improvement can be expected in

    A. a day or two

    B. one week

    C. one month

    D. two months

    E. four months

2. The skin protects against the multitude of bacteria that live on the epidermal surface and/or access to the dermis via "cuts," by all of the following EXCEPT
   A. the epidermis
   B. gland secretions
   C. variety of cells in the dermis
   D. vasculature of the dermis
   E. the lymphatics

3. Postganglionic adrenergic sympathetic nerves and sex hormones are involved in controlling secretions from
   A. sebaceous glands
   B. sudoriferous merocrine sweat glands
   C. sudoriferous apocrine sweat glands
   D. holocrine glands
   E. eccrine glands

4. Skin thickness refers to thickness of the
   A. epidermis
   B. dermis papillary layer
   C. dermis reticular layer
   D. tela subcutanea
   E. all the above

5. All the following may occur to skin after exposure to ultraviolet light, EXCEPT
   A. vitamin D forms
   B. beneficial in treating malignant melanoma
   C. pigmentation increases
   d. tyrosinase activity in melanocytes increases
   E. mitotic activity is inhibited

6. The body heat is conserved by
   A. vasodilatation of capillary loops in the dermal papillae
   B. vasoconstriction of the dermal papillae capillary loops
   C. stimulation of sudoriferous merocrine glands to secrete
   D. stimulation of sudoriferous apocrine glands to secrete
   E. none of the above

7. Aging of the skin shows all the following EXCEPT
   A. drying of skin
   B. increase in pigment spots
   C. loss of elasticity
   D. increase in subcutaneous adipose deposits
   E. loss of pigmentation of hair

8. All the following are parts of the nail EXCEPT
   A. corpus
   B. eponychium
   C. hyponychium
   D. root
   E. lanugo

9. The tela subcutanea (hypodermis) is the location of the
   A. panniculus adiposus
   B. arrector pili muscle
   C. arterio-venous anastomoses
   D. stratum papillare
   E. stratum lucidum

10. Elastic fibers
    A. occur in the epidermis
    B. are confined to the tela subcutanea
    C. are absent in the stratum papillare
    D. are absent in the stratum reticulare
    E. age by increasing in thickness

Explanatory Answers

1. C. The length of time involved in the process of renewal is 28 days (about one month). This information will prevent the patient from becoming overanxious and expecting immediate results.

2. E. The lymphatics do not bring anything to the skin, they remove tissue fluid. If anything they may provide a site of entrance. However, before that occurs the following stand in defense: the epidermis (A) provides a mechanical barrier; the secretions (B) of the sebaceous glands and the sudoriferous merocrine (sweat) glands contain bacteriocidal agents; the cells of the dermis (C) lymphocytes, neutrophils, and macrophages stand ready to attack bacteria that enter the epi-

dermis through a cut; and (D) the rich vasculature can deliver additional bacteria fighting cells if needed.

3. C. Of the other answers, (A) the sebaceous glands are not under nervous control, (B) the sudoriferous merocrine sweat glands are controlled by postganglionic *cholinergic* (not adrenergic as is the answer) sympathetic nerves, (D) the sebaceous glands are holocrine glands, and (E) eccrine glands are merocrine glands.

4. A. The terms "thick skin" and "thin skin" refer only to the thickness of the epidermis, and not any of the other layers. Epidermis that is 1 mm thick (palms, soles) is considered thick skin. All other areas are considered to be thin skin. The dermis is thicker on the posterior surface, and males tend to have a thicker dermis than females.

5. B. In controlled amounts, UV does inhibit mitoses of the mitotic epidermal cells. One might believe that treatment of carcinomas would be helped. However, only psoriasis has been helped by UV. UV in excess is known to be a factor in carcinomas and malignant melanomas. Pigmentation does increase by (1) darkening resident melanin, (2) stimulating dispersal of melanin pigment granules, and (3) increasing tyrosinase activity in melanocytes to produce more melanin.

6. B. Vasoconstriction of the dermal papillae capillary loops restricts blood flow, resulting in conservation of heat. Stimulating glandular secretion facilitates loss of body heat via evaporation of sweat.

7. D. Subcutaneous adipose deposits are lost, not increased. While pigment spots increase on the dorsum of the hand and face, pigmentation of hair decreases (graying). Decreasing the activity and number of sudoriferous glands results in drying of skin. Elasticity is lost due to fragmentation of elastic fibers and loss of flexibility of collagen fibers.

8. E. A through D are parts of the nail. *Lanugo* is the very smooth, almost woolly hair that covers a good part of the body of a newborn. The term **lunula** (a small moon) is the half-moon-shaped whitish area projecting under the proximal nail fold.

9. A. The panniculus adiposus is a fat pad of the tela subcutanea, which contributes to thermal regulation of the body. The arrector pili muscle and arterio-venous anastomoses normally reside in the dermis. The stratum papillare is a portion of the dermis below the epidermis, and the stratum lucidum (clear layer) resides between the stratum granulosum and straum corneum of the epidermis.

10. E. Loss of elasticity of aging skin results from an increase in elastic fiber thickness and subsequent fragmentation. There are no elastic fibers in the epidermis, and certainly they are not confined to the tela subcutanea. The majority of elastic fibers reside in the dermal stratum papillare. Though the stratum reticulare has some elastic fibers, the majority of fibers are composed of collagen.

16 The Digestive System

Introduction

I. *General:* Food is processed via a series of integrated anatomical and biological events. The entire process begins as a voluntary act and ends as a voluntary act, but all intervening biological events are involuntary.

A. Nutritional elements enter the *mouth* to be prepared for swallowing and digestion.

B. The *pharynx* and *esophagus* propel the *bolus* of food into the stomach, where it is churned and treated to facilitate absorption in the small intestine.

C. *Secretions* of various glands associated with the digestive apparatus assist in lubrication and digestion.

D. Unabsorbed food remnants are conveyed to the *large intestine*, where imbibed water and that added from glandular secretions is reabsorbed.

E. The *residue* is moved through the *rectum* and eliminated via the *anus.*

II. *Development* (Moore, 1988)

A. *General:* Most of the digestive apparatus derives from endoderm. Initially, a flattened endodermal layer forms a blind-ended tube. Starting from the midgut area, the tube grows cranially (toward the head) and later caudally (toward the tail). The midgut remains attached to the yolk sac for a period of time.

1. The blind cranial end of the endodermal tube fuses with the ectoderm of the invaginating stomatodeal ectoderm to form the *oropharyngeal membrane.*

2. Caudal to the yolk sac, the blind caudal end of the endodermal tube meets the invaginating ectoderm of the *proctodeum* (precursor of the anal canal) to form an *anal membrane.*

3. Rupture of the *oropharyngeal membrane* and the *anal membrane* results in an uninterrupted primitive digestive tube extending from the oral cavity through the anal canal.

B. *Parts of the embryonic digestive apparatus*

1. *Stomatodeum,* the embryonic oral cavity. Lined by ectoderm, gives rise to the

    a. *hypophysial sac* (Rathke's pouch),
    b. *primordium* of part of the *tongue,*
    c. *submandibular gland buds,*
    d. *sublingual gland buds,*
    e. *parotid gland buds,*
    f. *processes* of the maxillae, mandible, and palate,
    g. *lips, buccal cavity, gingivae,* and *teeth.*

2. *Pre-enteron* (foregut) of endoderm gives origin to the

    a. *primitive pharynx,*
    b. *primitive esophagus,*
    c. *primitive stomach,*
    d. *primitive duodenum,* which gives rise to
        (1) *hepatic diverticulum* (liver),
        (2) *hepatopancreatic duct,*
            (a) *ventral pancreas,*
            (b) *ventral pancreatic duct,*
        (3) ductus choledochus,
            (a) *hepatic duct,*
            (b) *cystic duct,*
        (4) *dorsal pancreas,*
        (5) *duodenum* (first part).

3. *Mesenteron,* or midgut, gives origin to the

    a. *duodenum* (remainder),
    b. *jejunum,*
    c. *ileum,*
    d. *cecum,*
    e. appendix vermiformis,
    f. *colon,* ascending,
    g. *colon, transverse* (first part).

4. *Metenteron*
  a. *colon, transverse* (remainder),
  b. *colon, descending,*
  c. *colon, sigmoid,*
  d. *rectum.*

5. *Proctodeum*
  a. *anal membrane,*
  b. *anal canalis,*
  c. *anus.*

The Oral Cavity

I. *Definition:* The *oral cavity* is the space confined by clinched teeth (the palate above and the floor supporting the tongue below). The *buccal cavity*, forming outside clinched teeth, is enclosed by the cheeks and closed lips.

II. *Components*

  A. The *lips* consist of three parts:

  1. Pars cutanea, the external cutaneous surface, is characterized by keratinized stratified squamous epithelium and hair follicles. The epidermis is penetrated by connective tissue papillae.

  2. Pars intermedia, which possesses lightly keratinized stratified squamous epithelium. These cells are sufficiently translucent that the color of underlying capillaries in the dermal papillae redden the lip. Since no glands open on this surface, they must be moistened by saliva to prevent drying (chapped lips).

  3. Pars mucosa, on the internal surface, is covered by moist stratified squamous epithelium that is penetrated by short connective tissue papillae. Opening onto the pars mucosa surface are the openings of short ducts of *labial glands*, whose secretions keep the epithelium moist. The secretory **acini** reside in the underlying connective tissue.

  a. The *seromucous acini* secrete two substances:
    (1) thin watery *serous fluid,* from *serous acini,*
    (2) thick viscous *mucus* (*mucus:* the noun).

  b. *Analogy:* A labial gland may be compared to a bunch of grapes that is half white and half purple.

    (1) Each white grape represents a group of *mucous* (the adjective) *cells* surrounding a small duct (the stem). These cells appear clear in preparations because *mucus* is extracted.

(2) Purple grapes represent *serous cells*, possessing large amounts of rER (basophilic).

4. The three forms of epithelium (keratinized, translucent, and moist) anchor into a connective tissue layer, supporting labial vessels and nerves and the **orbicularis oris** skeletal myocytes.

B. The mucosa of the *cheeks*, lacking a stratum granulosum and stratum corneum, does not undergo keratinization. Its connective tissue provides insertion sites for *buccinator* skeletal myocytes. Elastic fibers in connective tissue prevent the mucosa from being trapped by the teeth during chewing.

C. The *palate*, separating the oral from the nasal cavity, is composed of two parts, an anterior *hard* and a posterior *soft*.

1. The *hard palate* consists of bony processes of the maxillae and the palatine bones. A tough, resistant *mucoperiosteum* consists of *periosteum* adhering tightly to a **tunica mucosa** (mucosal coat) corrugated into ridges and valleys, which emit an elevated *median raphe*. The tunica mucosa consists of

a. self-renewing *keratinized, stratified squamous epithelium* on the inferior surface. The following are noted:

(1) basal epitheliocytes, squamous epitheliocytes, melanocytes, intraepidermal macrophages, tactile epithelioid cells, and taste buds. Neutrophils and/or lymphocytes move into the epithelium from the connective tissue below.

(2) a definite **stratum corneum** and **stratum granulosum** on the surface of the ridges are lacking in the valleys.

b. *three zones* of underlying connective tissue:

(1) **zona adiposa**, containing adipose tissue,

(2) **zona glandularis**, with mucous glands,

(3) **zona fibrosa** of dense fibrous tissue firmly attached to the periosteum.

2. The movable, nonbony *soft palate* extends posteriorly from the hard palate. From its free border, suspended between the oral cavity and the pharynx, hangs a median conical projection, the *uvula*. The intrinsic skeletal **musculus uvulae** elevates the soft palate during deglutition to close off the nasopharynx from the oropharynx during deglutition. The *soft palate* consists of

a. two surfaces:

(1) *nasopharyngeal surface*, covered by pseudostratified ciliated columnar epithelium,

(2) **oropharyngeal surface**, covered by nonkeratinized, stratified squamous epithelium.

b. three connective tissue layers:

(1) a **stratum elasticum:** a network of elastic fibers that provide elasticity,

(2) a **tela submucosa:** loose connective tissue with *palatine glands*, vessels, nerves, and some lymphoid tissue.

(3) a **lamina tendinomuscularis**, dense fibrous connective tissue, providing a place for the insertion of **musculus uvulae** skeletal myocytes.

D. Gingiva is formed by reflections of the mucosal epithelium of the cheeks onto the surface of the palatine extension bearing the upper teeth and onto the mandible bearing the lower teeth.

1. Moist stratified squamous epithelium of the gingiva appears red because of the tall underlying papillae bringing capillary loops almost to the surface. The epithelium attaches to the underlying basement membrane by hemidesmosomes. Anchoring fibrils attach the epithelium to the connective tissue (Susi, 1969).

2. There is no **stratum granulosum** or **stratum corneum**, and hence keratinization does not occur. This moist stratified squamous epithelium is tough enough to bear the continual trauma of eating rough foods and frequent brushing of teeth.

E. *Teeth* (Sicher, 1971)

1. *In babies, deciduous teeth* (temporary or milk teeth) begin to erupt at 6 to 7 months of age; by age 2, there are a total of 20. Though generally smaller, these teeth resemble the permanent teeth and have the same names. The *dental formula* (Table 16-1) lists the types of teeth, location, and eruption times (Clemente, 1985).

2. *Permanent teeth*, totaling 32, have the dental formula shown in Table 16-2).

3. The shape and number of roots of each tooth varies according to its function. However, for the sake of clarity, a simple one-cusp, one-root tooth will be presented.

a. The *dental alveolus* is a bony socket that encases each tooth in the mandible and the maxilla.

b. The **gingiva** (gum), composed of nonkeratinized stratified squamous epithelium on a vascularized bed of connective tissue, covers the bone. The **gingiva**, covering the underlying bone, surrounds the protruding portion of tooth.

c. The **periodontium**, a modified periosteum lining the alveolus, is continuous with the gingiva. The *tooth*, fitted into the

Table 16-1. Dental Formula of Deciduous Teeth*

Maxilla	Top right half					Top left half				
	M2	M1	C	Il	Ic	Ic	Il	C	M1	M2
Mandible	M2	M1	C	Il	Ic	Ic	Il	C	M1	M2
		Bottom right half					Bottom left half			

Name	Time of eruption (Variable)	
	Lower	Upper
Key: Ic = Incisor, central	6–9 mo.	8–10 mo.
Il = Incisor, lateral	15–21 mo.	15–20 mo.
C = Canines	16–20 mo.	16–20 mo.
M1 = First molars	15–21 mo.	15–21 mo.
M2 = Second molars	20–24 mo.	20–24 mo.

Number of teeth at what age?
1 year   6 teeth
1.5 years   12 teeth
2 years   16 teeth
2.5 years   20 teeth

*Usually the *deciduous teeth* are shed between 6 and 13 years of age. During that time the permanent teeth erupt and gradually replace the deciduous teeth.

Table 16-2 Dental Formula of Permanent Teeth

Maxilla	Top right half								Top left half same in reverse
	M3	M2	M1	PM2	PM1	C	Il	Ic	
Mandible	M3	M2	M1	PM2	PM1	C	Il	Ic	same in reverse
				Bottom right half					Bottom left half

Key to additional teeth:
  PM1 = first premolar
  PM2 = second premolar
  M3 = third molar

Eruption of permanent teeth
First molars   6th year
Two central incisors   7th year
Two lateral incisors   8th year
First premolars   9th year
Second premolars   10th year
Canines   11th to 12 year
Second molars   12th to 13th year
Third molars   17th to 25th year

alveolus, possesses a *crown* protruding above the gingiva and a *root* anchored to the peridontium by **cementum**, a substance similar to bone.

    d. Teeth have two tissue densities, hard and soft.

        (1) *Soft tissue*, in the central *pulp cavity* of the tooth, is composed of connective tissue, vessels, and nerves. *Pulpocytes (reticulocytes)* form the major connective tissue cell type.

        (2) Hard tissue forming the walls and roof:

            (a) *dentine*, surrounding the *pulp cavity*,

            (b) *enamel*, capping the dentine and forming the major portion of the *crown*,

            (c) **cementum**, surrounding the dentine in the alveolus.

    e. The *pulp cavity* narrows to a *root canal* in the dentine and opens via the *apical foramen* at the bottom of the tooth, where vessels and nerves may enter and exit. *Mesenchyme*, in the embryo, gives origin to cellular and fibrous elements of the pulp cavity.

        (1) *Dentinoblasts* (odontoblasts)

            (a) form a layer of mesodermally derived columnar cells between the dentine and the contents of the pulp cavity.

            (b) are anchored by apical processes, the *dentinal tubules*, extending into the dentine. While the elongated cell body possesses a rich endowment of cytoplasmic structures, these *tubules* are relatively devoid of any.

    f. *Dentine*, forming the wall of the root and roof of the pulp cavity, is an extremely dense material of approximately three-quarters inorganic salts and one-quarter organic proteins.

        (1) *Dentine* is recognized in sections by the presence of *dentinal tubules* radiating outward from the pulp cavity to the outer wall of the tooth. The *peritubular dentine* is extremely dense and refractile.

        (2) *Dentinoblasts*, when stimulated by wear and tear to the crown, mobilize and secrete additional dentine around their cell processes. The dentinoblast is a secretory-type cell, endowed with a well-developed granular endoplasmic reticulum and golgi complex.

    g. *Enamel* (Frank, 1979), in contrast to dentine, is almost totally composed of inorganic salts. Only about 1 to 3% is proteinaceous collagen-like substance.

        (1) *Enamel prisms*, oriented perpendicular to the dentine, comprise the unit of structure of enamel. Prisms together with intervening material are composed of hydroxyapatite crystals.

        (2) *Enameloblasts* (ameloblasts), during development, cover the crown as an epithelial sheet called the *prismatic membrane*.

(3) *Enamel* is deposited in waves, producing *incremental enamel lines* between *enamel lamellae.*

(4) Following completion of enamel deposition, the enameloblasts terminate, and *no further* deposition of enamel is possible. Erosion of enamel must be repaired by a dental "filling."

h. **Cementum**, covering the root of the tooth, contains collagen bundles that anchor to the **periodontium**. Like bone, cementum may be resorbed or increase in thickness by appositional growth.

F. *Salivary glands* (Mason and Chisholm, 1975) empty their products into the oral or buccal cavities.

1. *Cell types* found in salivary glands. Their location at the end of ducts forces them into pyramidal shapes. Their broad smooth bases lie against a basement membrane, surrounded by *myoepithelial cells* and numerous capillaries that provide the components to synthesize secretory products. Their apices increase surface area via microvilli projecting into duct lumen.

a. *Serous cells* produce a clear watery secretion.

(1) A *spherical nucleus* nidates in basilar rER covered by a well-developed golgi complex on its apical side.

(2) The apical cytoplasm contains electron-dense *zymogen granules* containing *ptyalin*, an enzyme that converts starch to soluble carbohydrates.

b. *Mucous cells* contain mucigen, the antecedent of mucin. The product is *mucin*, a glycoprotein that when hydrated forms the lubricant *mucus.*

(1) Electron-lucent mucin droplets, in the apical cytoplasm, are rarely discharged en masse.

(2) *rER* appears between mucin droplets.

(3) a well-developed *golgi complex* resides above the lumenal side of the nucleus.

2. *Major salivary glands* (Fig. 16-1)

a. *Parotid* glands, anterior to the external ear over the masseter muscle, are the largest salivary glands. They are composed of 100% serous cells in man, dog, rabbit, and cat. The intense pain associated with *mumps* results from stretching the very thick well-developed capsule.

(1) A *main duct*, the *parotid duct* (Stensen's duct), empties into the buccal cavity opposite the upper second molar tooth.

(2) The main duct branches into several *interlobar ducts* traveling in connective tissue between lobes.

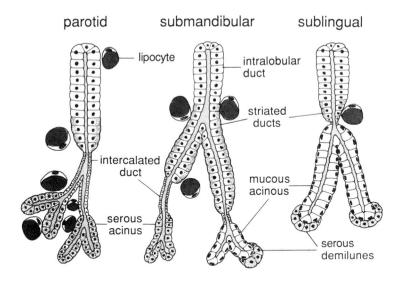

Figure 16-1 Characteristics of the major salivary glands.

(3) Interlobar ducts branch into *interlobular ducts,* which travel in the connective tissue septae of lobules (subdivisions of the lobes).

(4) Interlobular ducts branch repeatedly into *intralobular ducts* surrounded by the serous acini.

(5) The termination of the intralobular duct is represented by simple columnar epithelium (Fig. 16-1) leading into the low simple columnar or cuboidal epithelium of a *striated duct.* The *acidophilic striations,* formed by the *basal* invaginations of the plasmalemma, increase the basal surface area and compartmentalize mitochondria into columns perpendicular to the basement membrane.

(6) The striated duct leads into long, branching *intercalated ducts,* with simple cuboidal becoming simple squamous close to the acini.

(7) In Figure 16-1, adipocytes drawn around the duct branches represent relative numbers per gland. Compare the lengths of the striated ducts, intercalated ducts, and the types of acini.

b. The *submandibular glands,* one under each lateral mandible ramus, are enclosed by thin nonrestrictive *capsules.*

(1) The main *submandibular duct* (Wharton's duct) opens

anteriorly into the oral cavity, beneath the tongue, on one side of the frenulum. Its epithelium resembles that of the parotid duct: stratified or pseudostratified columnar.

(2) *Interlobular ducts* possess stratified columnar epithelium that is reduced to simple columnar closer to the intralobular ducts.

(3) *Intralobular ducts*, with simple columnar epithelium, are not as numerous in sections as in the parotid gland.

(4) *Striated ducts*, with simple columnar or simple cuboidal epithelium, are long and branching.

(5) Unbranched *intercalated ducts* may be short or long (Fig. 16-1).

(6) Although *serous* and *mucous acini* appear in a ratio of 50/50, serous cells are in the majority. Mucous acini are capped by a half-moon layer of serous cells, the *serous demilunes*. The serous secretion is delivered to the duct lumen between mucous cells.

c. *Sublingual glands*, one on either side of the midline under the body of the tongue, open via several ducts alongside the opening of the submandibular ducts. A delicate *capsule* does not interfere with tongue movements.

(1) *Main excretory ducts*, the sublingual ducts.

(2) *Interlobular ducts*, present in sections.

(3) *Intralobular ducts*, numerous and prominent.

(4) *Striated ducts*, short; not in all sections.

(5) *Mucous acini*, capped by serous demilunes.

(6) *Serous acini* occur occasionally.

3. *Minor salivary glands* are distributed throughout the oral cavity. Of these, three are named:

a. *Anterior lingual salivary glands* (glands of Nuhn) are *muco-serous* glands opening on the ventral surface of the tongue close to the apex. The acini are located in the tongue musculature.

b. Serous *glands* of the *vallate papillae* (of von Ebner) empty in the sulcus surrounding the vallate papillae. Serous fluid flows over the pores of taste buds to put crystalline substances into solution to facilitate taste.

c. *Mucous gland* acini, deep in the substance of the root of the tongue, may open

(1) in the **sulcus terminalis** (see tongue),

(2) between lymphatic nodules,

(3) into the crypts of the lingual tonsils.

G. The *tongue*

1. *Development*

a. The *body* (anterior two thirds), the freely movable portion concerned with mastication (chewing) and diction (speaking), develops from

(1) Two swellings on the pharyngeal floor corresponding to the site of union of the *first branchial arches.*

(2) This part grows anteriorly (forward) beyond the *oropharyngeal membrane* to acquire a coating of *ectodermally* derived stratified squamous epithelium.

b. The *root* (posterior one third) originates at the fusion site of the *second* and *third branchial arches* (primarily the second branchial arch).

(1) This part develops posterior to the oropharyngeal membrane (within the pharynx), where it acquires an *endodermally* derived moist stratified squamous epithelium.

(2) *Lymphocytes* from the underlying *lingual tonsils* penetrate the epithelium to the surface.

(3) The primary function of the *root* of the tongue is *deglutition* (swallowing).

2. *Tongue demarcation:* The embryological junction of oral ectoderm (the body) and pharyngeal endoderm (the root) is demarcated by a depression, the **sulcus terminalis.** Anterior to the **sulcus terminalis** are the *vallate papillae* arranged in a "V" pointing posteriorly to the **foramen cecum,** the site of origin of the thyroid.

3. *Structure:* The *body* of a fully formed tongue possesses

a. *skeletal myocytes* coursing longitudinally, transversely, and vertically. This arrangement facilitates delicate tongue movements for speaking, chewing, drinking, and swallowing. Ordinarily, skeletal myocytes are not branched; however, the tongue is the only site in the body possessing *branched skeletal myocytes.*

b. *Lingual papillae* on the upper surface have stratified squamous epithelium covering cores of connective tissue.

(1) *Filiform papillae,* the most numerous of the papillae, come to one or two thread-like points. They cover the tongue and impart its roughness.

(2) *Fungiform papillae,* scattered among the filiform papillae, have smooth domes resembling fungi (mushrooms). A vascular core of connective tissue imparts a red color.

(3) *Vallate papillae* (9 to 12) are arranged in a "V" at the junction between the *body* and the *root* of the tongue anterior to the **sulcus terminalis.** A smaller moat-like *sulcus* around each papilla receives secretions from ducts of *serous glands of the vallate papillae*

(von Ebner). Embedded in the epithelium of the lateral walls of the papillae are *taste buds* (see below). A core of connective tissue supporting vessels and nerves fill the papilla. Fine papillae protrude into the epithelium of the superior surface.

(4) Well defined in the rabbit, leaf-like *foliate papillae* with taste buds, on each side of the tongue (below the sulcus terminalis), are poorly defined in humans.

4. The *root of the tongue* has a rather smooth surface in contrast to the rough surface of the *body*. In place of papillae, only mucosal wrinkles occur. *Lingual tonsils*, in the underlying connective tissue **lamina propria**, are aggregates of lymphatic nodules characterized by a central invagination or *crypt* of moist stratified squamous epithelium. (A *tonsil* is a group of lymphatic nodules under an epithelium.) Lymphocytes migrate through the epithelium and mix with desquamated cells and detritus.

5. *Taste buds* are onion-like elongated epithelial structures embedded in epithelium.

a. *Location:* surface of the tongue, vallate papillae, sometimes the fungiform and foliate papillae, cheeks, palate, pharynx, palatoglossal and palatopharyngeal arches, epiglottis, larynx, and upper esophagus.

b. *Cell types:* Murray (1969) suggested the terms type I, II, and III for taste bud cells.

(1) *Type I, sensory epithelial taste cells.* These sensory "dark cells" of earlier microscopists (Kolmer, 1927) constitute 55% of about 50 cells in a taste bud.

(a) Murray (1986) presented evidence that type I cells are not sensory cells, but *sustentacular cells,* for they

[1] *occupy* the outer layer of the bud,

[2] *sheathe* nerve endings,

[3] *coat* "light" cells,

[4] *phagocytize* dead cells after denervation of taste buds (Fujimoto and Murray, 1970).

(b) Type I cells extend from the taste bud base to a space below the taste pore. Microvilli project into the glycoprotein-filled space (probably secreted by the cell). A dense slender nucleus is surrounded by fine cytoplasmic filaments interspersed between electron-opaque granules. The granules appear to be discharged in response to a taste stimulus. Granular ER profiles are more prominent in this cell than in others.

(2) *Type II,* a *sustentacular epithelial cell,* the "light cell" of

light microscopists, composes 35% of the taste bud cells. The *type II cell* is now considered a *sensory taste cell.*

(a) According to Murray (1986), these cells are "lighter" than type I or III cells because there are no cytoplasmic fibrils or polyribosomes.

(b) The abundant sER appears dilated.

(c) Type II cells are separated from one another by type I cells and end with microvilli in the glycoprotein space below the taste pore.

(d) Their nuclei are the largest and least defense of all taste bud cells.

(e) Contacts between these cells and nerve terminals are extensive, with mitochondria aggregating at the contact sites.

(3) *Type III.* Murray (1969) demonstrated a less numerous cell, the *type III* cell, with characteristics of a gustatory receptor cell. Slightly darker than type II, *type III* is a slender cell extending from the base and ending in the taste pore by a terminal process (microvillus?).

(a) Cytoplasmic vesicles, with dense material, are more concentrated in the basal part of the cell.

(b) rER (not as much as type I) and sER (not as prominent as type II) are scattered throughout the cytoplasm.

(c) Groups of synaptic vesicles crowd the point where nerves contact the basal part of the cell.

(4) *Type IV, epithelial basal cell,* at the base of the taste bud serves as the progenitor replacing the other cells.

c. Taste buds in certain locations can distinguish sweet, sour, bitter, or salty. The statement, "Only substances in solution can be tasted," is substantiated by the temporary loss in ability to distinguish sugar from salt with a dry tongue (caused by atropine).

H. *Tonsils:* Functionally, the tonsils provide new lymphocytes for the body and protect against foreign organisms. Years ago, it was customary to excise inflamed tonsils, at about the time a child entered first grade. Loss of appetite was dramatically restored following excision. Case histories revealed that appetite usually returned whether or not the tonsils were removed. Current practice avoids tonsillectomies, recognizing their important immunological role.

1. *Palatine tonsils*

a. *Development: Endoderm* of the second pharyngeal sacs grows laterally into the surrounding mesoderm. Numerous endodermal evaginations penetrate the mesoderm, like fingers into clay. The pharyngeal cavity, via these epithelial evaginations, continues into the *tonsillar crypts*. Mesoderm surrounding the crypts forms stroma and capsule.

    b. *Location:* Palatine tonsils fit in the arches formed by the palatoglossus and palatopharyngeus muscles at the junction of the oral cavity and the pharynx.

    c. *Tonsillar crypts* are invaginations lined by a thickened layer of moist stratified squamous epithelium. From the 10 to 20 lymphocytic nodules around the crypts, small lymphocytes arise to populate the epithelium. Desquamated cells, detritus, and bacteria plugging the crypts may become sources of inflammation.

    d. *Connective tissue* cells and fibers common to other lymphatic tissues are found in the tonsil. All sizes of lymphocytes, neutrophilic granulocytes, and plasma cells are present.

    2. *Pharyngeal tonsils*

    a. *Location:* On the roof of the nasopharynx, there is another mass of lymphatic tissue, the *pharyngeal tonsils* (adenoids).

    b. **Epithelium:** Instead of crypts, the epithelium is thrown into folds. The interior and surface of the folds are covered with pseudostratified ciliated columnar epithelium, while the periphery is protected by moist stratified squamous epithelium. Lymphocytes invading the epithelium impart a bizarre appearance.

    3. The *tubal tonsils* are one of the minor tonsils at the pharyngeal orifice of the *auditory* tube.

    4. *Lingual tonsils* reside in the root of the tongue.

    5. *Aging of tonsils*: Lingual, palatine, pharyngeal, and minor tonsils undergo gradual *aging involution*, noted by infiltrating connective tissue and adipocytes and diminution of nodular germinal centers. The tonsils are highly developed up to puberty, followed by gradual involution about the same time as the thymus. This curious fact may be related to hormonal and sexual development.

    6. *Immunological function:* The tonsils form an impressive immunological ring (Waldeyer's ring) of lymphatic tissue guarding the entrance to the pharynx.

The Tubes of the Digestive Tract

I. *Development* (Moore, 1988): The epithelium of the esophagus, stomach, and intestine develops from endoderm of the *archenteron* (primitive gut). The foregut and hindgut unite at the yolk stalk.

A. *Mesentery:* Reflections of peritoneal mesothelium from the dorsal wall suspend the primitive gut in a double layer of mesothelium, the *mesentery.* Vasculature, nerves, and connective tissue cells and fibers pass between the two mesothelial layers.

B. *Retroperitoneal:* Some portions of the developing gut are suspended by the mesentery, while others are covered by mesothelium on one surface. Viscera in the latter condition are referred to as *retroperitoneal* (Fig. 16-2).

II. *Layers common to all segments of the digestive tubes:* Despite anatomical modifications of the digestive tract, several components are common to each of the segments. Specifics will be considered with the segments. From inside to outside, the layers are described below (Fig. 16-2).

Figure 16-2 *A.* Layers of the digestive tube and associated glands. *B.* A retroperitoneal segment of the tube.

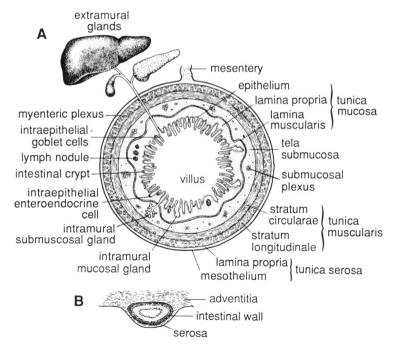

A. Tunica mucosa, the innermost layer facing the lumen of the tubes is composed of

1. **epithelium mucosae** (type of epithelium),

2. *basement membrane*, produced by the epithelium,

3. **lamina propria mucosae** (connective tissue conveying vasculature, lymphatics, and nerves),

4. **lamina muscularis mucosae,** composed of smooth myocytes.

B. Tela submucosa, a connective tissue layer conveying the major vasculature, nerves, and lymphatics. The *submucosal nerve plexus* (of Meissner) is housed in this layer.

C. Tunica muscularis, a bi- or trilayered muscle layer of skeletal striated or nonstriated (smooth) myocytes, depending on the segment.

1. **Stratum circulare,** the inner layer around the tela submucosa, composed of bundles of myocytes spiraled around the tube like a tightly wound spring.

2. *Myenteric nerve plexus* (of Auerbach) consists of several small ganglia situated between the stratum circulare and the stratum longitudinale.

3. **Stratum longitudinale,** the outer layer, is composed of loosely wound bundles of myocytes, resembling a stretched-out spring. An exception to this "spiraling" is the outer longitudinal **tenia coli** of the large intestine.

D. Tela subserosa is a thin layer of connective tissue separating the tunica muscularis from tunica serosa. Blood vessels, nerves, and lymphatics ramify through this layer.

E. Tunica serosa, enclosing the tube, consists of

1. **lamina propria serosae,** a connective tissue layer,

2. *basement membrane*, produced by mesothelium,

3. **mesothelium** of the mesentery suspending the gut. Tissue fluid from capillary networks in the lamina propria serosae crosses the mesothelium via micropinocytotic vesicles. The tissue fluid, a *transudate*, lubricates the mesothelial surface to enable intestines to glide against one another and prevent adhesions. Any mesothelium that transports a fluid is designated a *serous membrane*, thus **serosa**.

F. Tunica adventitia [fibrosa, Capsula]. If a tube is covered by a tunica serosa on one side only, then the opposite side must be protected by a layer of connective tissue, the **tunica adventitia** (examples: duodenum, ascending and descending colon). The esophagus and rectum have a complete tunica adventitia.

III. *Increasing the surface area of the digestive tubes*

A. *Coiling* of the intestines, to pack as long a tube as possible in the least available space.

B. *Intramural glands* (within the wall) originate from the surface epithelium and invaginate into the lamina propria mucosae or tela submucosa.

C. *Extramural glands* (outside the wall) originate from the intestinal epithelium, penetrate the layers, and develop outside the wall in associated mesenteries (liver, pancreas).

D. Plicae circulares, in the small intestine, increase surface area by fourfold.

E. Villi, evaginations of the tunica mucosa in the duodenum, jejunum, and ileum, increase the surface area by 10-fold.

F. *Submicroscopic modifications* for maximum absorption:

1. *microvilli* on the surface of intestinal cells,

2. *glycocalyx* on the microvilli.

IV. *Cell types of the digestive tubes*

A. Moist *stratified squamous cells* are characteristic of the esophageal epithelium. A stratum granulosum is absent. Cells desquamated every two or three days are replaced by cells dividing in the deeper layers.

B. *Superficial gastric epithelial cells* are columnar mucous surface cells of the stomach that discharge a carbohydrate-rich glycoprotein mucous blanket that protects the mucosa from the digestive action of acidic gastric juices. The mucin secretion is composed of electron-dense, membrane-bound granules. Surface cells are replaced by dividing cells in the isthmus of the gastric glands. The luminal surface of the cells is characterized by a few short microvilli with a filamentous glycocalyx.

C. *Cardiac exocrine cells* are mucous-secreting cells of the cardiac stomach.

D. *Undifferentiated epithelial cells,* confined to the neck of gastric glands, have the potential to develop into other cells of the gastric glands.

E. *Mucous neck cells* of gastric glands resemble the mucous surface cells, but their mucin granules are larger and not as electron dense.

1. The basal region is filled with dilated cisternae of rER. Mitochondria are dispersed throughout the cell. Toward the apical region, numerous mucin granules wait to be discharged.

2. In H & E preparations, *mucous neck cells* are difficult to distinguish from principal exocrine cells. To differentiate, PAS reagent or mucicarmine stain reveals the mucin mucopolysaccarides. Pathologists value this staining property when identifying poorly differentiated tumors.

3. *Mucous neck cells* appear in embryos between 11 and 12 weeks of gestation.

F. *Principal exocrine cells* (chief cells) comprise part of the epithelium of the walls of the *gastric glands*. Their apical cytoplasm is filled with *zymogen granules* containing *pepsinogen*.

1. In a low pH environment, created by HCl, pepsinogen is hydrolyzed to *pepsin*. Pepsin is an active proteolytic enzyme that splits large protein molecules into amino acids for absorption by intestinal cells.

2. Abundant rER, responsible for its basophilia, and a well-developed golgi complex confirm the cell's protein secretory capacity. Mitochondria are scattered in the cytoplasm. Short microvilli exist on the luminal surface, while longitudinal folds form the lateral cell surfaces.

G. *Parietal exocrine cells*, scattered along the epithelial walls of the gastric glands, produce HCl.

1. Differentiation of *parietal cells* occurs at 11 weeks of gestation, the earliest of all gastric mucosal cells.

2. In H & E preparations, these cells are strongly acidophilic. TEM reveals that the luminal surface is invaginated by branching *intracellular canaliculi*. Numerous fine microvilli protruding into the *canalicular lumen* increase the surface area of the cell membrane for exchange of sodium and hydrogen ions.

3. The energy required for the ionic exchange, in producing HCl, is provided by **mitochondria** occupying the available space between the nucleus and protoplasmic surface of the canalicular plasmalemma. Gastric HCl production is stimulated by the peptide hormone *gastrin*.

4. Smooth ER is required for the production of HCl. Thus rER is minimal and the golgi complex is not very prominent.

5. Parietal exocrine cells produce *gastric intrinsic factor*, a chemical substance necessary for the absorption of vitamin B_{12} in the ileum. Loss of parietal exocrine cells, by disease or surgery, results in the inability to absorb vitamin B_{12}, resulting in *pernicious anemia*. Recovery of the patient follows continued injections of vitamin B_{12}. Oral administration is ineffective because without intrinsic factor, the ileum can not absorb vitamin B_{12}.

6. *Aging:* Parietal cells decrease in number with age, resulting in an increased risk of pernicious anemia in the elderly.

H. *Gastrointestinal endocrine cells* occur in the lining epithelium of the stomach, small intestine, large intestine, respiratory apparatus, and the pancreas. Their metabolic conversion of amines, ie, *a*mine *p*recursor *u*ptake and *d*ecarboxylation, results in the acronym *APUD cells*. Old names are argentaffin cells, argyrophilic cells, and chromaffin cells, depending on the affinities of cytoplasmic granules for certain dyes.

1. *APUD cells* are intraepithelial endocrine unicellular endocrine glands. Prevailing evidence strongly indicates that these cells derive from the *neural crest*.

2. *History:* Only two types were recognized:

a. *argentaffin cells* reduce silver nitrate *directly*, without the need for pretreatment with extraneous reducing agents. This cell is the *enterochromaffin cell (EC cell)* because its granules stain intensely with fixatives using bichromate salts.

b. *argyrophil cells* required pretreatment with a reducing agent prior to treatment with silver nitrate.

c. Immunocytochemistry and TEM have accelerated the identification of additional cell types correlated with specific hormones. The number of cells identified to date establishes the gastrointestinal tract as the site of major endocrine activity.

3. Most hormones secreted by the gastrointestinal APUD cells are predominantly *polypeptides*. Not only can the APUD cells synthesize polypeptide hormones, but they can synthesize and secrete *biogenic amines*. Digestive apparatus nerves and CNS nerves share this ability.

4. *APUD cells*, distributed in the mucosal epithelium along the length of the gastrointestinal tract, are interspersed between the principal cells at the base of gastric glands and between the secretory cells of the intestinal glands.

a. All appear triangular in profile. The broad base rests on the gland basement membrane close to the basement membrane of surrounding capillaries.

b. Membrane-bound secretory granules are located, almost exclusively, in the basal cytoplasm close to the basement membrane. Electron microscopy facilitated identification of cell types based on granule shape, size, and disposition.

5. *Hormones of the APUD cells:* The number and variety of APUD cell types related to specific cell types and the hormones secreted is increasing as old methods improve and newer ones develop (Pearse, 1974; Pearse et al, 1977; Dawson, 1977; Gapp, 1986) (Table 16-3).

I. *Columnar epithelial cells* with microvilli are the absorptive cells lining the duodenum, jejunum, and ileum. These cells decrease in number as the colon is approached. Absorptive cells of the colon are surpassed in number by goblet cells.

1. The luminal surface is covered with **microvilli** to provide a large absorptive surface area (the old striated border of light microscopy). On the surface of cells capping the largest intestinal villi, microvilli may be 1 to 1.5 μm in length. The glycocalyx covering the microvilli may be 0.1 to 0.5 μm in thickness.

2. Some cells are more specialized for *lipid absorption* than others, since lipids enter columnar cells at the bases of microvilli via micropinocytosis. Actin-like filaments, occupying the core of the microvilli, not only serve a structural function, but also by contracting they "milk" emulsified lipids toward the base of the microvilli, where they enter as membrane-bound droplets.

3. Mitochondria, distributed throughout the cell, are more numerous in the basal portion. The *golgi complex* occupies a supranuclear position surrounded by the *sER*, which accounts for the slight acidophilia, and *rER* occupies an infranuclear position.

4. Microvilli contain important *enzymes* required for the final stages of absorption. Enzymes produced by individual cells appear at about the 10th week of gestation. Synthesis of *lactase* does not occur until just prior to birth, and then at very low levels. *Lactase deficiency*, causing milk intolerance in infants, may persist into adulthood.

J. *Goblet cells* are so named because they resemble a wine goblet.

Table 16-3. APUD Cell Hormones

Hormone	Cell*	Cell location	Hormone action
Cholecystokinin	I	resembles EG cells. duodenum, jejunum, and possibly ileum	contraction of gall bladder, induces bile flow, stimulates pancreas to secrete alkaline juices
Endorphin	?	wide distribution	morphine like
Enkephalin	?	wide distribution	stimulates smooth muscle contraction, inhibits pancreatic and gastric acid secretion
Enteroglucagon	EG	resemble α-cells. fundic glands, jejunum, ileum, colon. most numerous in ileum	reduces bowel motility to increase digestion time, stimulates growth of intestinal mucosa
Gastric inhibitory peptide (bombasin)	K	middle zone of glands in duodenum and jejunum	inhibits secretion of gastric acid and pepsin, stimulates insulin release
Gastrin**	G	pyloric antrum, basal duodenal glands, first part of jejunum	regulates HCl production by parietal cells of the stomach
Glucagon (pancreatic type)	A	stomach	hepatic glycogenolysis
Glucagon (gut type)	L	small intestine, colon resemble α-cells of pancreatic islets	antagonist to insulin by stimulating hepatic glycogenolysis
Histamine	?	pyloric glands, intestinal glands	Stimulate HCl production
Motilin	EC	duodenum, jejunum	contraction stomach musculature; acts in response to alkaline intestinal secretion
Neurotensin	N	ileum	inhibits gastric motor activity
Noradrenalin	EC	duodenum, jejunum, ileum	increases blood pressure, minimal effect on heart rate and cardiac output

Table 16-3. APUD Cell Hormones (*continued*)

Hormone	Cell*	Cell location	Hormone action
Peptide histidine isoleucine	?	wide distribution	similar to VIP (below)
Secretin***	S	duodenum, upper jejunum, maybe the ileum, bases of villi and upper crypts of glands	stimulates: pancreatic exocrine secretions, insulin release, pyloric musculature
Serotonin	EC	stomach, intestinal glands, appendix	stimulates smooth muscle, increases gut motility
Somatostatin	D	midzone gastric glands and intestinal glands, D cells of pancreas	inhibits release of growth hormone, paracrine regulatory action on closely associated cells
Substance P	EC	wide distribution	stimulates smooth muscle contraction
Vasoactive intestinal peptide (VIP)	D_1	fundus of stomach and intestines	similar to glucagon and secretin, dilates small intestinal arteries, raises blood glucose levels, stimulates exocrine pancreas

*Cell names are listed by letter. The *Nomina Histologica* has one generic name: **endocrinocytus gastrointestinalis.** Until there is general international agreement, the letters above will do. Most letters have meanings: EC = enterochromaffin, D = delta cell, A = alpha cell, etc.

**Four known forms of *gastrin* are named according to the number of amino acids in the polypeptide chain: *G-13* = little-little gastrin, *G-17* = little gastrin, *G-34* = big gastrin, a complete a.a. sequence, and *G-?* = big-big gastrin. It is possible that these may produce different forms of gastrin, with different actions.

***The S cells possess 100–150-nm electron-dense, membrane-bound granules. A halo between the granule and its membrane characterizes this cell type.

Mucus builds up and discharges en masse to coat the intestinal surface.

1. The apical cytoplasm is filled with mucin droplets that dissolve out in routine histological preparations. Special methods (ie, PAS method) for mucopolysaccharides are required to preserve the mucin.

2. The nucleus resides in the narrow basal portion of the cell (the

goblet stem). In early stages of droplet development, the nucleus may ascend along with other cytoplasmic structures. But as *mucus* accumulates, the nucleus and accompanying cytoplasmic structures are forced back into the stem.

3. *Goblet cells* first appear at the pyloro-duodenal junction and increase in number through the intestinal tract, reaching their greatest population in the large intestine. They are absent in the anal canal. In certain abnormal conditions they may appear in the stomach. The product, *mucus*, coats the entire epithelial surface.

K. *Columnar exocrine cells* of the intestinal gland epithelium are mucous producing cells. These cells dribble mucus rather than sudden discharge of the entire mass as in a goblet cell.

L. *Exocrine cell with acidophilic granules* (cells of Paneth) occupy the bases of the *intestinal glands* (crypts). This cell is an exocrine *serous* cell reaching its peak population in the ileum and the appendix (Erlandson and Chase 1972).

1. The secretory granules contain *lysozyme*, an enzyme that digests the walls of bacteria. It is presumed that these exocrine cells control the intestinal flora via antibacteriocidal action of lysozyme.

2. In inflammatory disorders, the *exocrine cells with acidophilic granules* may appear in other regions of the digestive tract.

3. TEM reveals electron dense membrane bound granules, extensive granular endoplasmic reticulum and a prominent golgi complex. The luminal surface is covered with microvilli.

Segments of the Digestive Tract

I. The *esophagus* is a relatively straight channel differentiated to conduct food to the stomach. The following layers are outlined:

A. Tunica mucosa

1. Epithelium mucosae is moist stratified squamous. While keratohyalin granules may appear in some superficial nucleated cells, keratinization *does not* normally occur.

a. *Development:* The embryonic esophagus is lined by simple columnar epithelium that becomes double layered with surface cilia after two months of intrauterine life. Between 2.5 and 3 months, the epithelium stratifies and loses its cilia. *Epithelial rests* of ciliated epithelium (rests are small islands of epithelium) may persist in infants and adults.

b. *Renewal:* The epithelial cells are constantly in the process of renewal, with mitotic figures appearing in the lower layers. Cells in the deepest layer are basophilic, attesting to the production of proteins in the granular endoplasmic reticulum. Differentiated cells in the superficial layers lose their ability to divide. An increase in keratohyalin granules imparts an acidophilia to the superficial cell layers.

c. *Anchoring:* The epithelium is anchored to the lamina propria mucosae by the *basement membrane* laid down by the basal cells. *Hemidesmosomes* anchor the epithelium to the basement membrane.

2. The **lamina propria mucosae** contains elements common to loose connective tissues.

a. *Ducts* of two types of esophageal glands pass through the lamina propria mucosae to empty their secretions onto the epithelial surface. Lymphatic nodules surrounding the ducts frequently assist in locating the ducts.

b. *Esophageal glands proper* are found in the **tela submucosa** and will be described with that layer.

c. *Esophageal cardiac glands* have secretory portions in the lamina propria mucosae. In man, these are branched tubular glands with mucous-secreting acini.

(1) *Esophageal cardiac glands* occur in

(a) the first part of the esophagus from the cricoid cartilage to the level of the fifth tracheal cartilage,

(b) the terminal portion of the esophagus close to the cardiac stomach.

(2) *Esophageal cardiac glands* have clinical significance, particularly if they possess aberrant parietal exocrine cells that produce HCl. Esophageal ulcers and various carcinomas have been attributed to the excessive activity of these deviate cells.

(3) *APUD cells* have been found occasionally in the lamina propria mucosae.

3. Lamina muscularis mucosae is composed of longitudinally oriented nonstriated (smooth) myocyte bundles and networks of elastic fibers. This lamina begins as a thin layer and thickens as it approaches the stomach.

B. The **tela submucosa** is a layer of dense irregular connective tissue, composed of bundles of collagen and elastic fibers, containing the esophageal glands proper.

1. The **tela submucosa** is thrown into temporary folds so that the lumen of the esophagus assumes a stellate shape. The elasticity of these folds facilitates enlargement of the lumen during swallowing and contraction to its original shape.

2. The *esophageal glands proper*, distributed randomly throughout the tela submucosa, are mucous, branched, tubuloalveolar glands.

    a. While generally confined to the submucosa, a cross section of the esophagus (midpoint of its length) might possess both esophageal glands proper in the lamina propria mucosae.

    b. This finding can be explained developmentally. During development, some esophageal glands proper (developing from esophageal epithelium) fail to penetrate the lamina muscularis and hence they settle permanently in the lamina propria mucosae.

3. *Lymphatic nodules*, as well as scattered lymphocytes, may be found in the tela submucosa.

4. A delicate *network* of *lymphatic vessels*, pervading the tela submucosa, accounts for the rapid spread of esophageal carcinomas. Also, major blood vessels and a *submucosal nerve plexus* of ganglion cells and nerves are found in this layer.

C. The **tunica muscularis:** Consider the esophagus in three somewhat unequal, variable regions: *upper*, *middle*, and *lower*. Through its length, it increases in thickness from 0.5 to 2.5 mm.

    1. Two muscle layers are easily distinguished:
        a. inner **stratum circulare** (a tight spring),
        b. outer **stratum longitudinale** (a loose spring).

    2. In the *upper region* of the esophagus, both strata consist of striated skeletal myocyte bundles.

    3. In the *lower region* (closer to the stomach), the muscle is all nonstriated (smooth) muscle.

    4. The *middle region* contains both nonstriated and striated muscle. Closer to the upper region, smooth muscle appears while toward the lower portion skeletal muscle disappears.

    5. A *myenteric plexus* of nerve fibers and ganglion cells exists between the two muscle layers to control the peristaltic muscular movements of the esophagus during deglutition.

    6. The existance of a rich network of *lymphatic vessels* within the muscle layers, as well as the tela submucosa, encourages the spread of esophageal carcinoma.

D. Tunica adventitia [fibrosa]: The esophagus is not suspended by a mesentery from the posterior thoracic wall, and hence is totally retroperitoneal. At one small point the pleural somatic mesothelium may be interpreted as a bit of esophageal serosal lining (Amenta, 1987). It can be generalized that there is no **tunica serosa**. Instead, a thick layer of connective tissue joins the esophagus to surrounding structures (example: trachea).

II. The *stomach* stores food and begins the process of digestion by the action of its powerful muscular walls and activity of its gastric glandular secretions. Solid foods are churned to an acidic fluid, the *chyme*, which is intermittently squirted into the duodenum.

    A. Three parts are considered:

      1. Part I, the *cardia*, is a region about 25 mm long (range: 5 to 40 mm) commencing at the junction with the esophagus.

      2. Part II consists of

        a. the *fundus*, the dome-like portion to the left of the cardia. Usually filled with air, it is detected readily in x-rays.

        b. the *body*, which comprises the bulbous first two thirds of the stomach.

        c. the *intermediate portion*, which is the narrow canal of the body, leading to the pyloris.

      3. Part III, the *pyloris*, a region about 5 cm long, connects the stomach to the first part of the *duodenum*.

    B. Part I of the stomach, the *cardia*

      1. The *esophageal–cardiac junction* is marked by an abrupt change of epithelium from stratified squamous to simple columnar.

      2. An SEM view of the mucosal surface reveals mucous cells with numerous mucus droplets pinching off. These cells are the *superficial gastric epitheliocytes*, commonly called mucous surface cells. Normally, there are no goblet cells in the epithelium.

      3. Surface openings, the *gastric foveolae*, lead into the mucous-secreting *cardiac glands* residing in the lamina propria mucosae. These are branched, tubuloalveolar, mucous-secreting glands, distinguished from the pyloric glands by the length of the necks:

        a. *cardiac glands* have short necks, occupying one quarter the thickness of the mucosa.

        b. *pyloric glands* have long necks, occupying one half the thickness of the mucosa.

    C. Part II of the stomach: Commencing in the *fundus* and continuing throughout the body, the cardiac glands give way to long (up to 1.5 mm) forked-type *gastric glands proper* with short necks. The neck connects to two, three, or more long straight tubular gland portions that do not coil or branch.

1. *Mucous surface epithelium* and *mucous neck cells* are fairly uniform throughout the stomach.

a. The mucous surface cells form simple columnar epithelium that dips into the *gastric foveolae* (sometimes preferred to as gastric pits). The *mucous surface cells* continuously produce a neutral glycoprotein that protects the entire tunica mucosa from constant exposure to the harsh activity of gastric acidic juices.

(1) For this reason it is not surprising that this epithelium undergoes continual renewal. The life span of a mucous cell is about 3 days.

(2) New cells migrate onto the surface from mucous neck cells and mucous surface cells protected in the gastric foveolae (LeBlond, 1981).

b. *Mucous neck cells* are those forming the neck below the gastric foveolus and extend to the upper part of the gastric gland. In the latter location they may be interspersed with the principal exocrine cells.

(1) The secretion is an *acidic* glycoprotein, in contrast to the neutral glycoprotein of the mucous surface cells.

(2) The rER confers a more basophilic appearance than the mucous surface cells, and the golgi complex accordingly is larger. In contrast to the surface cells, the larger mucous droplets are more spherical and less dense.

2. *Fundic* and *body glands* are characterized by the appearance and increasing numbers of parietal exocrine cells, principal exocrine cells, and occasional APUD cells.

a. *Parietal exocrine cells* produce a 0.1N solution of HCl. Ordinarily this concentration would destroy any living cell. This cell type is characterized by the following features:

(1) several *intracellular canaliculi*, lined by microvilli to increase the surface area. HCl is produced along this vast surface. Along the bottom and lateral surfaces are receptors for acetylcholine, gastrin, and histamine, required to initiate production of HCl and bicarbonate.

(2) a rich tubular sER. During acid secretion the sER subsides and the microvilli increase in size and number. When acid is not being produced, sER builds up and microvilli subside.

(3) an acidophilia, due to mitochondria and sER. Mitochondria, packed between the intracellular canaliculi, are required for the high energy requirements involved in producing HCl.

b. *Principal exocrine cells*, with zymogen granules, are characteristic protein-secreting cells. These cells, elaborating *pepsinogen*, compose the major population of the gastric glands.

D. Part III, the *pyloris*, contains the long-necked *pyloric glands* (about one half the depth of the mucosa), which begin in the *intermediate portion* where the *gastric glands* end. The pyloris occupies one ninth of the entire stomach.

E. *Layers of the stomach*

1. Tunica mucosa (0.25 mm in the pars cardica to 1.5 mm in the pyloris)

a. Epithelium mucosae, considered above with glands.

b. Lamina propria mucosae houses the glands of the stomach, which are surrounded by scattered lymphocytes, plasma cells, and loose connective tissue. The plasma cells secrete immunoglobulin type A (IgA), which is important in combatting infectious agents that may invade the epithelium. A *subepithelial capillary network* resides in this layer, along with a *subepithelial lymphocapillary network*.

c. Lamina muscularis mucosae lies under the bases of the glands of the stomach. Bundles of nonstriated (smooth) myocytes are arranged into

(1) a *inner circular layer* sends slips of myocytes between the glands up to the epithelium. Their contraction pulls the epithelium down to assist the expression of the glandular contents.

(2) an *outer longitudinal layer*.

(3) an *outer circular layer* may appear in some areas.

2. Tela submucosa is a connective tissue layer thrown into folds that form the gastric **rugae**. Lymphoid aggregates occur as well as diffusely spread lymphocytes and plasma cells. Located here are the

a. *submucosal nerve plexus,*

b. *submucosal lymphatic plexus,*

c. *submucosal arterioles,*

d. *submucosal venous plexus.*

3. Tunica muscularis is composed of three layers that are quite difficult to define, since they are lacking in some areas. The disposition of smooth muscle around curvatures and areas of thickening compound the problem.

a. Inner *oblique fibers*. Since this is an incomplete layer, it is designated simply as oblique fibers of smooth myocytes.

b. Middle **stratum circulare** is a complete layer that increases in thickness in the pyloris, especially where it forms the muscle of the *pyloric sphincter*.

   c. The outer **stratum longitudinale** continues from the longitudinal stratum of the esophagus.

   d. The myenteric nerve plexus is distributed between the two strata.

   4. Tunica serosa: The stomach is covered by simple squamous mesothelium resting on a basement and a **lamina propria serosae** over the outer stratum longitudinale of the **tunica muscularis.**

   F. *Pyloro-duodenal junction:* In the transition from the pyloris to the duodenum, the following changes are noted:

   1. The epithelium changes abruptly from simple columnar mucous surface cell type to *simple columnar epithelium.* The latter, distinguished by lumenal **microvilli** (the striated border of light microscopy), is specialized for absorption.

   2. *Goblet cells* characterize the epithelium of all the intestines and appear first at the abrupt change of epithelium.

   3. At the pyloric junction, the thickened tunica muscularis forms an annular sphincter. On contraction it "squirts" chyme into the duodenum.

   4. In the duodenum, the tunica muscularis of nonstriated (smooth) myocytes returns to the typical bilayered type.

   5. Villi appear on the duodenal side of the junction. *Intestinal glands* (of Lieberkuhn) empty into *intestinal crypts* at their bases.

   6. Lymphatic nodules occur at the pyloroduodenal junction, similar to those occurring at the esophageal–cardiac junction.

   7. Appearance of *submucosal duodenal glands* (Brunner), which in man may protrude back into the submucosa of the pyloris.

III. The *small intestine* is about 6 meters long (20 feet). The **tunica muscularis** is composed of an inner **stratum circulare** and an outer **stratum longitudinale**, sandwiching the *myenteric nerve plexus.* The tunica muscularis is responsible for *peristalsis*, a wave-like contraction that moves intestinal contents down the small intestine a few centimeters a second. Isolated lymphatic nodules, in the lamina propria mucosae, occur throughout the intestinal tract, increasing in number toward the colon.

   A. The **duodenum**, the retroperitoneal first segment of the small intestine, embraces the head of the pancreas. It measures about two and a half hand widths, or 12 finger breadths, named by the ancient method of measuring with hands and fingers.

1. The first 5 cm of the lumenal surface appears relatively *smooth*, being lined only with large leaf-like **villi**. Via SEM, the villi appear like closely packed cactus leaves. The surface of villi is covered by intestinal columnar cells with microvilli.

2. The remainder of the duodenum has a striking wrinkled appearance. These wrinkles are permanent, spirally oriented folds, the **plicae circulaers**, which are covered with villi. Both the tunica mucosa and tela submucosa are drawn into the plicae circulares.

3. The straight first portion of the duodenum curves sharply around the head of the pancreas. About midway in the arch, the *duodenal papilla* appears as the united terminus of the pancreatic duct and the bile duct. From the pyloric sphincter to the duodenal papilla lies a distance of 7.5 cm.

4. *Duodenal glands* occupy the submucosa from the pyloris to the duodenal papilla. Thereafter they diminish in size until they disappear. These glands distinguish this part of the duodenum.

a. The terminal submucosal portions are highly coiled branching tubules arranged in lobules 0.5 to 1.0 mm in diameter. The ducts penetrate the **lamina muscularis mucosae** and empty into the *intestinal crypts* (Lieberkuhn).

b. The duodenal glands probably secrete zymogen granules in addition to mucus. Mucus in the first part of the duodenum protects the tunica mucosa from the acidic gastric contents.

5. The **lamina propria mucosae** contains networks of lymphocapillaries that commence in the villi as blind-ended *lacteals*. Accommodation of absorbed emulsified fats in the lacteals is an important function of these lymphatics.

B. Jejunum (Latin: empty). The beginning of the *jejunum* is difficult to delineate. To the surgeon it is the site where the duodenum exits its retroperitoneal position and acquires a mesentery for the next 8 feet of intestine. If the histological section preserves the tunica serosa and **plicae circulares** are present, together with longer narrower villi, identification is enhanced.

C. Ileum (Greek: to roll up or twist). The ileum is the remaining 12 feet of coiled small intestine.

1. Villi are long and narrow, like those of the jejunum.

2. Absorptive cells, fewer; goblet cells, more.

3. *Aggregated lymphatic nodules* (Peyer's patches), with up to 40 nodules in a row in the lamina propria mucosae, are unique to the ileum. Over nodules, villi are smaller or absent. The epithelium is filtrated with lymphocytes.

IV. *Large intestine:* 1.5 m long (5 ft)

   A. *Colon:* Striking differences exist between the small intestine and the colon. The entire wall is thinner and feels like parchment in *sacculations* (outpouchings) between the **tenia coli.**

     1. Tunica mucosa: Villi are absent.

      a. Goblet cells are more numerous.

      b. Superficial columnar cells, fewer in number, have smaller and fewer microvilli.

      c. Intestinal glands (crypts) are deeper.

       (1) Undifferentiated cells replace surface cells.

       (2) Many more goblet cells.

       (3) Columnar mucous cells fewer.

       (4) *No* exocrine cells with acidophilic granules.

      d. APUD cells occur as described above.

     2. Tunica muscularis: Most of the stratum longitudinale is gathered into three equidistant bands, the **tenia coli.**

     3. Tunica serosa surrounds the transverse colon, but the ascending and descending colon are frequently retroperitoneal, with serosa covering only the surface facing the peritoneal cavity. It is not unusual for the ascending and descending portions to acquire a mesocolon (a mesentery) so that a serosa covers all surfaces.

     4. Tunica adventitia protects the surface opposite the tunica serosa if the ascending and descending segments of the colon are retroperitoneal.

     5. Appendices epiploicae are lobules of adipose tissue, surrounded with serosal mesothelium, hanging from the free surface of the colon opposite the mesocolon or the adventitia.

   B. *Vermiform* (worm-shaped) *appendix*, appended to the base of the *cecum* (first part of the colon), ranges from 2 to 18 cm in length. A *mesoappendix* suspends it in the lower right quadrant of the abdominal cavity. The appendix is an important component of the immune system, in a sentry position at the first part of the colon.

     1. Tunica mucosa: Epithelium is composed of columnar cells with microvilli and only a few goblet cells. Villi are lacking, and the lamina muscularis mucosae is poorly developed.

      a. Five to 10 APUD cells and exocrine cells (with acidophilic granules) occupy an intestinal gland. A predominant APUD cell is that which secretes *serotonin*. *Argentaffinomas*, carcinoid tumors of the appendix, produce excessive amounts of serotonin.

    b. Most characteristic are the lymphatic nodules arranged in a ring in the lamina propria mucosae. Nodules can increase in size to such a degree that the angular lumen may be occluded, causing the inflammation known as *appendicitis*.

    2. The **tunica submucosa** is a thickened connective tissue layer supporting numerous blood vessels, lymphatics, and nerve plexuses.

    3. Tunica muscularis: The three bands (tenia coli) of the stratum longitudinale come together at the base of the cecum to form a thin continuous layer. A complete stratum circulare appears slightly thicker.

    C. The *rectum* (12 cm long) resembles the colon.

    1. Tunica mucosa

    a. *Intestinal glands* are straight, like long test tubes lined almost exclusively with goblet cells.

    (1) APUD cells may be found, and exocrine cells with acidophilic granules, though generally absent, may appear in some inflammatory disorders.

    (2) Toward the end of the rectum, the intestinal glands decrease in length and gradually disappear.

    b. The tunica mucosa evaginates into several longitudinal *rectal columns* (Morgagni).

    c. The **lamina muscularis mucosae** thins out and becomes interrupted until it disappears.

    d. In the united **lamina propria mucosae** and **tela submucosa** the veins are more flaccid and thin walled. These vessels are prime targets of varicosities or dilatations, resulting in *hemorrhoids*.

    2. Just before the anal canal, the rectal columns disappear, and at about 3 cm above the anal orifice the columnar epithelium changes abruptly to moist stratified squamous. Proctologists recognize this as the **linea anorectalis** (white line of Hilton). Lymphatic nodules may be present, as in other junctions.

    D. *Anal canal* (4 cm long): External to the anal orifice, the stratified squamous epithelium becomes keratinized, and hair follicles appear. This is the **linea anocutanea.**

    1. Large *circumanal sudoriferous glands* (up to 5 mm in diameter) in the subcutaneous connective tissue discharge their secretions in plasmalemma membranous envelopes.

2. The **tunica muscularis** is modified as follows:

a. The stratum longitudinale (nonstriated muscle) shortens to cause bulging of the mucosa as *transverse circular folds.*

b. At the anal canal, the stratum circulare (nonstriated muscle) thickens to form the internal sphincter of the anus.

c. The external sphincter is composed of striated skeletal muscle.

Extramural Glands of the Digestive Tract

I. Pancreas (Greek: all flesh): The ancient Hebrews called it the "finger of the liver" and noted it in the Talmud. The name **pancreas** was coined by Ruphas of Ephesus about A.D. 100. Some 400 years earlier, Herophilus made the earliest known anatomical description.

A. *Development:* The pancreas is a major digestive gland that develops from endoderm of the duodenum.

1. During the fifth week of gestation, dorsal, followed by ventral, evaginations of endoderm grow into the loose connective tissue of the dorsal and ventral mesenteries.

2. During the sixth week, rotation of the gut brings the ventral mass around to fuse with the dorsal portion, resulting in

a. the duct of the ventral mass becomes the main *pancreatic duct,*

b. the duct of the dorsal mass atrophies or persists as an *accessory duct.*

3. Continued growth of the ducts gives rise to two portions of the pancreas:

a. an *exocrine* portion with secretory cells surrounding the duct ends,

b. an *endocrine* portion in which the blind ends of the proliferating ducts give rise to isolated *pancreatic islets* (Langerhans).

(1) Though the ducts to the islets atrophy or never develop lumena, they may be traced (following appropriate staining techniques) to their termini to count the islets.

(2) The number of islets, varying from 200,000 to 1,800,000, increase in number and concentration toward the tail.

4. Following rotation of the gut, the pancreas lies against the posterior abdominal wall covered on its anterior surface with mesothelium. The posterior surface lies against an adventitial connective tissue bed. Thus, the pancreas is *retroperitoneal.*

B. *General structure*

1. *Capsule:* A gossamer capsule surrounds the entire pancreas, rendering the pancreas vulnerable to invasive diseases.

2. *Duct system:* The large main duct through the head and body, surrounded by a dense layer of connective tissue, provides the only internal structural integrity. Stripped of exocrine cells and islets, the duct system resembles a fish skeleton.

3. *Lobulation:* Connective tissue between the duct branches provides *interlobular septae*. **Lobules** can be seen with the naked eye, through the transparent capsule, as pink fleshy units.

4. *"The hidden gland"* is the name given by diagnosticians. Because of its retroperitoneal position and its cover of stomach and transverse colon, it cannot be palpated as readily as the liver and the spleen. Thus, lesions can only be discovered when far advanced. The enormous reserve of islet tissue makes insulin deficiency difficult to detect until a large number of islets are destroyed.

C. The *exocrine pancreas* (Sarles, 1977)

1. *Pancreatic acinus* (Greek: acinar means grape, recall the comparison of serous cells as purple grapes!)

a. From the main ducts, progressively smaller ducts continue branching until the smallest ducts insert into *pancreatic acini*. A section through the acini reveals an important feature of the exocrine pancreas, the *centroacinar epithelial cells*, distinguished by a paucity of cytoplasmic structures. The pyramidal-shaped *pancreatic exocrine cells* making up the acinus surround the lumen of the smallest duct, the *intercalated duct* (review the parotid gland).

b. Refractile granules fill the apex of the pyramidal acinar cells, while mitochondria in the base line up parallel to the longitudinal cell axis in the base. The supranuclear zone (toward the lumen) is occupied by a very well-developed golgi complex. The basal and lateral portions of the nucleus are packed with rER.

2. *Pancreatic exocrine cell* zoning reveals the cytological pathway of typical protein synthesis:

a. *Zone 1:* the subnuclear and lateronuclear area occupied by rER. Polyribosomes manufacture protein-digestive enzymes and transfer them into the ER cisternae.

b. *Zone 2:* the supranuclear area occupied by the golgi complex is the packing and condensing zone. The secretory products are concentrated in condensing vacuoles.

c. *Zone 3:* the apical zone, characterized by stored *zymogen granules* that originated from the condensing vacuoles. Zymogen protein granules ultimately are released into the lumen of the intercalated duct through the free surface of the cell. While enclosed in membranes, the enzymes cannot digest the pancreatic cells.

3. *Products:* Continued activity throughout the day results in more than a liter of digestive juice, containing the following enzymes:

    a. *Proteases* and *nucleases* break down *proteins.*

    b. *Amylases* break down *carbohydrates.*

    c. *Lipases* break down *fats.*

4. Two *hormones* are secreted by the duodenal APUD cells following stimulation by the acidic chyme.

    a. *Secretin* influences the pancreatic exocrine cells to secrete a voluminous serous fluid with an alkaline pH. The function of this solution is to neutralize the acid chyme and elevate the pH above the neutral point so the pancreatic enzymes may function optimally.

    b. *Pancreozymin* stimulates the pancreas to secrete digestive enzymes. Acting with secretin, they cause the release of large amounts of alkaline digestive juice.

D. The *endocrine pancreas* (Cooperstein and Watkins, 1981) is spread out as islets of cells attached to atrophied vestiges of the duct system. Islets measure from 100 to 200 μm in diameter and contain several hundred cells.

1. *General:* Almost all laymen are familiar with the control of *diabetes mellitus* and recognize *insulin.* The discovery of insulin ranks as a major landmark of modern medicine.

2. *Pancreatic endocrine cells* (Erlandsen, 1980)

    a. *Alpha (μ) endocrine cells* constitute 20% of the islet cell population, usually located at the periphery of the islet.

        (1) The *alpha granules*

            (a) *LM:* the *acidophil* polygonal *granules* are best preserved by alcohol fixatives (contrast with beta granules) and stain red with Mallory-Azan.

            (b) *TEM:* measure 250 nm in diameter. The membrane-bound granule contains an eccentric, spherical, electron-dense core surrounded by a less dense matrix.

        (2) Other *cell structures*

            (a) An eccentric *nucleus* may be indented at one or more places.

            (b) The *golgi complex* is fairly well developed, but not as large as that of the beta cell.

(c) Oval to elongate *mitochondria* are less numerous than those of the beta cell.

(d) *rER* has shortened flat cisternae and almost no vesicles.

(3) *Product: glucagon*, a hormone that elevates blood sugar should it fall below a normal titer. Alpha cells working in concert with beta cells balance glucose levels in the circulating blood. In *target organs*, such as the liver (as well as several other tissues), glucagon breaks down glycogen and promotes gluconeogenesis.

b. *Beta (β) endocrine cells* (also: insulinocytes), comprising about 70% of the islet cell population, assemble in the center of the islet.

(1) The *beta (β) granules*

(a) Via *LM* the basophilic granules stain brownish orange with Mallory-Azan. Alcohol fixatives are avoided because the granules are extracted in alcohols.

(b) Via *TEM*, the outstanding feature is an abundance of membrane-bound *beta granules* containing eccentric electron-dense crystals. Depending on the species, crystals may be spherical, rectangular, or polygonal, surrounded by a clear space. In *humans*, the granules measure about 300 nm in diameter with a loose-fitting membrane surrounding one or more angular crystals of *insulin*, complexed with zinc.

(2) Other *cell structures*

(a) The spherical nucleus has a smooth surface and is rarely indented (compare with alpha cell).

(b) A well-developed golgi complex capping the nucleus is smaller than that of a pancreatic exocrine cell.

(c) Sparse rER, with short flattened cisternae or vesicles studded with polyribosomes, is distributed evenly throughout the cytoplasm. Basophilia is due to rER.

(d) Numerous large mitochondria and polyribosomal granules populate the cytoplasm.

(3) *Product: Insulin* lowers blood glucose levels, speeds up glycogenesis, and promotes the storage of unused nutrients. Primary *target organs* are those specialized to store energy, ie, liver, muscle, and adipose tissue.

(4) *Diabetes mellitus:* Failure of *beta cells* to synthesize insulin results in the disease diabetes mellitus. Blood glucose as such cannot be utilized by the body cells and cannot be converted to usable glycogen. Unconverted glucose is eliminated in the urine, a major diagnostic feature of the disease. Administration of insulin to the

patient circumvents the diabetic syndrome by converting glucose to glycogen.

(5) *Insulin granule production:* It should be apparent that beta cell morphology depends upon the phase of granule production. Insulin granules are released via *exocytosis* into the circulatory system whenever the concentration of blood glucose is elevated or when there are increased levels of amino acids such as leucine or arginine. Depletion of intracellular membrane-bound insulin granules initiates production of new granules, as follows:

(a) *Production:* rER produces a single polypeptide chain, *proinsulin.*

(b) *Packaging:* In the golgi complex, proinsulin is packaged in a membrane and then split by proteolytic cleavage into one molecule of insulin and one molecule of C peptide.

(c) *Transport:* Vesicles containing the insulin crystal migrate toward the cell surface next to a capillary.

(d) *Discharge of insulin*
[1] The vesicle membrane fuses with beta cell plasmalemma,
[2] An opening appears at the fused site of the plasmalemma,
[3] Crystal fragments are expelled.
[4] The empty transport vesicle evaginates as a microvillus.

(e) *Discharged crystals pass through*
[1] beta cell basement membrane,
[2] endothelial cell basement membrane.
[3] capillary endothelium.

c. *C cells* appear to be undifferentiated cells. The letter "C" represents its chromophobic nature, as it does not stain. A lack of granules in large clear vesicles is characteristic. The golgi complex is diminutive. C cells represent undifferentiated reserve cells for either alpha or beta cells in the guinea pig. C cells have not been reported in humans.

d. *D cells* resemble the alpha cells in H & E preparation. Variable in shape and often elongated, they can occur anywhere in the islet.

(1) *LM:* The least abundant cells in an islet, they are distinguished from alpha cells by the Mallory-Azan technique: *Alpha* cells stain *red,* D cells stain *blue.*

(2) *TEM:* The membrane-bound granules, 325 nm in diameter, have a homogeneous matrix of a moderate to low electron density.

(3) *Product:* somatostatin, a 14-amino-acid polypeptide. In the pancreatic islet, this hormone inhibits the secretion of insulin and glucagon. Somatostatin influences the exocrine pancreas by decreasing pancreatic exocrine secretion. Hypothalamic somatostatin functions as a somatotrop(h)ic hormone release-inhibiting factor (SRIF).

    e. *PP* cells (also termed F, X cells) occur in the islet and appear scattered throughout the exocrine pancreatic acini.

    (1) Via *TEM,* granules are membrane bound, 175 nm in diameter, spherical, of variable density, and surrounded by a wide electron-lucent area.

    (2) *Product:* The hormone produced is termed *pancreatic polypeptide* (hence the *PP* cell name). Although its function in humans is unknown, experimental evidence suggests that it

        (a) stimulates gastric enzyme secretion,

        (b) inhibits intestinal motility,

        (c) relaxes the gallbladder,

        (d) inhibits pancreatic exocrine secretion.

    f. Immunocytochemical studies have identified two additional cell types:

    (1) a D-type argyrophilic cell, with 175 nm granules that secrete *vasocactive intestinal polypeptide* (VIP), which stimulates pancreatic exocrine secretion.

    (2) an EC (enterochromaffin) cell type, with granules that vary widely from 175 to 400 nm in diameter, which secretes *serotonin.*

II. *Liver:* The superb diagrams and masterful colored plates by Hans Elias should be referred to in Elias-Pauly's *Histology and Human Microanatomy,* 5th Edition, pp 314–341 (Ed. P.S. Amenta).

    A. *General:* The liver, an extramural digestive gland, is the largest gland in the body, weighing about 1500 g (2% of adult body weight). It is situated in the upper right quadrant under the diaphragm.

    B. *Development* (Moore, 1988)

    1. The liver develops from duodenal *endodermal* epithelium as a *pouch* that evaginates into the ventral mesentery. The endodermal duct uniting the pouch and duodenal endoderm remains patent. The tip in the duodenum develops as the *duodenal papilla.*

    2. From the extramural *duct* leading to the pouch, a lateral bud develops that forms the anlage of the *gallbladder.*

    3. Growth of the duct forms the *right* and *left hepatic ducts.* Each of these continues branching dichotomously until they are blind-ended tiny ducts. The terminal buds will form the parenchymal *liver epithelial cells.*

4. Bile produced by the liver cells is directed via the duct system to the gallbladder, where it is concentrated. When needed, and on stimulation, the bile will be released and delivered to the duodenum.

C. *General structure:* The liver interposes itself in the vascular system between the portal vein and the inferior vena cava. The portal vein carries blood from the digestive tract and the spleen.

1. The *hepatic portal vein* delivers blood through the **porta hepatis** and divides repeatedly into smaller branches, ultimately leading to the *hepatic lobules*, composed of parenchymal *liver epithelial cells (hepatocytes).* The terminal branches of the portal vein from *sinusoidal vessels* whose basement membranes contact, but do not fuse with those of the *liver cells.*

2. The *perisinusoidal space* (of Disse), a potential space between the sinusoidal endothelium and the liver cell, provides an avenue for the voracious phagocytic appetite of *stellate macrophages* (Kupffer cells), which are derived from monocytes. When enlarged, they may prevent blood from leaving the sinusoids, thus controlling blood flow through the liver. Stellate *perisinusoidal lipocytes* (Ito and Shibasaki, 1968) may store lipids, differentiate into fibroblasts, or engage in turnover of vitamin A. The rat has another cell, the *pit cell*, function unknown. Its existence in humans has not been reported.

3. The *sinusoidal vessels* deliver liver cell products into the blood and transfer nutrients from portal blood to liver cells.

D. The *liver lobules*

1. The *classic liver lobule* explains the general structure and relationship of vessels to the liver cells. This lobule model, exemplified by the lobules of the pig liver, has been used to introduce generations of students to the complexities of liver structure. The *classic* lobule is composed of liver cells arranged so that in sections they appear to converge upon a central hub. All cells form a three-dimensional sponge-like lobules with the spaces occupied by sinusoidal vessels.

a. *Delivery of venous blood* to the classic lobule

(1) Imagine the *lobule* resembling a long six-sided prism with a rounded top and bottom.

(2) *Portal vein* smallest branches run longitudinally along the six corners of the "prism" lobule. The portal vein brings blood originating from capillary plexuses in the intestinal mucosa and from the spleen.

(3) From portal vein branches, *interlobular veins* connect each of the portal veins so that it appears as if these are perilobular veins. In fact, the old name was "perilobular vein."

(4) *Sinusoidal vessels* with fenestrations up to 2 μm branch from interlobular veins and converge upon a "hub" where the *central vein* is located. Digested substances in the venous blood are delivered to the *liver* cells for processing.

(5) The *central veins* of neighboring lobules empty into a *sublocular vein.*

(6) The *sublobular veins* empty into the *hepatic veins*, which ultimately drain into the *inferior vena cava.*

b. *Delivery of arterial blood* to the classic lobule

(1) *Hepatic arteries* accompany the portal vein branches directly to the lobules where they branch into *interlobular arteries.*

(2) Small branches of the *interlobular arteries* empty directly into interlobular veins and sinusoidal vessels.

c. Thus, liver lobules receive a dual blood supply.

(1) *Venous blood* from the hepatic portal veins brings products of digestion and splenix products (iron).

(2) *Arterial blood* brings oxygen and usable metabolic substances.

d. The concept of the classic lobule helps to understand endocrine functions and explain necrotic changes produced by toxic substances (eg, carbon tetrachloride).

2. Please examine Figure 16-3 to compare the classic hepatic lobules with *portal lobules* and the *portal acinus* (Rappaport, 1958). Whereas classic lobules, as in the pig liver, are surrounded by connective tissue, human liver has connective tissue only around the portal veins and hepatic arteries. Walls of liver cells from adjoining lobules appear to bridge from one lobule to the other, hence the *portal acinus* is another way to study the liver. The concept of the *portal cinus* helps to

a. explain gradient zonation in lobule,
b. understand regeneration patterns,
c. understand liver cirrhosis.

E. The *liver epithelial cell (hepatocyte)* has an incredible capacity to divide and replace lost cells. While the general population is stable, lost portions of the liver (from carbon tetrachloride) may be completely regenerated in a relatively short period of time.

1. *Structure:* a three-dimensional polygonal cell.

a. LM shows a relatively large nucleus, usually with a single

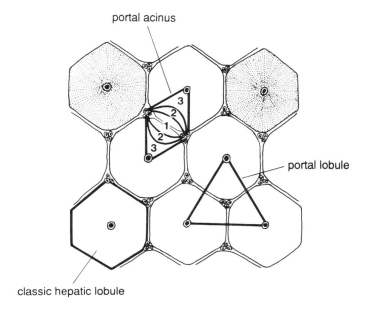

Figure 16-3 Diagrammatic representation of the *classic liver lobule*, the *portal acinus*, and the *portal lobule*.

nucleolus and fine granular mitochondria, via the vital stain Janus green B.

    b. TEM shows (Fig. 16-4)

        (1) oval mitochondria with leaf-like cristae. Circular profiles of some cristae suggest the existence of tubular cristae.

        (2) abundant glycogen granules with a fair distribution between membranes of ER. Single glycogen particles are referred to as *alpha particles.*

        (3) lysosomes, which catabolize effete cytoplasmic structures and exogenous substances to repair and maintain liver cells.

        (4) profiles of rER that can transform to sER. The sER is involved in the synthesis of cholesterol, albumin, and fibrinogen; in the detoxification of drugs and steroids; and in the formation of triglycerides.

        (5) a well-developed golgi complex.

    2. *Functions:* The liver is involved in multiple functions, both exocrine and endorcrine.

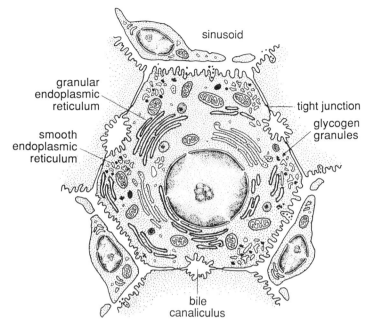

granular endoplasmic reticulum

smooth endoplasmic reticulum

sinusoid

tight junction

glycogen granules

bile canaliculus

Figure 16-4 The liver epithelial cell (hepatocyte) and its relationship to other liver cells to form bile canaliculi. Note relationship to sinusoidal vessels.

    a. *Synthesis and secretion of bile*
        (1) 90% of the bile acids (phospholipids, cholesterol, bilirubin) are absorbed from the intestine, brought to the liver via the portal blood, and recirculated.
        (2) 10% of the bile acids are synthesized de novo in the sER.
        (3) Bilirubin, a bile pigment or dye, is formed by macrophages (including the stellate macrophages) and brought to the liver epithelial cells for disposition.
        (4) Dyes (ie, sulfobromophthalein) are eliminated by the liver cells, an attribute used as a liver function test.
    b. *Synthesis of protein*
        (1) *Protein for self-maintenance:* Polyribosomes synthesize proteins for use by the liver epithelial cells.
        (2) *Protein for export:* Rough ER synthesizes the plasma proteins: albumin, fibrinogen, prothrombin, and lipoproteins. They

are released as formed into sinusoids. As such, this is considered an endocrine activity.

c. *Detoxification and inactivation* of drugs, insecticides, and other toxic substances occurs in the sER. Among substances inactivated are antihistamines, steroids, and barbiturates.

d. *Storage* of blood in sinusoids to extract substances brought by the blood and to deposit liver cell products. *Storage* of carbohydrates and fats as glycogen and triglycerides. *Storage* of vitamins, especially vitamin A.

e. *Metabolism: Gluconeogenesis* converts lipids and amino acids to glucose, to maintain blood glucose levels. *Deamination* of amino acids, forms urea.

f. *Hemocytopoesis* in the embryo and extramedullary in the adult in cases of extreme need.

g. *Filtration of blood*-borne foreign materials, a phagocytic activity involving the stellate macrophages.

h. *Conversion* of T4 to T3.

i. *Immune functions:* sequester IgA and deliver it to the intestine.

F. *Bile ducts*

1. The *liver epithelial cell* walls possess a crease, so that when any two liver cells align opposing creased surfaces, a partial *bile canaliculus* is formed. Along the union site, a zonula occludens forms to prevent bile from passing between liver cells back to the sinusoids. Such a condition would lead to jaundice. The canaliculi are lined by microvilli serving to increase surface area.

2. Many liver cells in tandem will form a complete *bile canaliculus* carrying bile to the periphery of the lobule. Liver cells toward the periphery decrease in size, until they become small cuboidal cells of the small *bile ducts*. This schema confirms the embryological development of the ducts and terminal liver acinar portions.

3. Union of several peripheral bile duct portions from the bile ducts located in the connective tissue at the lobule periphery and which travel with the longitudinal portal veins and hepatic arteries.

4. Bile ducts emanating from the liver form the *hepatic duct*, which receives the *cystic duct* from the gallbladder to become the *common bile duct*.

a. The epithelium of these ducts commences at the liver lobule as short cuboidal cells, and as the ducts increase in size, so do the cells. The extrahepatic ducts possess tall columnar epithelium, which may secrete an atypical mucus.

b. Mucosal folds characterize the duct lumen.

5. The tunica muscularis is arranged as *sphincters* at appropriate points, particularly at the entrance of the duodenum.

a. Generally, the main pancreatic duct joins the common bile duct, and at these union sites, smooth muscle sphincters develop to prevent backflow of bile into the pancreas or flow of pancreatic juices into the bile duct.

III. Vesica biliaris, the *gallbladder*

A. *General:* This viscus is attached to the ventral surface of the liver. It consists of a bulbous end, the **fundus**, a body, the **corpus** and a neck, the **cervix**. The gallbladder can be filled with up to 50 cc of bile.

B. *Histological organization*

1. The **tunica mucosa** may be thrown into complex folds that disappear when the gallbladder is empty.

a. **Epithelium** of simple tall columnar cells with junctional complexes, and desmosomes along the lateral plasmalemmae. A basement membrane anchors the epithelium to the underlying connective tissue. The cells contain

(1) supranuclear golgi complex,

(2) granular ER,

(3) membrane-bound granules,

(4) small, but numerous mitochondria,

(5) superficial microvilli covered with fine *filiform appendages* rather than a filamentous glycocalyx.

b. **Lamina propria mucosae** is the connective tissue layer with numerous blood vessels, nerves, and lymphatics. Glands reside in this layer, particularly in the neck region. These mucous-secreting glands, with interspersed goblet cells, proliferate in patients with chronic inflammation.

c. A **lamina muscularis mucosae** is absent, and therefore there is no **tela submucosa**.

2. The **tunica muscularis** consists of at least three layers of non-striated muscle separated by elastic fiber networks.

3. The free surface of the gallbladder is covered by **tunica serosa**, with a thick underlying **lamina propria serosae**. Major blood vessels nerves and lymphatics run through this layer. On the surface opposed to the liver parenchyma, only a thin layer of **tunica adventitia** intervenes.

C. *Functions:* The gallbladder stores and concentrates bile by absorbing water and inorganic ions. The musculature responds to the influence of cholecystokinin. Ingestion of fat or meat initiates contraction of the musculature, aiding in expelling and delivering the bile contents to the duodenum.

D. In pathological conditions, the luminal epithelium may evaginate through the lamina propria mucosae and tunica muscularis to form *Rokitansky-Aschoff pouches.* These pouches (sinuses, crypts, or diverticulae) may harbor bacteria, leading to serious inflammatory conditions that weaken the wall.

Questions

DIRECTIONS: For each of the items in this section, one or more of the numbered options is correct. Select
  A if only *1, 2, and 3* are correct
  B if only *1 and 3* are correct
  C if only *2 and 4* are correct
  D if only *4* is correct
  E if *all* are correct

1. The pars mucosa of the lip is kept moist by the secretions of
  1. sebaceous glands
  2. mucous glands
  3. sudoriferous glands
  4. serous glands

2. The gingiva lacks a stratum
  1. basalis
  2. corneum
  3. spinosum
  4. granulosum

3. Dentinoblasts (odontoblasts)
  1. mobilize and secrete dentine
  2. are anchored into the dentine by dentinal tubules
  3. are derived from mesoderm
  4. have a well-developed golgi complex and rER

4. Which of the glands below (normal average situation) contain mucous acini?
   1. Submandibular
   2. Sublingual
   3. Anterior lingual
   4. Parotid

5. In the adult, the junction between the posterior one third and anterior two thirds of the tongue is marked by location of the
   1. sulcus terminalis
   2. foramen cecum
   3. vallate papillae
   4. submandibular duct

6. Taste buds are found in the epithelium of the
   1. cheeks
   2. palate
   3. epiglottis
   4. vallate papillae

7. The pharyngeal tonsil
   1. is covered entirely by stratified squamous epithelium
   2. has epithelium thrown into folds rather than crypts
   3. develops from the second pharyngeal sac
   4. resides on the roof of the nasopharynx

8. Parietal exocrine cells are characterized by
   1. intracellular canaliculi lined by microvilli
   2. acidophilic granules containing lysozyme
   3. abundant mitochondria
   4. rough endoplasmic reticulum

9. Principal exocrine cells of the stomach
   1. are part of the gastric gland epithelium
   2. have an apical cytoplasm filled with zymogen granules
   3. have an abundant basal rough ER
   4. produce intrinsic factor

		Directions Summarized		
A	**B**	**C**	**D**	**E**
1,2,3	1,3	2,4	4	All are
only	only	only	only	correct

10. Gastrointestinal endocrine cells
   1. are predominantly polypeptides
   2. are neural crest descendants
   3. have electron-dense secretory granules at the cell base
   4. are distributed singly in mucosal epithelium

11. In H & E preparations, distinction between the mucous surface cells and mucous neck cells in the stomach is difficult. Histochemical and special stains can distinguish them:
   1. Mucous surface cells produce a neutral glycoprotein.
   2. Mucous surface cells undergo division to produce gland cells.
   3. Mucous neck cells produce an acidic glycoprotein.
   4. Mucous neck cells no not undergo division.

12. Esophageal glands proper can occur in the
   1. lamina propria serosae
   2. lamina propria mucosae
   3. tunica muscularis
   4. tela submucosa

13. Duodenal glands (Brunner's)
   1. occupy the submucosa
   2. secrete zymogen granules as well as mucus
   3. diminish in size and number past the duodenal papilla
   4. resemble pyloric glands

14. Aggregated lymphatic nodules appear in the following sites:
   1. ileum
   2. appendix
   3. palatine tonsils
   4. thymus

15. At the linea anorectalis these epithelial types are noted:
1. simple columnar
2. stratified columnar
3. stratified squamous, moist
4. stratified squamous, keratinized

16. Endoderm gives rise to the anlage of the
1. gallbladder
2. liver
3. endocrine pancreas
4. exocrine pancreas

17. The pancreatic exocrine cells has the following structures
1. subnuclear and lateronuclear rER
2. supranuclear golgi complex
3. apical zymogen granules
4. peripheral beta granules

18. Pancreatic alpha endocrine cells
1. have loose membranes around angular crystals
2. constitute 70% of all islet cells
3. have smooth-surfaced, rarely indented nuclei
4. are usually located at the periphery of an islet

19. The classic liver lobule receives blood from the
1. central vein
2. hepatic artery
3. sublobular vein
4. portal vein

20. The liver epithelial cell is characterized by
1. oval mitochondria with leaf-like cristae
2. alpha particles
3. smooth endoplasmic reticulum
4. lysosomes

21. The gallbladder
1. responds to cholecystokinin
2. lacks glands
3. is lined by an epithelium of tall simple columnar cells
4. lacks a tunica muscularis

22. The bile canaliculi form
    1. between liver cells
    2. from simple squamous cells
    3. from endoderm
    4. the bile

Explanatory Answers

1. C. 2 and 4 are correct. Mucous and serous glands secrete onto the epithelial surface of the pars mucosa. The sebaceous glands and sudoriferous glands, if present, would secrete on the pars cutanea. No glands empty onto the pars intermedia, and hence they have a tendency to dry out if not moistened.

2. C. 2 and 4 are correct. The gingiva, though lacking both the granulosum and corneum is exceptionally tough. The lack of these two layers signifies that the gingival epithelium does not undergo keratinization.

3. E. All are correct. The apical processes of dentinoblasts are termed dentinal tubules, which extend into the dentine. The peritubular dentine is secreted by these cells and hence they are endowed with a well-developed golgi complex and rER befitting a protein secreting cell.

4. A. 1, 2, and 3 are correct. The submandibular is a mixed gland, containing about a 50/50 proportion of mucous and serous acini. Serous cells predominate because almost all the mucous acini are capped by serous demilunes. The sublingual gland is composed predominantly of mucous acini, but is capped by serous demilunes. Occasional serous acini are found. The anterior lingual salivary gland is a mucoserous gland. The only gland without mucous acini is the parotid.

5. A. 1, 2, and 3 are correct. The sulcus terminalis is the trench behind the "V"-shaped row of vallate papillae. The apex of the "V" points directly at the foramen cecum, site of origin of the thyroid gland. The submandibular duct opens on the floor of the oral cavity, in an area difficult to delineate as the junction.

6. E. All are correct. In addition to these sites, taste buds have been found in the larynx, upper esophagus, pharynx, sometimes the fungiform and foliate papillae, surface of the tongue, and the palatoglossal and palatopharyngeal arches. The greatest concentration is on the tongue.

7. C. 2 and 4 are correct. Answers 1 and 3 describe the palatine tonsil.

8. B. 1 and 3 are correct. The parietal cell is specialized to secrete HCl. The large surface area of the microvilli-studded intracellular canaliculi, smooth endoplasmic reticulum (rather than rough), and the abundant mitochondria make this cell an especially productive cell. The acidophilic granules with lysozyme characterize another exocrine cell (Paneth cell).

9. A. 1, 2, and 3 are correct. The protein-secreting parietal exocrine cell produces pepsinogen, which is hydrolyzed to pepsin in the low pH environment created by HCl. Intrinsic factor is produced by the parietal exocrine cell.

10. E. All are correct. These cells are also called APUD cells (*A*mine *P*recursor *U*ptake and *D*ecarboxylation), enterochromaffin cells (EC cells), and argentaffin cells. The increasing number and distinctions of cells make the GI tract an important member of the endocrine system. Secretory granules almost always accumulate on the side (the base) of the cell closest to a capillary.

11. B. 1 and 3 are correct. Distinctions are best made by the identification of the cellular product. The sequence of cellular proliferation is from the gland to the surface, and not vice versa. Hence the surface cells are fully differentiated. It is true, however, that when the glands are first formed, at some 11 to 12 weeks of gestation, the surface epithelium invaginates to form the glands.

12. C. 2 and 4 are correct. The esophageal glands proper are usually distributed randomly in the tela submucosa, but they can occur in the lamina propria mucosae if they fail to penetrate the lamina muscularis mucosae. This situation could only be recognized in the middle portion of the esophagus. In the beginning and the end, they would be interpreted as esophageal cardiac glands.

13. E. All are correct. The duodenal gland secretions together with those of the pyloric glands produce an abundant mucus that protects the duodenal mucosa from the acidic gastric chyme.

14. A. 1, 2, and 3 are correct. Aggregated lymphatic nodules appear under an epithelium. In the first three, lymphatic nodules aggregate in a variety of ways: in the ileum up to 40 line up under the columnar epithelium opposite the mesentery; in the appendix they form a ring around the lumen; in the palatine tonsils, the nodules form between the crypts. The thymus has a cortex of T lymphocytes, but no discrete nodules.

15. B. 1 and 3 are correct. There is no stratified columnar epithelium at this site. Keratinized stratified squamous epithelium appears at the anal orifice.

16. E. All are correct. The liver enters the ventral mesentery, while the pancreatic buds enter the dorsal and ventral mesenteries. Rotation of the gut brings them into correct positions. Both exocrine and endocrine portions derive from the same endoderm. Cell differentiation changes their courses. The gallbladder forms terminal buds that form the hollow vesicle. The other bud continues proliferating into terminal buds that form the liver acinus.

17. A. 1, 2, and 3 are correct. The answers reflect the zonation of the exocrine cell, wherein rER manufacture the zymogen granules, the golgi complex packs them, and they wait in the apical cytoplasm to be discharged into the duct lumen. The beta granules occur in the beta pancreatic endocrine cell.

18. D. 4 is correct. The items in 1, 2, and 3 are specific for the pancreatic beta endocrine cell, which tends to concentrate in the islet center area. The membrane-bound granules have a clear space around the insulin crystals. Alpha cells produce glucagon.

19. C. 2 and 4 are correct. The liver lobule receives a dual supply: the portal vein, carrying venous blood loaded with substances absorbed by the intestines and products from the spleen (eg, from old erythrocytes-iron) and oxygenated blood via the hepatic artery. The central vein drains the lobule into the sublobular vein, and eventually the blood is carried away from the liver by the inferior vena cava.

20. E. All are correct. The alpha particles are single glycogen particles. Some cristae may be oval, resembling the smooth endoplasmic reticulum. The sER is involved in the detoxification of drugs and steroids, among others. Lysosomes assist in repair and maintenance of the liver by catabolizing effete cytoplasmic structures and exogenous substances.

21. B. 1 and 3 are correct. The tunica muscularis responds to the influence of cholecystokinin to expel the contents. The tunica muscularis consists of at least three layers of smooth muscle separated by elastic fiber networks. The lamina muscularis mucosae is lacking. The tall columnar cells possess microvilli covered by filiform appendages and not the usual glycocalyx.

22. B. 1 and 3 are correct. When the surfaces of two liver cells with minute creases join the canaliculus is formed. Along the junction site, a zonula occludens (tight junction) forms to prevent bile from leaking back into the sinusoidal vessels. When that happens, the patient appears jaundiced. Bile formed in the liver epithelial cell is passed into the canaliculus lined by microvilli for delivery to the gallbladder. What may appear like a capillary tube lined by simple squamous cells is not so. The canaliculus is a lumen between the surfaces of two liver epithelial cells.

17 The Respiratory System

I. *Introduction:* Breathing is an activity that every human must perform to sustain life. Cessation of respiration necessitates emergency measures, because oxygen deficiency profoundly affects the vital organs.

A. *Oxygen* is inhaled into the lungs to be transferred to the circulatory system for distribution to the body cells.

B. *Carbon dioxide* from the body cells is conveyed via the circulatory system to the lungs for expiration.

II. *Development* (Boyden, 1971): The lining of the tracheobronchial tree develops from a bud of evaginating endoderm, originating from the floor of the pharynx at the midpoint between the left and right sixth branchial arches.

III. *Definitions*

A. The *nasal cavity* is the gateway of the respiratory system.

B. The *nasopharynx* conducts air from the nasal cavity to the larynx.

C. The cartilaginous **larynx**, connecting the pharynx to the trachea, "plays" the vocal cords to produce sounds when air pressure causes them to vibrate. Proximity of the esophagus requires precise coordination of laryngeal movements to prevent food from entering the lung.

D. The *tracheobronchial tree* is a system of tubes strengthened by cartilaginous rings, which conduct oxygen (in the air) to the *alveoli* and carbon dioxide from the **alveoli**.

E. The *respiratory unit* is the terminal unit supporting the *alveoli* which actually perform the intricacies of gaseous exchange.

IV. *The nasal cavity:* the major entrance and exit of the respiratory system is via the *anterior nares* (nostrils) of the nose. Three regions are recognized: *cutaneous, respiratory,* and *olfactory.*

346

A. The *cutaneous region* is covered with keratinized stratified squamous epithelium continuous with the skin.

1. The cavity, known as the *nasal vestibulum*, is divided into a right half and a left half by the *nasal septum*.

2. Replacing the keratinized epithelium is a moist stratified squamous epithelium, which lines the lateral and medial walls of the vestibulum.

3. Vibrissae (long hairs), associated with sebaceous and sudoriferous glands at the openings, participate in the initial filtration of air to remove large particulate matter.

B. The *respiratory region*, the posterior part of the nasal cavity, is divided by a continuation of the nasal septum. The floor is formed by the hard palate, the roof by bones of the cranial cavity, and the lateral walls by three shelf-like **conchae** projecting into the nasal cavity. Lateral to the conchae are the large maxillary sinuses in the maxillae (bones) lined by respiratory epithelium. Serous fluid produced in the sinuses drains into the nasal cavity through **foraminae** located under the conchae.

1. A **tunica mucosa respiratoria** covers a **lamina propria mucosae** attached directly to the underlying hyaline cartilage or bone. There is *no* tela submucosa and *no* tunica muscularis.

a. Pseudostratified ciliated columnar epithelium is interspersed with goblet cells.

b. The lamina propria mucosae harbors a luxurious vasculature, nerves, and lymphatic in a special stratum, the **stratum cavernosum**, containing all connective tissue cell types.

2. The **stratum cavernosum** is distinguished by large plexuses of veins, the **plexus cavernosus concharum**, bearing a remarkable resemblance to erectile tissue (Cauna and Hinderer, 1969), except that the connective tissue septae lack nonstriated myocytes. Nevertheless, they are capable of considerable engorgement, which alternately block the right and left halves of the nasal cavity and the sinus foraminae located under the conchae. The "stuffy nose" of a cold or allergic reaction is attributed to venous engorgement.

a. The rich venous plexuses warm and moisten the incoming air. To fully appreciate the significance of the location of these plexuses, try breathing very cold air through the nose, then through the mouth.

3. *Inhaled air* is cleaned initially, by the *vibrissae* of the nasal vestibule followed by the ciliary activity of the respiratory epithelium in the nasal cavity. Goblet cells and *nasal glands* located in the lamina propria mucosae deliver copious mucus and serous secretions to the epithelial surface (Ladman and Mitchell, 1955).

a. Cilia whip the mucus, at a rate of over 1000 lashes per minute, toward the *posterior nares* (opening into the pharynx). Particulate matter trapped in the mucous blanket drips back into the pharynx and is swallowed.

b. 95% of all particulate material is removed by the nose. The remaining 5% is eliminated by the mucous blanket moving upward (by ciliary activity) in the tracheobronchial tree, up through the larynx and transferred to the esophagus for disposal. Particles managing to penetrate the mucous blanket and epithelium are phagocytized by macrophages of the lamina propria mucosae.

C. The *olfactory region*, a 500-mm^2 area specialized to distinguish seven to ten primary odors, is structurally similar to the respiratory area. The **tunica mucosa olfactoria** supports a 50-μm-thick *olfactory epithelium* consisting of the following cell types (Wolstenholme and Knight, 1970):

1. Bipolar *olfactory neurosensory epitheliocytes*, with nuclei settled at different levels.

a. The apical part of each cell is a modified cylindrical *dendrite*, terminating in a *dendrite bulb* that protrudes above the epithelial luminal surface.

(1) Several extremely long **cilia**, protruding from the dendrite bulb, are embedded in a serolipid secretion produced by *olfactory glands* in the underlying lamina propria (cf 4 below). The cilia appear to be essential components of these olfactory cells. (Like taste buds, the substance to be "smelled" must be in solution.)

b. The proximal portion tapers into an *axon* (olfactory neurofiber) that penetrates the basement membrane, lamina propria, and the bony cranial floor, and finally the *olfactory bulb* of the *brain*.

2. *Sustentacular epitheliocytes*, supporting cells, are tall columnar cells whose nuclei are situated closer to the luminal surface than nuclei of the bipolar neurons. The apical region of the cells are filled with mucous droplets.

a. Long microvilli bathe in the mucous cover and intermingle with the olfactory cilia.

b. The cell bases spray out into several processes that encircle the axons of the olfactory cells and anchor to the basement membrane.

3. *Basal epitheliocytes*, rounded basal cells with stellate processes, surround the olfactory cell axons. Irregularly shaped nuclei comprise the first nuclear layer (of the olfactory eoithelium) closest to the basement membrane. Whether these cells are progenitors of other cells has not been established.

4. *Olfactory glands* (branched, tubuloalveolar) in the lamina propria possess ducts that empty onto the epithelial surface. Two cell types characterize these glands, *light* and *dark*.

    a. *Light cells*, pyramidal in shape, are distinguished by a large central nucleus and dilated cisternae of rough endoplasmic reticulum. The secretion of these cells is *serous* (aqueous) in nature. Odiferous materials could only be registered in solution, and serous fluid provides this milieu.

    b. *Dark cells* possess low-density secretory granules and nongranular (smooth) endoplasmic reticulum that occasionally whirls into tightly formed concentric rings. These cells provide a lipid component of the glandular secretion, especially for odiferous substances that are more soluble in a lipid medium.

5. The **organum vomeronasale**, an auxilliary olfactory organ, occupies a portion of the floor of the nasal cavity along each side of the nasal septum. In lower mammals, this organ assists in attracting males to females (Powers et al, 1979). In primates this organ appears only during embryonic life.

V. *The* **pharynx**, the common receptacle for the oral cavity and the nasal cavity, comprises three continuous regions of similar structure and function, the *nasopharynx*, *oropharynx*, and *laryngopharynx*:

A. The *nasopharynx* is the superior region of the pharynx. Air entering the nasopharynx passes into the pharynx and is channeled to the larynx.

B. The *oropharynx* is the region between the nasopharynx and the laryngopharynx. The oral cavity communicates directly with the oropharynx. Food is propelled into the esophagus by contraction of the pharyngeal muscles.

C. The *laryngopharynx* is the inferior funnel-shaped zone above the entrance to the larynx and esophagus. It funnels air into the larynx, and nutrients into the esophagus.

D. *Structure:* The pharynx possesses a tunica mucosa and, in some areas, a rather loose submucosa. The tunica mucosa is lined by respiratory-type epithelium, except in those regions subjected to friction, eg, where the free edge of the soft palate "slaps" against the posterior pharyngeal wall during deglutition. In these areas, the epithelium is modified to the protective stratified squamous type.

E. *Function:* Activity in one pharyngeal zone involves the others. The pharynx is shaped like a "V," with the narrow end aimed inferiorly, and is flattened in the anteroposterior dimension. During deglutition, elevation of the soft palate separates the nasopharynx from the oropharynx, thereby preventing food or liquids from entering the nasal cavity.

VI. *The laryngeal cavity* is the superior cavity of the **larynx** above the vocal cords (Fink, 1975). Below the vocal cords, the *infraglottic cavity* communicates with the trachea. The larynx, housing the vocal cords, consists of

A. *Muscle components*

1. *Extrinsic skeletal muscles* position the larynx for various functions, such as deglutition, by elevating it as a whole.

2. *Intrinsic skeletal muscles* move cartilage components and indirectly control the position of the vocal cords, which can then be oscillated at different frequencies, by air, to produce sound with pitch.

B. *Cartilage components*

1. *hyaline cartilage*
   a. thyroid
   b. cricoid
   c. arytenoids

2. *elastic cartilage*
   a. tips of arytenoids
   b. corniculate
   c. cuneiform
   d. epiglottis

C. *Bone,* the hyoid bone

D. *Connective tissue membranes,* thyrohyoid, quadrates, cricovocal.

E. The **tunica mucosa** lining the interior of the larynx forms two folds projecting from the lateral walls. A narrow space between the folds provides the necessary access to the trachea below.

1. The upper fold, the *false vocal cords,* are separated from the lower folds, the *true vocal cords,* by chambers or *vestibules.*

2. The *thyroarytenoideus muscle* (of *skeletal muscle myocytes*) parallels the lateral borders of the true vocal cords.

3. The pseudostratified ciliated columnar epithelium lining most of the interior of the larynx is interspersed with goblet cells.

4. The epithelium of the epiglottis and the superior surface of the vocal cords is moist stratified squamous.

VII. *Tracheobronchial tree*

A. *The basic plan:* From the larynx, the **trachea** descends into the thorax where it bifurcates into **bronchi**, one for each lung. The bronchi divide dichotomously into *lobar bronchi* and *segmental bronchi*. A *bronchopulmonary segment* is the lung tissue plus associated bronchial branches that can be surgically divided via connective tissue septae. The smallest bronchial branches, the bronchioles, end in terminal bronchioles.

B. The *basic tissue layers* of the tracheobronchial tree are the **tunica mucosa, tela submucosa, tunica fibromusculocartilaginea**, and the **tunica adventitia**. A serosa is not found in usual conditions.

C. The *trachea*

1. Tunica mucosa respiratoria
   a. Epithelium: pseudostratified ciliated columnar, including four distinctive cell types: ciliated columnar epitheliocytes, columnar cells with microvilli, goblet cells, and basal cells.
   (1) *Ciliated columnar epitheliocytes* attach to the basement membrane and reach the lumenal surface.
   (a) Smoking evokes a cough reflex. Constant insult of smoke components (especially carbon monoxide) suppresses ciliary motility, with subsequent stagnancy of the mucous blanket.
   (b) A chronic cough may initiate *metaplasia*, that is, conversion of pseudostratified ciliated columnar epithelium to stratified squamous epithelium. The latter is far more adapted to protection from abrasive activity. Change to a malignant cell type is the next step.
   (c) Substantial evidence since the first warnings by the Surgeon General's Office and the American Cancer Society has necessitated strengthening the statement from a warning to a declaration that smoking is a major cause of lung cancer.
   (2) Some *columnar cells* with microvilli.
   (3) *Goblet exocrine cells.*
   (4) *Basal cells*, capable of differentiating into any of the above cells, never reach the lumen.

b. The basement membrane appears more prominent by the thickness of the underlying layer of elastic fibers.

c. Lamina propria mucosae consists of

(1) loose connective tissue that may have diffuse lymphocytes or lymphatic nodules,

(2) an underlying **lamina fibrarum elasticarum** (a feltwork of elastic fibers separating the tunica mucosa from the tela submucosa.

2. The **tela submucosa** consists of a layer of connective tissue supporting the secretory portions of *tracheal glands* with mucous and serous portions. Their ducts may be lined with ciliated cells. *Tracheal lymphatic nodules* appear in the tela submucosa.

3. Surrounding the tela submucosa is the **tunica fibromusculocartilaginea**, consisting of three parts:

a. The hyaline *tracheal cartilages*, in the shape of C or Y rings, form the anterior and lateral walls of the trachea and provide rigidity to the trachea to prevent collapse.

b. The *tracheal muscle*, of smooth myocytes, completes the flat posterior wall of the trachea, filling in the gap between the cartilages. During inspiration, the trachea expands, and during expiration the tracheal muscles contract to pull the cartilages back.

c. The *annular ligament* provides connective tissue support for the tracheal muscle and cartilages.

4. Paries membranaceus is a fibroelastic membrane continuous with the perichondrium of the hyaline cartilage.

5. Tunica adventitia unites with that of the esophagus, that is, the posterior wall of the trachea binds to the anterior wall of the esophagus.

D. Two extrapulmonary **bronchi** form by bifurcation of the trachea. Anatomical features resemble those of the trachea, that is, the posterior surface appears flattened. Hyaline cartilage C rings are connected posteriorly by connective tissue and muscle.

E. Intrapulmonary **bronchi** appear more cylindrical because the C rings are replaced by O rings of hyaline cartilage. *Bronchopulmonary branches* of the bronchi are presented in Table 17-1.

F. The segmental bronchi divide dichotomously into subsegmental bronchi. With successive branches the bronchial branches are reduced in size.

1. Cartilage rings are smaller and are replaced by irregular cartilaginous plates in segmental bronchi.

Table 17-1 Bronchopulmonary Branches of the Bronchi

Branches	Left lung	vs	Right lung
Extrapulmonary branches			
Main bronchi	1		1
Intrapulmonary branches			
Lobar bronchi	2		3
Segmental bronchi, upper lobe	5		3
middle lobe	no middle lobe		2
lower lobe	5		5

2. Cartilage plates disappear in the subsegmental bronchi.

3. Bronchial ciliated columnar epithelium is gradually reduced to cuboidal at the ends of the subsegmental bronchi.

4. Goblet cells diminish in number and finally disappear.

5. Submucosal glands also diminish at the ends.

6. The lamina propria mucosa is delineated by a prominent basement membrane. Loose connective tissue and elastic networks housing a variety of tissue cells reside in this layer. *Elastic fibers* increase in prominence as the connective tissue decreases in the smaller tubes.

G. *Bronchioles*, following the smallest bronchi, are 11th to 16th generation branches of the bronchi, with diameters of 0.5 mm to 0.2 mm. There are no goblet cells or cartilage plates in the bronchioles.

1. The epithelium consists of
   a. *ciliated cuboidal cells.* Positioning of ciliated cells below the point where goblet cells ceased is significant. The cilia catch any mucus and prevent it from draining into the **alveoli.** Alveoli loaded with mucus are incapable of efficient gaseous exchange.

   b. *bronchiolar exocrine cells* (formerly the *Clara cells*), are bulbous cells with a few short microvilli confined to the bronchioles (Massaro, 1988). They are characterized by the presence of electron-dense cytoplasmic granules of unknown chemical nature. Some investigators suggest a surfactant-like role for these granules. An abundant supranuclear sER suggests the possibility of a role in detoxification, as reported in the liver.

2. **Tunica submucosa** glands decrease in size and number and finally disappear before the bronchioles divide to become *terminal bronchioles.* Mucous acini are negligible. Substances trapped in serous fluid are moved away from the alveoli.

3. The **tunica muscularis** forms an inconspicuous, incomplete muscular ring. However, contraction of the smooth myocytes that are present constricts the bronchiole lumen quite effectively.

H. Some 65,000 *terminal bronchioles* divide to form about 130,000 *respiratory bronchioles*, usually less than 0.2 mm in diameter. These divide repeatedly for three more times, resulting in a total of about 530,000 branches.

1. The ciliated cells diminish in number and disappear for the most part in the alveolar ducts.

2. The distinction between a terminal bronchiole and a respiratory bronchiole rests on the presence of "blebs" or little sacs in the latter. The sacs are **alveoli** where gas exchange occurs. As **alveoli** increase numerically, the respiratory bronchiole is transformed to an *alveolar duct*.

I. *Alveolar ducts* are branched extensions of the respiratory bronchioles. A *duct* can be discerned only in properly aligned tissue sections. Smooth myocytes and some ciliated cuboidal cells may appear in sections. There are some 4 million ducts.

J. **Alveoli** are the terminals of the pulmonary tree. There are 300 million alveoli divided between the two lungs. Alveoli may be compared to a bag of ping-pong balls, or on a smaller scale a berry or a drupe (acinus) composed of druplets, the *alveolar sacs*.

1. Space between alveoli is filled with loose connective tissue and capillary networks, forming the *interalveolar septum*.

2. An *alveolus* can be compared to a basketball in the net. The net represents the capillary plexus.

3. Communicating channels, the *alveolar pores*, from one alveolus to the other appear between capillaries of the alveolar wall. Usually a small amount of surfactant plugs the pore.

a. *Pores* facilitate collateral circulation of air, which might otherwise result in *atelectasis* (alveolar collapse).

b. *Pores* also facilitate spread of bacteria.

K. *Interalveolar septum.* The septum consists of the segment of one *respiratory epitheliocyte* and a segment of **endothelium** separated by basement membrane material (Fig. 17-1).

1. Components of the septum (Fig. 17-2)

a. The *respiratory epitheliocyte* (type I cell, alveolar cell) is a highly specialized simple squamous epithelium, with a nucleus bulging into the alveolar space.

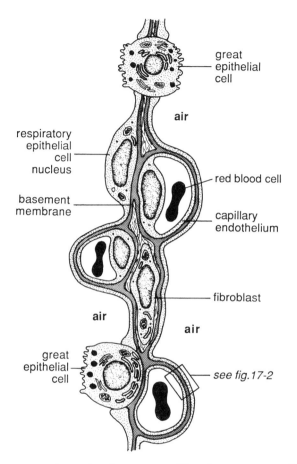

Figure 17-1 The interalveolar septum. The clear areas on either side of the septum represent two adjacent alveolar spaces. The rectangular area is represented by the TEM of Figure 17-2.

    (1) The flattened part of the cell (without the nucleus) is so attenuated (less than 0.2 μm) that it is difficult to distinguish in light microscopic histological sections.
    (2) These cells attach to one another and to *great epitheliocytes*.
    b. Fused *basement membranes* of the respiratory epitheliocyte and the capillary endothelium.

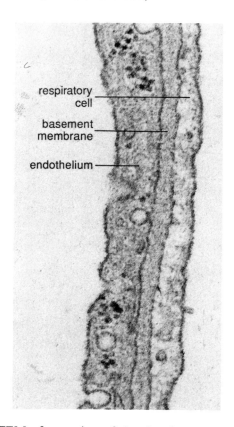

respiratory
cell

basement
membrane

endothelium

Figure 17-2 TEM of a portion of the alveolar septum (cf Fig. 17-1, rectangular area). Capillary endothelium is to the left and the respiratory epitheliocyte is the right separated by a basement membrane (3 × 168,000×).

    c. *Capillary endothelium*, characterized by micropinocytotic vesicles.

    d. *Great epitheliocytes* (type II cells, granular pneumocytes, septal cells), punctuating the interalveolar septum at intervals (Rooney, 1985), produce *surfactant*.

        (1) *Great epitheliocyte* locations (Fig. 17-1):

            (a) attached to the basement membrane between the peripheral edges of two respiratory alveolar cells.

(b) insinuated in the interalveolar septum, surrounded at the equatorial plane by

[1] the peripheral edges of adjacent respiratory epitheliocytes on one side,

[2] basement membrane,

[3] peripheral edges of adjacent respiratory epitheliocytes on the opposite side (cf Fig. 17-1).

(2) *Great epitheliocyte structure*

(a) These are cuboidal-like cells with short microvilli on the surface(s) facing the alveolar lumen.

(b) Electron micrographs (Fig. 17-3) reveal electron-dense lamellated bodies in the cytoplasm, which are the principal source of the active phospholipid *pulmonary surfactant*. When released, the surfactant decreases surface tension in the alveoli.

2. Other components of the interalveolar septum

a. *Alveolar macrophages* (dust cells) are mononuclear cells that can maneuver onto the lumenal surface of the respiratory epitheliocytes (Harmsen et al, 1985).

(1) These 45 μm-diameter cells exhibit voracious appetites for all inhaled particulate matter.

(2) Alveolar macrophages originate from *monocytes*, which develop in bone marrow and migrate to the interalveolar septum via the capillary network.

(3) Though the ER is sparse, lysosomes containing large numbers of hydrolytic enzymes populate the cytoplasm.

(4) Functional aspects

(a) In smokers and in city dwellers, carbon accumulates in the macrophage cytoplasm as indigestible remnants (Pratt et al, 1971).

(b) In cardiac patients with pulmonary congestion, *hemosiderin granules* from phagocytized erythrocytes accumulate in the cytoplasm.

b. An abundance of septal elastic fibers restores the alveolus to its original shape after inhalation of air.

c. Collagen fibrils and fibroblasts are also found.

d. There are no smooth myocytes, no lymphatic capillaries, and no nerve fibers within the interalveolar wall.

VIII. *APUD cells* (neuroendocrine cells), scattered along the tracheobronchial epithelial lining, resemble the APUD cells of the gastrointestinal tract (Sorokin and Hoyt, 1988).

A. Spherical dense-core, membrane-bound granules, 120 nm in diameter, populate the cytoplasm.

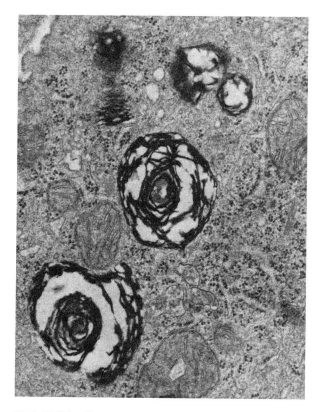

Figure 17-3 TEM of a great epithelial cell. The lamellated bodies contain surfactant (×38,000).

B. Aggregated APUD cells, the *neuroepithelial bodies*, are prominent in the fetus and the newborn. They are confined to the intraepithelial bronchial branches, particularly at bifurcations.

C. While the precise function of these cells is not known, speculations relate them to lung development and neonatal adaptation.

IX. The *pleura* (Wang, 1974)

A. *Visceral pleura* consists of

1. *simple squamous mesothelial cells*, closely applied to the outer (visceral) lung surface, which are characterized by intricate intercellular junctions and microvilli covered surfaces (protruding into the pleural cavity).

2. The basement membrane attaches to a layer of fibrous connective tissue.

3. A deeper connective tissue layer, under the previous one, possesses an abundance of elastic networks interspersed with tissue basophils (mast cells).

4. Blood is supplied by bronchial artery branches.

B. *Parietal pleura* consists of

1. *simple squamous mesothelial cells* (similar in nature).

2. A basement membrane attached to a thicker connective tissue layer with far fewer elastic fibers. The number of adipocytes is increased substantially.

3. Blood is supplied by vessels in the body wall.

Questions

DIRECTIONS: Select the best answer to the question or incomplete statement. There may be other options that are partially correct, but there is only one best answer.

1. The lining of the tracheobronchial tree develops from
   A. pharyngeal endoderm
   B. branchial mesoderm
   C. stomodeal ectoderm
   D. parietal mesothelium
   E. visceral mesothelium

2. The stratum cavernosum of the nasal cavity respiratory region is distinguished by
   A. an auxilliary olfactory organ
   B. vibrissae
   C. large plexuses of veins
   D. sebaceous and sudoriferous glands
   E. alveoli

3. Olfactory neurosensory epitheliocytes possess all the following EXCEPT
   A. cilia
   B. nuclei residing at different levels
   C. apical dendrite bulb
   D. axon
   E. mucous droplets in the apical regions

4. The epithelium of the trachea consists of all the following cell types EXCEPT
   A. ciliated columnar epitheliocytes
   B. columnar cells with microvilli
   C. goblet exocrine cells
   D. dark cells
   E. basal cells

5. Intrapulmonary bronchi have all the characteristics of extrapulmonary bronchi EXCEPT
   A. circular cartilage rings
   B. tracheal muscle
   C. submucosal glands
   D. tunica adventitia
   E. lymphatic nodules in the tela submucosa

6. Bronchioles possess all the following EXCEPT
   A. goblet cells
   B. cuboidal ciliated cells
   C. bronchiolar exocrine cells (Clara cells)
   D. tunica muscularis
   E. submucosal glands

7. Which cell type is confined to the bronchiolar epithelium?
   A. Light cell
   B. Bronchiolar exocrine cell (Clara)
   C. Goblet cell
   D. Great epitheliocyte
   E. Respiratory epitheliocyte

8. All the following are components of the interalveolar septum
   EXCEPT
   A. respiratory epitheliocyte
   B. fused basement membranes
   C. capillary endothelium
   D. great epitheliocytes
   E. sustentacular epitheliocytes

9. Atelectasis is prevented from occurring by the presence of
   A. interalveolar septum
   B. alveolar macrophages
   C. hemosiderin granules
   D. alveolar pores
   E. surfactant

10. APUD (neuroendocrine) cells are thought to be involved in
    A. mucus
    B. serous fluid
    C. lung development
    D. production of surfactant
    E. phagocytosis

Explanatory Answers

1. A. The entire tracheobronchial tree lining develops from a bud of evaginating endoderm originating from the pharyngeal floor at the midpoint between the right and left sixth branchial arches. The branchial mesoderm gives origin to muscles, bone, and connective tissues. Stomodeal ectoderm (oral cavity) gives origin to structures associated with the oral cavity and the hypophysis. Visceral mesothelium covers the external surfaces of the lung, while parietal mesothelium covers the body wall facing the pleural cavity.

2. C. These veins, the plexus cavernosus concharum, bear a strong resemblance to erectile tissue, except that there are no smooth myocytes in the connective tissue septae. Vibrissae are long hairs associated with sudoriferous and sebaceous glands at the cutaneous region of the nasal cavity. Alveoli are the terminal functional components of the tracheobronchial tree.

3. E. The olfactory neurosensory epitheliocytes are bipolar neurons, and as such are expected to possess axons and dendrites. Cilia are involved in stirring up the liposerous solution containing the substance to be "smelled." The nuclei at different levels give the impression of pseudostratification. Mucous droplets fill the apical regions of the sustentacular (supporting) epitheliocytes.

4. D. The dark cells characterize the olfactory glands in the lamina propria of the olfactory region. These cells provide the lipid moiety to the glandular secretion, especially for those odiferous substances that are more soluble in a lipid medium. All the other cells comprise respiratory pseudostratified ciliated columnar epithelium.

5. B. The bronchi possess all the structures listed except the tracheal muscle. In extrapulmonary bronchi, cartilaginous rings are C or Y shaped. The posterior segment of the "C" is filled in with the tracheal muscle. (The Y ring is simply a forked C ring.)

6. A. There are no goblet cells to produce mucus that could drain back to the alveoli. Most particulate material has been trapped prior to reaching the bronchioles. Cilia move serous fluid up to where mucous glands and goblet cells are prevalent. Submucosal glands have a negligible population of mucous acini.

7. B. The bronchiolar exocrine cell, formerly the Clara cell, is confined to bronchioles. A precise function has not been clarified as yet. Some investigators suggest that it produces surfactant-like substance; others, intrigued by the abundant smooth ER, suggest a role in detoxification. There is no goblet cell and no light cell. The latter occurs in olfactory glands, where it contributes a serous fluid to dissolve substances to be "smelled." The great epitheliocyte and respiratory epitheliocyte occur in the alveoli.

8. E. Sustentacular epitheliocytes occur in the olfactory epithelium as supporting cells. Components of the interalveolar septum do not require cells as large as the sustentacular cells. Gaseous exchange occurs through the anuclear parts of the squamous respiratory epitheliocyte and the anuclear parts of the squamous capillary endothelium and through the fused basement membranes sandwiched between the two. The great epitheliocytes are the surfactant producing cells.

9. D. Communicating alveolar pores, between alveoli, facilitate collateral circulation of air, which otherwise might result in alveolar collapse. Alveolar macrophages clean the alveoli and frequently may devour erythrocytes to account for the presence of hemosiderin granules. Surfactant decreases alveolar surface tension and may contribute to preventing collapse of alveoli. However, the pores are especially dedicated to fulfilling this role.

10. C. While the precise function of the APUD cells is not defined, current speculations relate them to lung development and neonatal development. As endocrine cells, they are not involved in exocrine production of mucus, serous fluid, or surfactant. Phagocytosis is a function of the alveolar macrophages.

18 The Urinary Organs

I. The urinary organs form an excretory system consisting of the *kidneys*, which excrete urine, *ureters*, which convey urine to the *urinary bladder* for temporary storage, and the *urethra*, which conducts urine to the exterior.

    A. *The kidneys* (Brenner and Rector, 1976)

        1. *Statistics*

            a. Each kidney houses from 1 to 3 million *renal corpuscles* (glomerulus + capsule).

            b. The filtration surface of all renal corpuscles in both kidneys averages 1.5 m^2, approximately equal to the surface area of the skin (cf integument).

            c. A **glomerulus** (consisting of fenestrated capillaries) is covered by a bilayered epithelial *glomerular capsule* leading to a 30- to 35-mm-long tubule, the *nephron.*

            d. Placing all nephrons end to end would form a straight line 40 to 50 miles long.

            e. Kidney diseases account for 10% of all deaths.

        2. *Kidney functions*

            a. *Excretion* of

                (1) *waste products* from protein metabolism,

                (2) *salts,*

                (3) *foreign substances,*

                (4) *toxic substances.*

            b. *Maintenance* of extracellular fluid volume.

            c. *Regulation of*

                (1) *salt balance:* amounts and types of salts to be retained or excreted.

                (2) *fluid balance* (total body water): the volume and composition of all body fluids according to the changing needs in health and disease.

    (3) *acid-base balance.*
    (4) *blood pressure.*

  3. *Structural considerations* (Fig. 18-1)
    a. *Location:* retroperitoneally in the posterior abdominal wall, to the right and left of the vertebral column.
    b. *Packing:* the surrounding loose connective tissue and adipose tissue permits the kidney to move with diaphragmatic excursions. Some degree of stability is offered by the large renal artery and renal vein.
    c. *Vasculature* (Fig. 18-1C): The vasculature is organized to provide blood to the cortical lobules via the *interlobular arteries.*

Figure 18-1 Organization of the kidney. (A) Gross structure, (B) coronal section through an entire kidney, (C) vasculature.

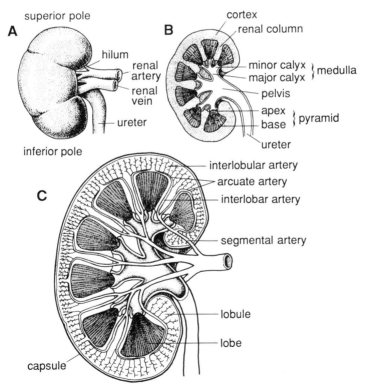

(1) These give rise to *afferent glomerular arterioles,* which enter the capsules to form glomeruli.

(2) Blood is drained from the glomeruli via *efferent glomerular arterioles.*

(3) The efferent arterioles give rise to

(a) complex *cortical peritubular capillary networks* that continue into the medulla as

(b) *medullary peritubular capillary networks* following the path of the nephrons.

(c) descending straight vessels looping to form ascending straight vessels. These are called the **fasciculus vascularis** or **vasa recta.**

(4) The vasa recta ascend into the cortex to empty into *interlobular veins,* which drain blood from the kidney into exiting veins corresponding to supplying arteries.

d. *Surfaces:* the bean-shaped *kidney* is flattened in the antero-posterior dimension.

(1) *Superior pole:* the upper surface.

(2) *Inferior pole:* the lower surface.

(3) *Convex surface:* faces laterally.

(4) *Concave surface:* the **hilum,** faces medially.

e. *Measurements*

(1) *Height:* 12 cm (superior to inferior).

(2) *Width:* 6 cm (medial to lateral).

(3) *Thickness:* 3 cm (anterior to posterior).

(4) *Weight:* 130 to 175 g

4. *Kidney components:* A median coronal plane through the superior and inferior poles divides the kidney into an anterior half and a posterior half. In this type of section the following structures can be recognized (Fig. 18-1):

a. *fibrous capsule* of dense fibrous connective tissue

(1) The capsule is loosely adherent to the underlying parenchyma.

(2) If bound tightly by adhesions, prior inflammatory disease (nephritis) is suspect.

(3) A more delicate layer of connective tissue, with fewer collagen fibers and some elastic fibers, lies under the fibrous capsule, providing access for vessels and capillary beds.

b. *renal cortex,* dark red color is attributed to a rich vasculature supplying and draining glomeruli.

c. *medullary rays* consist of numerous bundles of *renal collect-*

ing tubules, arranged perpendicularly to the convex surface. Medullary rays reaching into the cortex produce striations.

    d. *renal medulla* composed of 8 to 18 *renal pyramids.*

        (1) *Pyramid base* abuts against the renal cortex.

        (2) *Renal papilla* (apex) aims at the hilum.

            (a) The *renal papilla* is the focus where all *papillary ducts* terminate as *papillary foramina* (Fig. 18-3).

            (b) Up to 20 papillary foramina comprise the **area cribrosa** (Latin: *cribrum*, sieve).

        (3) Medullary striations form two zones:

            (a) **zona externa** (basilar half of pyramids),

            (b) **zona interna** (apical half of pyramids).

    e. *renal columns* of cortical tissue surround the periphery of the renal pyramids.

    f. *renal pelvis*, the expanded end of the ureter in the hilum, "funnels" urine into the ureter.

        (1) The renal pelvis branches into three smaller divisions, the *major calyces.*

        (2) Each *calyx* in turn branches into at least four *minor calyces*, which cup tightly against the *renal papilla.*

        (3) One, two, or three *papillary ducts* drain into each minor calyx.

            (a) *Papillary ducts* penetrate the substance of the renal papilla and

            (b) branch several times within the pyramid to form the *renal collecting tubules.*

    g. *renal lobe* is an entire pyramid plus associated cortical tissue.

        (1) Cortical tissue is that capping the base of the pyramid (up to the capsule), *plus* half the width of a renal column adjacent to the walls of the associated pyramid.

        (2) Thus, 8 to 18 renal lobes are in each kidney.

    h. *cortical lobule*

        (1) All *nephrons* draining into one *renal collecting tubule* of a medullary ray form one *cortical lobule.*

        (2) Since there is no demarcation surface other than the medullary rays, the number of collecting tubules in the cortex equals the number of lobules in one kidney (about 20,000).

    5. *Development* (Moore, 1988) (Fig. 18-2)

    a. The *nephrogenic cord* is a longitudinal orientation of the intermediate mass of paraxial mesoderm, forming a

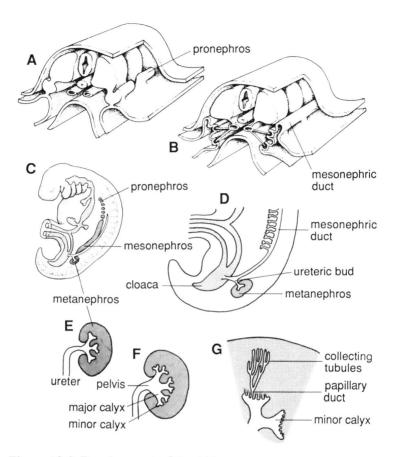

Figure 18-2 Development of the kidney.

(1) *pronephros*, which appears early in the fourth week of development, but is rudimentary and nonfunctional.

(2) *mesonephros*, appearing later in the fourth week caudal to the degenerating pronephros, serves as the excretory organ of the embryo until a permanent kidney is established. The *mesonephric duct* forms from the nephrogenic cord.

(3) *metanephros* appears early in the fifth week of development, surrounds the collecting ducts, and differentiates into components of the nephrons.

b. A permanent kidney arises from two mesoderm sources:
    (1) *metanephric diverticulum* (ureteric bud), which gives rise to
        (a) ureter,
        (b) renal pelvis,
        (c) calyces,
        (d) papillary ducts,
        (e) renal collecting tubules,
        (f) renal arcuate tubules.
    (2) *metanephric mesoderm*, which gives rise to metanephric vesicles:
        (a) the proximal end is invaginated by capillaries forming the *corpuscles.*
        (b) the distal end elongates to form the tubules of the *nephron.*

6. *Microscopic orientation*
    a. *Introduction* to the *nephron:* English nomenclature and relationships (Fig. 18-3). Each nephron has the following segments:
        (1) *Renal corpuscles*, consisting of **glomeruli** and *glomerular capsules*, reside at all levels of the cortex. Three nephron sizes, based on tubule length, are distinguished.
            (a) *Short nephrons*, close to the fibrous capsule, send their tubules into the **zona externa** of the medulla and loop back into the cortex to terminate in collecting tubules.
            (b) *Long nephrons*, near the base of the renal pyramids (medulla), send their tubules deep into the **zona** *interna* of the medulla.
            (c) *Intermediate nephrons* send tubules into the medulla at relative depths between the short and long nephrons.
        (2) The *proximal convoluted tubule*, a thick, highly coiled tubule commencing at the tubular pole of the renal corpuscle, which eventually straightens out to become the
        (3) *proximal straight tubule*, a thick descending tubule traveling from the cortex and into the medulla to about the junction with the inner stripe of the external zone, where it becomes the
        (4) *thin tubule.* In intermediate and long nephrons the thin tubule consists of
            (a) a *descending part*,
            (b) a *loop of the nephron*, and
            (c) an *ascending part* that reaches the junction of the internal zone and external zone, where it becomes the

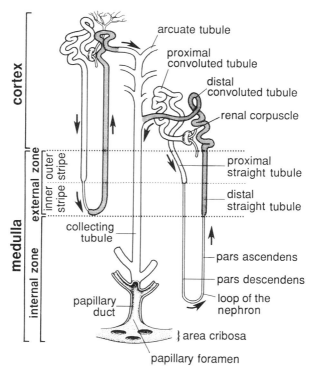

Figure 18-3 The nephron.

(5) *distal straight tubule*, a thick segment ascending into the cortex, close to the corpuscle of origin, to become

(6) the *distal convoluted tubule*. After several convolutions, it straightens out to join a renal arcuate tubule.

    b. *Structure of the renal corpuscle:* English nomenclature (Fig. 18-4).

        (1) *Renal corpuscle* consists of the *glomerular capsule* + a **glomerulus**.

            (a) The *glomerular capsule*, with an *external wall* and an invaginated *internal wall*, confines a narrow space, the *capsular lumen*. Two polar ends are discerned:

                [1] a *vascular pole*, through which vessels enter and leave,

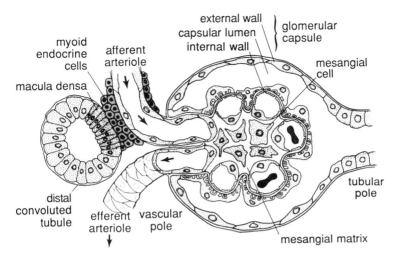

Figure 18-4 The renal corpuscle. The vacant space, associated with the juxtaglomerular complex (between the afferent and efferent arterioles), is occupied by the extraglomerular mesangium.

[2] a *tubular pole*, directly opposite, which gives origin to the proximal convoluted tubule begins.

(b) The **glomerulus** (Latin: *glomus*, a ball) consists of a *glomerular capillary network* suspended from the *vascular pole* by two arterioles:

[1] an *afferent glomerular arteriole*, which delivers blood to be filtered into the glomerular capillaries.

[2] an *efferent glomerular arteriole*, which transfers filtered blood into the arterial circulation.

7. *Cells of the glomerular capsule* (Fig. 18-5)

a. The *external wall*

(1) *Simple squamous epithelium* adheres to its basement membrane, which attaches to the surrounding connective tissue stroma. The epithelial cells are characterized by

(a) nuclei bulging into the capsular lumen.

(b) the surface **plasmalemma** facing the capsular lumen:

[1] over the nuclear bulge, it bears a single cilium and a few short microvilli.

[2] over the cell periphery, it bears large numbers of short microvilli.

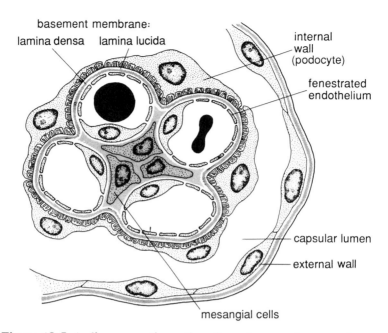

Figure 18-5 A diagrammatic section through a renal corpuscle.

(2) At the *tubular pole* (Fig. 18-4), the epithelium changes abruptly from simple squamous to simple columnar of the proximal convoluted tubule.

b. The *internal wall*

(1) After invagination of the renal corpuscle, the embryonic, simple squamous epithelium transformed to low cuboidal and then to columnar.

(2) *Podocytes*, complex branching cells with foot processes, are produced after further differentiation (Fig. 18-6). Repetitive branching forms:

(a) *primary, secondary,* and *tertiary foot processes.*

(b) *pedicels*, terminal branches extending at right angles from tertiary foot processes. Pedicels, clasping the capillaries, interdigitate so precisely that the entire outer surface of every capillary is covered.

(3) *Filtration slit membrane*, a 25-mm slit bridging interdigitating pedicels.

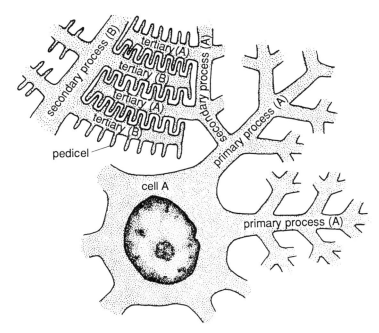

Figure 18-6 The interdigitation of pedicels of podocyte A and part of podocyte B.

    (a) In profile this membrane appears as thin as a diaphragm covering a capillary fenestration.

    (b) Pedicel and filtration slit membrane integrity is dependent on a thick coating of *sialic acid*.

    8. The **mesangium** (literally, "between vessels")

    a. *Mesangial cells* are embedded in an extracellular matrix "between vessels" of the glomerulus. Extraglomerular mesangium "between" afferent and efferent arterioles contributes to the juxtaglomerular complex (Barajas and Lata, 1967).

    b. *Capillaries*, forming at least four lobule-like loop structures in each glomerulus, are supported by the cellular **mesangium**.

    (1) At least one half to three quarters of the capillary outer surface faces the *capsular lumen*.

    (2) The remaining one or one quarter of the capillary surface is in intimate contact with the **mesangium**.

    c. The stellate-shaped *mesangial cells*
      (1) are voracious, active phagocytes,
      (2) provide structural support to the lobules,
      (3) maintain the structural integrity of the *glomerular basement membrane* (Fig. 18-5),
      (4) may participate in the formation of *renin*.
    9. *Glomerular capillaries* (Beeuwkes, 1980)
      a. The majority of the endothelial *fenestrae* (50 nm in diameter) lack diaphragms.
      b. Branched thickened regions (lacking fenestrae) provide structural support for the thinner fenestrated portions. The thickened regions bear various forms of microprojections of unknown nature.

    10. The *glomerular basement membrane (GBM)*, between capillary endothelium and podocytes, is thicker than basement membranes in most epithelial tissues. The *GBM* is composed of three identifiable *laminae* (Fig. 18-7).
    a. *Laminae* of the *GBM*
      (1) lamina lucida interna, a 10-nm-thick, electron-lucent layer in contact with the fenestrated endothelium.
      (2) lamina lucida externa, a 10-nm-thick, electron-lucent layer in contact with the pedicels of the podocytes.
      (3) lamina densa, a thicker (20 to 50 nm) electron-dense layer sandwiched between the two laminae lucidae, represents the fused product produced by podocytes and endothelial cells.

Figure 18-7 The glomerular basement membrane between capillary endothelium and tips of the podicyte pedicels.

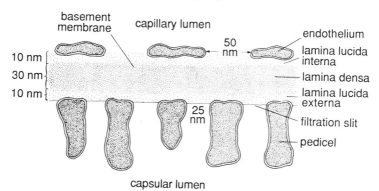

b. *Formation* of the *GBM*

(1) The lamina lucida interna + one half of the lamina densa are produced by the capillary endothelium.

(2) The lamina lucida externa + the other half of the lamina densa are products of the podocytes.

c. *Location* of the *GBM*

(1) The GBM (Fig. 18-5) covers the external endothelial surface (facing the capsular lumen) of all capillaries.

(2) There is *no* basement membrane on the external mesangial surface of the capillaries. The juxtacapillary mesangial matrix appears to possess adequate basement membrane properties.

d. *Maintenance* and *integrity* of the *GBM*

(1) The phagocytic *mesangial cells* maneuver through the mesangial matrix to remove foreign substances.

(2) Deteriorated portions of the lamina densa are removed by phagocytic activity of mesangial cell processes.

(3) New basement membrane material may be produced by the mesangial cells.

e. *Chemical nature* of the *GBM*

(1) *Fibronectin* and *laminin* occur in the lamina lucida externa and lamina lucida interna. Both have strong binding properties (Madri et al, 1980).

(2) *Type IV collagen* occurs in the lamina densa.

(3) Mesangial cells (in vitro) produce type IV collagen and fibronectin, suggesting participatory potential in structuring the GBM.

(4) Laminin production by mesangial cells has not been verified.

11. *The filtration barrier* consists of

a. *glomerular fenestrated capillaries*

(1) *Fenestrations* permit molecules up to 70,000 mw to pass through.

(2) *Albumin*, the principal plasma protein, with a 70,000 mw is retained in the circulation.

b. *glomerular basement membrane*

(1) is the major unit of this barrier.

(2) prevents necessary plasma proteins from leaking out.

c. *pedicel filtration membrane*

(1) The contributions of this part of the barrier are not considered as great as once proposed.

(a) Prior attributes were based on high mw cationic proteins (myeloperoxidase and horseradish peroxidase) passing through and binding to negatively charged epithelial cell surfaces and the laminae lucidae.

(b) This finding suggested that endothelial fenestrae were 100 nm in diameter.

(2) However, anionic tracers (native ferritin, catalase, IgG, or endogenous albumin) and neutral tracers do not penetrate beyond the lamina lucida interna. These findings

(a) confirm morphological studies that endothelial fenestrae are more in the range of 50 nm in diameter,

(b) designate the **lamina densa** as the major component of the filtration barrier (Farquhar, 1975).

12. *Structural details of the nephron tubules*
a. *Proximal convoluted tubules* are highly coiled, measuring under 15 mm in length, and 60 μm in diameter. They make up the greater mass of the cortex.

(1) The *epithelial cells* range from simple cuboidal to simple columnar, with a single spherical nucleus.

(a) The *luminal surface* is covered by long, tightly packed, branched microvilli (the old "brush border"), increasing the absorptive surface by 20×. In routine preparations, the long microvilli project into the lumen and frequently obscure it.

(b) The *basal* and *lateral* surfaces are invaginated by numerous folds that

[1] provide narrow cytoplasmic columns to accommodate the rod-like mitochondria.

[a] The aligned acidophilic mitochondria produce striations in the basal cytoplasm, resembling those of the salivary gland striated ducts.

[b] Mitochondria provide the high energy required for active transport of fluids.

[2] prevent visualization of the lateral borders of the cells in routine preparations.

(c) *Junctional complexes* unite the luminal edges, thereby preventing filtered fluid from passing between cells. Fluid to be absorbed must be processed intracellularly, before reentering the circulation.

(d) The *golgi complex* caps the luminal surface of the nucleus.

(2) *Capillary plexuses:* To provide for the return of fluids and absorbed substances to the circulation, rich capillary plexuses surround the proximal convoluted tubules.

(a) A thin basement membrane separates the capillary endothelium from the base of the absorbing epithelial cell.

(b) These capillaries possess fenestrations, closed by a single-layered diaphragm with a thickened central knob.

(3) *The filtrate*

(a) 1300 ml of blood flows through both kidneys, per minute.

(b) 125 ml filtrate forms in the capsular lumen.

(c) 124 ml is resorbed in the nephron tubules.

(d) *result:* 1 ml urine/min is excreted.

(4) *The proximal convoluted tubule* and the *proximal straight tubule* account for the reabsorption of

(a) 85% of the NaCL, or 3 lb/day,

(b) 85% cf the water,

(c) 100% of the glucose, or 0.5 lb/day,

(d) 100% of the acetoacetic acid and ascorbic acid.

(5) Other portions of the nephron remove the remainder of fluids and other molecules.

b. The *thin tubule*, about 15 μm in diameter,

(1) forms a loop consisting of

(a) a *descending part*,

(b) an *ascending part*.

(2) Distinctive cell types have been reported in rats and in animals with unilobular kidneys. Some similarities exist between humans and these animals, particularly the height of the cells and the quality of the tight junctions (Kriz et al, 1980).

(a) Type I: characteristic of short nephrons

[1] thin squamous epithelium, sparse microvilli,

[2] no cellular interdigitations,

[3] tight junctions consist of up to four junctional strands.

(b) Type II: found in the descending portion of long nephrons, up to the beginning of the internal zone of the medulla.

[1] cells are about three times the thickness of type I cells and have some interdigitations,

[2] numerous microvilli,

[3] nuclei do not appear as frequently as other cell structures,

[4] luminal junctional tight junctions have only two junctional strands.

(c) Type III: found in the remaining descending portion through the internal zone and part of the loop.

[1] cells are about one half the thickness of type II cells,

[2] composed of noninterdigitated cells, with some microvilli,

[3] several (more than four) strands occur in the tight junctions.

(d) Type IV: the remainder of the loop and the ascending part of the thin tubule, ending at the junction with the external zone of the medulla. Here it widens into the distal straight tubule.

[1] thin squamous epithelium,

[2] many cell interdigitations, and only minimal microvilli,

[3] the tight junctions have only one or two strands.

c. *Distal straight tubule*, the thick portion about 9 mm long, enters the cortex and approaches its renal corpuscle of origin. There it adheres to the *afferent arteriole* to become a component of the *juxtaglomerular complex* (Barajas and Latta, 1967), consisting of

(1) differentiated *smooth myocytes* of the afferent arteriole at the contact site, the *myoid endocrine cells* (juxtaglomerular cells). These cells are probably the source of the enzyme *renin*.

(a) a basophilic cytoplasm due to an abundant granular endoplasmic reticulum,

(b) cytoplasmic membrane-bound granules with a crystalline internal structure (probably the source of *renin*).

(2) the **macula densa**, a thickened region of tall columnar cells of the *distal straight tubule* at the contact site with the myoid endocrine cells.

(3) a thin *basement membrane* separating the myoid endocrine cells from the macula densa, which are considered to be functionally related.

(4) The enzyme *renin* may form in response to fluid in the lumen of the tubulus rectus distalis at the macula densa. Extraglomerular *mesangial cells*, part of the juxtaglomerular complex, participate in the production of renin.

(a) *Renin* is released by the juxtaglomerular complex in response to a decrease in extracellular fluid volume.

(b) *Renin* acting on *angiotensinogen* produces an inactive decapeptide, *angiotensin I*.

(c) *Angiotensin I* (via action of a converting enzyme) is converted to the octapeptide *angiotensin II*, which is also a vasoconstrictor.

(d) *Angiotensin II* stimulates the suprarenal gland zona glomerulosa to release *aldosterone*.

(e) *Aldosterone* acts on the cells of the collecting ducts to resorb *Na* ions in exchange for *H* or *K* ions.

d. The *distal convoluted tubule*, beginning at the macula densa, is characterized by a wide lumen lined by simple cuboidal epithelium. After straightening out it connects to the *renal arcuate tubules*.

(1) A few short microvilli, and some "bald" cell surfaces, distinguish this segment from the proximal convoluted segment.

(2) The basal surface of the cells is highly compartmentalized by invaginations of the plasmalemma and filled with numerous long vertically oriented mitochondria.

(3) The golgi complex capping the luminal side of the nucleus is small. The rER is scattered among free polyribosomes.

(4) One small cilium arising from a single centriole (basal body) may project from the free surface.

(5) Tight junctions are weak, suggesting that water and solutes may pass between cells as well as through them.

13. *Renal collecting tubules* originate as blind-ended tubules and travel a total of some 20 mm from their origin in the cortex to their exit at the *papillary duct*. Three portions may be distinguished (Fig. 18-3):

a. *Arcuate renal tubules* in the cortex arch over to meet the terminus of the distal convoluted tubule. These are about 1 mm long and 30 μm in diameter. Lightly acidophilic simple cuboidal epithelium lines the lumen.

b. *Straight collecting tubules* extend from the cortical medullary rays to the external zone of the medulla. Simple cuboidal epithelium with large cells surround a lumen twice the diameter of the arcuate tubules.

c. *Papillary ducts* 10 to 12 mm long (formerly: the ducts of Bellini), formed by the union of several collecting tubules, are lined by simple columnar epithelium. The lumen gradually increases to a diameter of 200 μm at the area cribrosa leading into a minor calyx.

14. *The calyces*

a. From the *papillary ducts*, *urine* flows successively into the minor calyx, major calyx, renal pelvis, and finally into the ureter for conveyance to the urinary bladder.

b. The *minor calyx*

(1) In the portion attached to the renal papilla, the epithelium is stratified columnar (continuous with the simple columnar of the papillary duct).

(2) The luminal free walls are lined with transitional epithe-

lium, over a thin lamina propria, characteristic of the remaining portions of the urinary apparatus.

c. The *major calyx* is like the free portion of the minor calyx, in which the transitional epithelium may be up to three cells thick.

(1) A tunica muscularis is represented by

(a) an *internal longitudinal stratum*,

(b) an *external circular stratum*.

[1] A sphincter of circular smooth myocytes rings the union of the major calyx to the renal pelvis. Muscular contractions "squirt" urine into the renal pelvis.

(2) The outer tunica adventitia consists of layers of collagen fibers.

15. The *renal pelvis*

a. is the flattened funnel-shaped end of the ureter in the hilum of the kidney that branches into *major calyces* and *minor calyces.*

b. offers no remarkable differences from the calyces, other than a thicker transitional epithelium and a thicker tunica muscularis.

B. *The ureter* is a tube with a stellate-shaped lumen, extending from the renal pelvis to the urinary bladder, a length from 25 to 34 cm.

1. The *ureter* is divided equally into

a. a retroperitoneal portion,

b. an abdominal portion,

c. a pelvic portion.

2. Three layers compose the wall of the ureter:

a. tunica mucosa

(1) transitional epithelium, increased in thickness up to 5 cells.

(2) lamina propria (connective tissue, with vessels and nerves).

b. tunica muscularis (nonstriated myocytes)

(1) *internal longitudinal stratum.*

(2) *circular stratum* (between strata). This layer does not exist in the termination of the ureter.

(3) *external longitudinal stratum* appears close to the urinary bladder and blends into its external layer.

(4) The advantage of two longitudinal layers is that on contraction (shorten the tube) within the wall of the urinary bladder, the lumen of the ureter dilates to release urine. Since smooth circular myocytes are absent in the termination of the ureter, only contraction of the bladder musculature closes the lumen of the ureter terminus.

c. tunica adventitia of connective tissue.

C. *Urinary bladder:* The urinary bladder is structurally similar to the ureter, but possesses thicker layers.

1. Tunica mucosa

    a. *Transitional epithelium* of specially adapted cells to accommodate repeated filling and voiding.

        (1) *Surface characteristics* of transitional cells facing the lumen:

            (a) numerous crests scallop the external surface of the plasmalemma.

            (b) a thick feltwork of cytoskeletal fibrils is layered under the cytoplasmic surface of the plasmalemma.

            (c) invaginations and interdigitations of the plasmalemma surfaces of deeper cells.

            (d) relatively few desmosomes connect the cells, thus permitting them to glide over one another to facilitate and increase the number of intercellular invaginations when the bladder is filling. This results in thinning the epithelium of the distended bladder. The reverse increases epithelial thickness.

        (2) *Fusiform vesicles:* Within the feltwork and deep cytoplasm of cells facing the lumen, numerous fusiform vesicles possessing walls with the same structure as the plasmalemma.

            (a) It is suggested that the vesicles form from the fusion of opposing crests of the plasmalemma.

            (b) After pinching off from the surface, they migrate through the feltwork into the deeper cytoplasm where they apparently are destroyed by lysosomes.

            (c) This mechanism gradually replaces the surface plasmalemma worn out by constant exposure to hypertonic urine.

        (3) *The basement membrane* is extremely thin, by TEM standards. In fact, light microscopists questioned its existence. Thin-walled venules in the underlying connective tissue abut against the basement membrane, so that if trauma loosens the epithelium, invariably there will be blood in the urine.

    2. Tunica muscularis: three smooth muscle layers

        a. internal longitudinal stratum

        b. circular stratum (between strata)

        c. external longitudinal stratum

    3. Tunica serosa: covers the superior external surface with peritoneal mesothelium over a connective tissue **tela subserosa.**

    4. Tunica adventitia: covers the other external surfaces.

D. *Urethra*

   1. The *male urethra* is characterized by the anatomical regions it traverses:

      a. *prostatic part:* about 3 cm long, is lined by transitional epithelium.

      b. *membranous part:* about 1 cm long, is lined by stratified or pseudostratified columnar epithelium. This part perforates the urogenital diaphragm which contributes skeletal myocytes to form the *urethral sphincter.*

      c. *spongiosa part:* about 15 cm long, passes through the corpus spongiosum of the penis. It is lined by stratified squamous epithelium. Mucous-type *urethral glands* residing in the lamina propria, and sometimes in the spongiosum, empty on the surface epithelium.

   2. The *female urethra:* only 3 cm long

      a. Epithelium:

         (1) stratified squamous epithelium with

         (2) occasional patches of pseudostratified columnar epithelium.

      b. Lamina propria: resembles the male corpus spongiosum with its venous plexuses.

      c. *Urethral mucous glands* empty onto the epithelial surface.

Questions

DIRECTIONS: For each of the items in this section, one or more of the numbered options is correct. Select

   A if only *1, 2, and 3* are correct
   B if only *1 and 3* are correct
   C if only *2 and 4* are correct
   D if only *4* is correct
   E if *all* are correct

  1. The renal pelvis connects directly with the
    1. urethra
    2. ureter
    3. pyramid base
    4. three major calyces

2. The total number of cortical lobules equals the number of
   1. renal pyramids
   2. medullary rays
   3. minor calyces
   4. renal collecting tubules

3. The permanent kidney arises from
   1. metanephric diverticulum
   2. mesonephros
   3. metanephric mesoderm
   4. mesonephric duct

4. The renal corpuscle consists of
   1. glomerular capsule
   2. proximal convoluted tubule
   3. glomerulus
   4. distal convoluted tubule

5. Podocytes
   1. develop from internal wall cells of the glomerular capsule
   2. are complex branching cells
   3. possess interdigitating pedicels
   4. form the filtration slit membrane

6. The mesangium
   1. consists of stellate phagocytes in an extracellular matrix
   2. occurs between the afferent and efferent arterioles
   3. may participate in the formation of renin
   4. occurs between glomerular capillary loops

7. The glomerular basement membrane receives contributions from
   1. endothelial cells
   2. podocytes
   3. intraglomerular mesangial cells
   4. macula densa

8. The glomerular filtration barrier consists of the
   1. fenestrated capillaries
   2. basement membrane
   3. pedicel filtration membrane
   4. extraglomerular mesangial cells

		Directions Summarized		
A	**B**	**C**	**D**	**E**
1,2,3	1,3	2,4	4	All are
only	only	only	only	correct

9. The juxtaglomerular complex consists of differentiated
   1. mesangial cells
   2. smooth myocytes
   3. tubular epithelial cells
   4. endothelial cells

10. Characteristics associated with the surface plasmalemmma of transitional epithelial cells of the urinary bladder are
    1. scalloped crests
    2. cytoskeletal fibrils
    3. invaginations and interdigitations
    4. relatively few desmosomes

11. The urethra is characterized by
    1. stratified squamous epithelium
    2. a tunica muscularis
    3. mucous glands
    4. a tunica serosa

12. A thin tubule of a nephron is separated into four types, based on
    1. number of strands in the tight junction
    2. cell interdigitations
    3. microvilli
    4. height of cells

Explanatory Answers

1. C. 2 and 4 are correct. The three major calyces reach deeper into the hilum and give rise to the minor calyces, which in turn cup against the renal papilla (apex of the pyramid). The pyramid base contacts the renal cortex. The urethra makes no contact with the renal pelvis. The terms urethra and ureter are used. The question could be, "What is the difference between the ureter and urethra?"

2. D. 4 is correct. Renal collecting tubules plus all the nephrons draining into them compose a cortical lobule. The medullary rays consist of bundles of renal collecting tubules, thus counting bundles would not provide an answer. The renal pyramids plus all associated cortical tissue make up a lobe (not a lobule). Counting minor calyces into which the apices of the pyramids fit also provides the number of lobes.

3. B. 1 and 3 are correct. The metanephric diverticulum gives rise to tubules from the ureter up to the renal arcuate (collecting) tubules. The metanephric mesoderm gives origin to the renal corpuscles plus the tubules of the nephron. The mesonephros and its ducts serve as an excretory organ until the permanent kidney is established.

4. B. 1 and 3 are correct. The associated convoluted tubules belong to the nephron.

5. E. All are correct. The filtration slit membrane is a 25-nm slit bridging interdigitating pedicels. Pedicels are the terminal branches extending at right angles from tertiary processes.

6. E. All are correct. The mesangium forms the intraglomerular support of the capillary loops. They are not only phagocytic, but also assist in repair and maintenance of the basement membrane. An extraglomerular mesangial mass between the afferent and efferent arterioles contributes to the formation of the enzyme renin.

7. A. 1, 2, and 3 are correct. The endothelial cells produce the lamina lucida interna plus one half of the lamina densa, which is fused to the lamina densa produced by the podocytes. The podocytes also produce the lamina lucida externa. Contributions to the maintenance and repair of the basement membrane is a function of the intraglomerular mesangial cells. The macula densa is involved with the juxtaglomerular complex.

8. A. 1, 2, and 3 are correct. Each of the components are important, but the glomerular basement membrane is the major unit. The capillary fenestrations retain molecules larger than 70,000 mw. The extraglomerular mesangial cells do not contribute to this filtration barrier.

9. A. 1, 2, and 3 are correct. The smooth myocytes of the afferent arteriole transform to myoid endocrine cells, which may be the source of renin. A second component of the juxtaglomerular complex is a thickened region of tall columnar cells of the distal straight tubule at the contact site with the myoid endocrine cells. A third component, albeit indirect, is the mesangium. Mesangial cells do participate in the production of renin. Endothelial cells are only involved by virtue of their relative positions.

10. E. All are correct. The external surface plasmalemma of superficial cells show scalloped crests. The cytoplasmic surface of the plasmalemma is lined by a thick feltwork of cytoskeletal fibrils. Invaginations and interdigitations of all plasmalemma surfaces appear on deeper cells. The relatively few desmosomes give more freedom to the cells, permitting them to glide over one another to accommodate filling of the bladder.

11. B. 1 and 3 are correct. The male urethra also has transitional epithelium in the prostatic portion and some pseudostratified columnar epithelium. The female urethra has only some patches of pseudostratified columnar epithelium in addition to the stratified squamous epithelium. Urethral mucous glands in the male and female urethrae empty onto the epithelial surface. There is no tunica muscularis as in the ureter. The abdominal and pelvic portions of the ureter have a tunica serosa, but the urethra that is housed in spongiosum does not.

12. E. All are correct. Tabular form compares the characteristics:

Cell type	Tight junctions	Interdigitations	Microvilli	Cell height
Type I	4− strands	no	sparse	thin squamous
Type II	2 strands	yes	many	thick squamous
Type III	4+ strands	no	some	thick squamous
Type IV	2− strands	yes	minimal	thin squamous

19 The Genital Apparatus

I. The *male genital organs* (Fawcett, 1976) consist of *primary* and *accessory organs*. The **testis** is the only primary organ. Accessory organs consist of the **epididymis, ductus deferens,** *seminal vesicle, prostate, bulbourethral glands,* and the **penis.** Sperm developing in the testis are conveyed to the exterior through a series of tubes (the accessory organs). During passage, various contributions by the accessory organs nourish the sperm, make them more motile, and counteract the acidity of vaginal fluids.

 A. Testes (sing. **testis**) are two bean-shaped organs residing outside the body cavity in the scrotum. A prolongation of the peritoneal tunica serosa extends through the inguinal canal into the scrotum and clasps the testis in a mitten-like sac (Fig. 19-1).

 1. The sac, **tunica vaginalis,** consists of an inner *visceral lamina* and an outer *parietal lamina.* Generally, the sac is sealed off from the peritoneal cavity. Should a patency occur, it is possible for a loop of intestine to herniate through the *inguinal canal* and into the sac of the tunica vaginalis.

 2. The testis proper is encased in a thick, white collagenous capsule, the **tunica albuginea,** except at the concave **hilum,** where it is much thicker. This area is the **mediastinum testis.** The visceral lamina of the tunica vaginalis contacts the tunica albuginea.

 3. From the mediastinum testis, connective tissue *septulae* radiate outward to the convex surface to divide the testis into approximately 250 *compartments.*

  a. Each compartment contains *testicular lobules* composed of 70-cm-long convoluted *seminiferous tubules,* packed in loose connective tissue. In any one compartment, there may be from one to four convoluted seminiferous tubules, which may be independent of one another or randomly interconnected. Consider for the sake of rapid

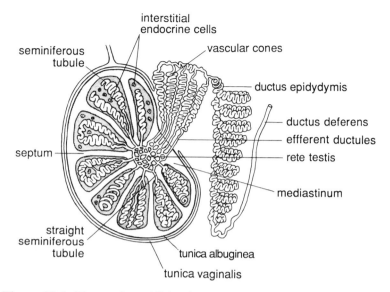

Figure 19-1 The testis, epididymis, and ductus deferens.

calculation, two seminiferous tubules per lobule at an average length of 50 cm each. For 250 compartments, there would be 50,000 cm of seminiferous tubules for both testes, or about the length of five or six football fields.

    b. Spermatogenesis, occurring within the seminiferous tubules, is a process whereby spermatogonia are transformed into spermatozoa.

    (1) Three phases characterize this process:

        (a) *Spermatocytogenesis:* In this process, mitosis of **spermatogonia** occurs, giving rise to more diploid spermatogonia, some of which become *spermatocytes.*

        (b) Meiosis is the process in which two successive maturation divisions reduce the human chromosome number from the diploid 46 to the haploid 23 of *spermatids.*

        (c) *Spermiogenesis* consists of a series of maturation changes whereby spermatids mature into **spermatozoa.**

    (2) Two major cell types characterize the continuously proliferating seminiferous tubule epithelium:

        (a) *spermatogenic cells,* the parenchymal cells in the process of sperm formation. *Phase I* occurs close to the basememt membrane surrounding the seminiferous tubule. *Phase II* occurs in the mid region of the epithelium. *Phase III* occurs at the luminal surface. The tails or flagella of the spermatozoa wave in the lumen while the head (nucleus) appears embedded in the luminal surface.

(b) *sustentacular epitheliocytes* (formerly the Sertoli cells), tall columnar cells reaching to the lumen (Dym, 1973).

[1] *Nuclear characteristics:* The nuclear membrane is indented in several places. Most striking is the nucleolus, comprising an acidophilic center flanked by two spherical basophilic accessory nucleoli.

[2] *Basal cytoplasm:* Smooth ER is abundant, with scattered patches of rough ER. A golgi complex and elongated/spherical mitochondria are surrounded by lipid droplets, glycogen granules, and thin filaments. Membrane-bound vesicles of varying electron densities occur.

[3] *Supranuclear* and *lateronuclear* areas contain rod-shaped mitochondria and longitudinally aligned fibrils.

[4] **Zonulae occludens** near the base join adjacent sustentacular cells to form an effective *blood–testis barrier*, which appears to prevent "foreign" proteins (androgen-binding protein, ABP) produced in the haploid cells from gaining access to the vascular system. These tight junctions also compartmentalize the developing spermatozoa: *basal compartment* (basement membrane to the tight junction) supports the spermatogonia in various stages of development; *adluminal compartment* (luminal side of the junction) supports the more mature haploid stages.

[5] *Spermatid nuclei* are buried in the indented apical plasmalemma of the sustentacular cells. Fine filamentous material and smooth flattened endoplasmic reticulum of sustentacular cells lie in a row around the spermatid nucleus. Crystalloids of parallel filaments close to the nucleus are found in man, but not in other species. Sustentacular columnar cells provide nutrition and flanking support for developing spermatozoa.

[6] *Ionizing radiations* delivered to the testes produce temporary sterility by destroying advanced differentiating stages of spermatocytes. However, the sustentacular cells are radioresistant and remain intact.

[7] *Functions:* formation of a blood–testis barrier, phagocytosis of degenerating cells, production of a fluid component to accompany the spermatozoa, provision of support and nutrition until spermatozoa are released.

(3) The **spermatozoön** consists of (Fawcett, 1975)

(a) the *head* (4 μm) has a **nucleus** hooded by an *acrosome* (a thin membranous bag containing several enzymes) surrounded by a tightly adhering plasmalemma. When the head touches the ovum, an *acrosomal reaction* occurs in which the membrane of the acrosome fuses at several points with the plasmalemma (quite similar to protein secretion). At these points, *pericephalic perforations* allow a first wave of enzymes out to disperse the protective cells (*follicular epitheliocytes*) around the ovum. Release of a second wave of enzymes facilitates penetration of the sperm.

(b) **cervix** (neck), a thin short segment (1 μm) attached to the *tail* (flagellum).

(c) *tail* (55 μm long) divided into three parts:

[1] the 4-μm-long **pars intermedia** contains a *mitochondrial sheath* and a demarcation **annulus** at the distal end,

[2] a 45-μm-long **pars principalis** with its *fibrous sheath*. Dense *external fibrillae* reside around the inner flagellum, resembling 9 + 2 typical cilia structure,

[3] a 6-μm-long **pars terminalis** (end piece) with no fibrillae under plasmalemma.

c. *Interstitial endocrine cells* of the testis (formerly the Leydig cells) reside in the loose connective tissue packing of the seminiferous tubules. They are spherical- or polyhedral-shaped cells (Christiansen, 1975).

(1) These 20-μm-diameter endocrine cells produce the hormone *testosterone* after stimulation by *ICSH*. Testosterone mediates the development and maintenance of male reproductive organs and secondary male characteristics (hair distribution, voice, bone structure, etc). The interstitial endocrine cells aggregate in patches along capillaries to facilitate transfer of testosterone into the circulatory system.

(2) The *interstitial endocrine cell* possesses a large golgi complex and an abundant tubular sER, with profiles varying from small circles to long ovals according to the plane of section. The sER forms concentric whorls around lipid droplets. Mitochondria display the tubular (and occasional leaf-like) cristae. Prominent *crystalloids* (formerly: crystals of Reinke) of varying sizes and shapes populate the cytoplasm (Sohval et al, 1971). The external cell surface is covered with numerous small microvilli.

4. *Straight seminiferous tubules:* As the convoluted seminiferous tubules of each compartment converge upon the mediastinum, they form *straight seminiferous tubules,* lined with simple columnar epithelium. In the dense connective tissue of the mediastinum, the *straight seminiferous tubules* branch repeatedly into the **rete testis**, a network of irregularly shaped tubules. A basement membrane is not resolvable by light microscopy and the lamina propria is indistinct. The cuboidal epithelium of the rete testis has a luminal surface with a sparse covering of microvilli. Some cells may project a single long flagellum.

B. Epididymis (pl. *epididymides*), the first extratesticular accessory organ, consists of *efferent ductules* and **ductus epididymidis** wrapped in connective tissue (Hamilton, 1975).

1. *Efferent ductules of the testes*, some 12 or more about 5 mm in length, exit the rete testis at the concave mediastinum. An equal number (12) first become convoluted and then coil to form 10-mm-long *vascular cones*, which ascend in increasingly larger coils (forming a "cone") to the level of the superior pole of the testis. A maze of capillary plexuses and loose connective tissue surround the vascular cones.

a. A pseudostratified columnar epithelium consists of the following cell types:

(1) *basal epitheliocytes,*

(2) *ciliated columnar cells*, in groups of short and tall cells, give a scalloped outline. Ciliary motility moves the immature spermatozoa toward the ductus epididymidis. Cytoplasmic organelles are sparse.

(3) *nonciliated columnar cells*, shorter in height, are distinguished by intracellular lysosomal granules. A glycocalyx coats the short luminal microvilli. That these cells are involved in fluid absorption is attested to by three zones of vesicle development in the apical cytoplasm: apical pits (at the bases of the microvilli), apical vesicles (pinched off from the pits), and various sized vacuoles (formed by the fusion of the vesicles).

b. The lamina propria of the straight efferent ductules contains a few circularly oriented smooth myocytes. The efferent ductules forming the coiled vascular cones are surrounded by a thicker muscular layer.

2. Ductus epididymidis (translation: duct of the epididymis. Note: epididymi*des* is the plural form; epididymi*dis* is the singular genitive).

a. At the larger ends of the vascular cones, the convoluted efferent ductules unite to form a single **ductus epididymidis**. From the level of the superior pole of the testis to the inferior pole of the testis, the *5-m-long* ductus epididymidis is tortuously convoluted and compressed into a 5 cm length. At the terminus, it straightens out for 50 cm.

b. The epithelium of the tall columnar cells in some sections appears pseudostratified. The luminal cell surfaces are covered with tall branched microvilli (formerly: stereocilia). A large golgi complex occupies the apical cytoplasm, and tubular sER fills the cytoplasm. The basement membrane rests on a network of capillaries and a circular layer of smooth myocytes.

C. **Ductus deferens:** the muscular excretory passage for sperm.

1. The most impressive feature of this tube is the massive size of the muscular wall compared to the lumen. Of the 2.5 mm diameter, 0.5 mm = lumen, 2.0 mm = nonstriated (smooth) muscle. Despite its small size, the ductus deferens is the most muscular tube in the body. Three muscle layers exist: *internal longitudinal stratum*, middle *circular stratum*, and *external longitudinal stratum*.

2. Though most of the ductus deferens is covered by a tunica adventitia, some portions are covered by a tunica serosa.

3. The low-profiled epithelium is gathered into longitudinal folds by the lamina propria.

4. The ductus deferens (covered by adventitia) exits the scrotum by ascending to the inguinal ring, passes through it into the pelvic cavity, and travels lateral to the bladder, where it may acquire a tunica serosa. It arches over the ureters and just prior to penetrating the substance of the prostrate gland, it dilates into the **ampulla ductus deferentis** (Fig. 19-2).

D. *Seminal vesicles.* The exiting duct of the **ampulla ductus deferentis** is joined by the duct of the *seminal vesicle.* (Note: Fig. 19-2, that one end is a blind sac.) The *seminal vesicles* are elongated pouches honeycombed by primary, secondary, and tertiary folds. Three layers comprise the wall:

1. **Tunica mucosa:** The columnar epithelium is generally pseudostratified. Yellow pigment appearing at puberty is found in apical vacuoles. Primary, secondary, and tertiary folds are composed of connective tissue of the tunica mucosa.

2. **Tunica muscularis:** This is a thin layer of muscle myocytes separated from the tunica mucosa by a thin lamina propria containing many elastic fibers.

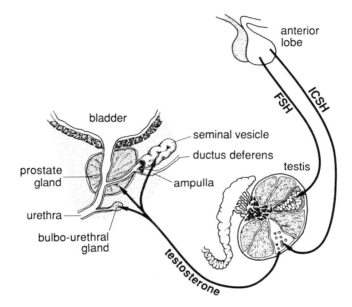

Figure 19-2 The testis and major hormonal relationships.

3. **Tunica adventitia** covers most of the surface. A **tunica serosa** may occur in some areas.

E. The *prostate gland* (McNeal, 1973): The prostate gland, about the size of a horse chestnut, is a mass of glandular tissue surrounding the urethra, after it emerges from the bladder.

1. The 50 composite glands (located anteriorly, posteriorly, and laterally) pass their secretions through 25 excretory ducts, some of which unite or empty directly alongside the small hill of tissue in the posterior wall of the prostatic urethra, the **colliculus seminalis.**

2. The glands are grouped concentrically around the urethra in three layers: tunica mucosa, tela submucosa, and in the fibromuscular layer. The latter is surrounded by a thick connective tissue capsule.

3. The glands have irregular lumina surrounded by elastic and collagen fibers. The epithelium, resting on an indistinct basement membrane, varies *from* squamous and low cuboidal in larger glandular alveolar cavities *to* pseudostratified columnar in most places. Nu-

merous membrane-bound secretory granules occupy the cytoplasm of the glandular epithelial cells.

4. The gland lumina frequently contain small, spherical, lamellated acidophilic bodies, the *prostatic concretions*, which can increase in number and size (up to 2 mm) after age 40. Small concretions may be added to the seminal fluid at the time of ejaculation. Large concretions may block exiting ducts, causing enlargement of the prostate. Severe enlargement may compress the prostatic urethra causing difficult urination.

F. *Bulbourethral glands* (Fig. 19-2) in the urogenital diaphragm empty into the proximal portion of the penile urethra. About the size of a pea, the glands discharge a mucous-like lubricant. Unlike mucus of salivary glands, this mucus fails to precipitate with acetic acid.

G. The **penis** serves dual functions: copulation and urination.

1. Three cylindrical elongate bodies are comprised in the penis: a right and a left **corpus cavernosum** and a **corpus spongiosum**. The urethra, conducting either seminal fluid or urine, travels through the corpus spongiosum.

a. Each corpus is sheathed by **tunica albuginea** and loose connective tissue, the **fascia penis**. The outermost covering of the penis is the **cutis penis**, thin skin with bundles of smooth myocytes in the dermis.

b. *Erectile tissue* is a plexus of collapsed veins, which when engorged with blood under elevated pressure results in penile erection. The portions between the endothelial walls contain fibromuscular septae of connective tissue interspersed with nonstriated (smooth) myocytes (Goldstein et al, 1982).

c. The **glans penis** is the conical enlargement crowning the terminal portion of the urethra. It is a continuation of the corpus spongiosum, but lacks a tunica albuginea. A thin stratified squamous epithelium is firmly attached to the underlying erectile tissue.

2. *Functions* and *contributions* of the male excretory ducts and accessory glands: The sum total of spermatozoa plus contributions of the ducts and accessory glands yields the ejaculate.

a. The **testes** produce about 200 to 300 million spermatozoa in a saline fluid. Counts may exceed 300 million (up to 500 million) or be reduced as low as 20 million. A 50 million sperm count is considered low fertility, while a 20 million count equates to sterility. A 20% to 25% amount of abnormal sperm is not unusual in a 2- to 6-ml ejaculate.

b. The *efferent ducts* forward spermatozoa and some fluid via the activity of ciliated cells. Most of the fluid is absorbed by the nonciliated columnar cells.

c. The **epididymis** is so long that it may take one month for sperm to make the journey. During this time, the sperm mature and lose the last bit of cytoplasm attached to the sperm head and middle piece. Smooth myocytes in the walls contract rhythmically during ejaculations to move the sperm along. The contribution of the epididymis secretory epithelium is a *viscid, nutritive substance.* Among the many components are sialic acid, glycoproteins, and some steroids.

d. The **ductus deferens** does not store sperm or make any substantial contribution to the seminal fluid. Its primary and probably only function is rapid propulsion of sperm during ejaculation.

e. The *seminal vesicles* produce a *yellowish, sticky, thick liquid* containing *globulin* and *fructose* (an energy sugar). The yellow lipochrome pigment *flavin* is identified by its *fluorescence,* an important medicolegal component of seminal fluid. *Prostaglandins* synthesized in the glandular epithelium not only act as regulators of smooth myocyte activity, but also influence transit of spermatozoa and implantation of the fertilized ovum. The secretion is slightly alkaline.

f. The *prostate* discharges large quantities of fluid to dilute the previous viscid secretions and stimulate sperm activity.

(1) The *thin milky emulsion* identified by its *opalescence* contains proteins and fine lipid droplets in suspension.

(2) This secretion, containing the *polyamine phosphate* of *spermine,* is the only secretion possessing the strong characteristic odor of semen. All other secretions in the male reproductive organs are odorless.

(3) Prostatic secretions, though slightly acid (pH 6.5), counteract the more acidic vaginal fluids. The prostate secretes continually, and not just at the time of ejaculation. Consequently, some of its components (zinc, citric acid, and acid phosphatase) are present in urine.

(a) High concentrations of acid phosphatase exist in the 0.5 ml to 2.0 ml/day prostatic secretion. Prostatic function is assessed quite reliably from the concentration of acid phosphatase:

[1] if *higher* than normal, prostatic carcinoma may be indicated.

[2] if *lower* than normal would indicate cessation of activity, as in senility.

(b) Prostatic proteolytic enzymes aid in identifying semen. The most important one, fibrinolysin, assists in the liquefaction of semen.

g. The *bulbourethral glands* and *urethral glands* contribute mucous-like substances to the semen.

H. *Basic hormonal interrelationships* (Fig. 19-2)

1. *ICSH + FSH* stimulate the interstitial endocrine cells of the testis to secrete *testosterone.*

2. *Testosterone + FSH* is required for development and maintenance of the seminiferous tubules.

3. *Testosterone* influences secondary characteristics and maintains the accessory glands.

I. *Aging:* Although spermatogenesis continues well into senility, the seminiferous tubules do involute, and eventually may show no spermatogenic cells. Within acceptable limits, in all age groups, some degeneration of spermatogenic cells occurs.

II. The *female genital organs* consist of a right and left *ovary,* right and left *uterine tube,* a single *uterus, vagina,* and *external genitalia* (Ludwig and Metzger, 1976).

A. The *ovary* (Peters and McNatty, 1980) measures 5 cm × 3 cm × 1.5 cm and weighs 8 g.

1. The *superficial epithelium* covering the ovary is generally torn loose in routine preparations. It consists of a single layer of cuboidal mesothelial cells bearing microvilli. The view that this was a "germinal epithelium" producing **ovogonia** is no longer espoused. The epithelium rests on a basement membrane, which in turn adheres to a layer of dense fibrous connective tissue, the **tunica albuginea** (similar to that encasing the testes).

2. A longitudinal section through the ovary reveals two distinct zones under the tunica albuginea: an outer parenchymal **cortex ovarii** and a central vascular **medulla ovarii** (Fig. 19-3).

a. The **cortex** consists of a connective tissue stroma bearing the parenchymal *ovarian follicles* containing **ova** (eggs) in varying developmental stages. Some **ovogonia** enter the process of **ovogenesis** on their way to becoming an **ovum.** **Ovogenesis** follows developmental stages corresponding to **spermatogenesis.** The sequential stages are: (1) the **ovogonium** develops into a *primary ovocyte* + a *primary polocyte,* which atrophies and dies, (2) the primary ovocyte forms a *secondary ovocyte* + a *secondary polocyte* (which atrophies and dies), (3) the secondary ovocyte forms a haploid **ovum.**

(1) *Primordial ovarian follicles* (primitive follicles) consist of small quiescent **ovogonia** enveloped by a monolayer of squamous

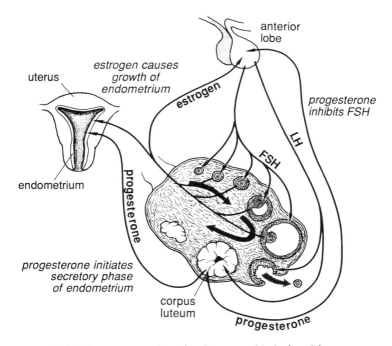

Figure 19-3 The ovary and major hormonal relationships.

follicular epitheliocytes. Active mitosis of ovogonia continues through fetal life, producing thousands of primitive ovogonia. After birth, ovogonia are no longer produced. Prenatally, some 2 million ovogonia enlarge to become *primary ovocytes.* Acquisition of one or more layers of cuboidal follicular cells changes the primordial follicle to a *primary ovarian follicle.*

(2) *Primary ovarian follicles* containing *primary ovocytes* are enveloped by one or two layers of cuboidal or columnar follicular epitheliocytes. Maternal gonadotrop(h)ins during pregnancy may stimulate some primary follicles to develop; however, the remaining are quiescent until puberty. Mesenchymal stromal tissue surrounding the follicle form a few concentric layers of fibroblast-like cells, which will differentiate into the *theca of the follicle* (specialized endocrine cells that will produce *estrogen*). Hormonal interactions between the hypophysis and the ovary and their effects on differentiation of follicular epitheliocytes is introduced and will be built on in subsequent courses (Richards, 1980).

(a) The large spherical *primary ovocyte*, identical to the ovogonium, measures about 45 μm and possesses a large vesicular nucleus with a single nucleolus. Cytoplasmic structures include a complex juxtanuclear structure referred to at one time as Balbiani's vitelline body. Electron microscopy reveals that this complex body consists of (1) spherical mitochondria, (2) multiple golgi complexes, bundles of fine wavy filaments attached to the nuclear membrane, (3) vesicles, (4) compound aggregates (membrane-bound structures containing lipid droplets among other substances), (4) ER, and (5) the *annulate lamellae* (Kessel, 1968), parallel stacks of membranes formed from the nuclear membrane. The latter are involved in nucleocytoplasmic relationships.

(b) *Follicular epitheliocytes* have rER surrounding a large nucleus, distinguished by heterochromatin along the nuclear membrane (Amenta et al, 1973). Lipid droplets and dense *aggregates* resembling those of the ovocyte accumulate in the cytoplasm.

(3) The *maturing ovarian follicle* involves growth of the ovocyte and surrounding follicular cells. Changes in the primary ovocyte are reflected mainly in increasing size and complexity of organelles. The golgi complex becomes widely dispersed throughout the cytoplasm, while sER and free polyribosomes increase in quantity.

(a) The *secondary ovarian follicle* continues growth by adding layers of *follicular epitheliocytes* and a developing *follicular theca*.

(b) The *tertiary follicle* consists of a large primary ovocyte enveloped by *follicular epitheliocytes*. Rapid cell division forms a stratified *follicular epithelium* (stratum granulosum).

[1] The *ovocyte* grows to a diameter of about 150 μm. The diameter of the entire follicle is about 10 mm.

[2] Between the ovocyte and follicular epitheliocytes appears the **zona pellucida**, a space filled with acidophilic refractile carbohydrate-rich materials. Both ovocyte and follicular epitheliocytes contribute to its formation. Long anchoring microvilli from the inner lamina of follicular epitheliocytes penetrate the zona pellucida and intermingle with the smaller anchoring microvilli from the ovocyte.

[3] The *growing follicle* is shrouded by concentric layers of connective tissue cells, known as the *theca of the follicle*. These fibroblast-like cells differentiate into a highly vascularized **theca interna** of cuboidal cells and a **theca externa** of cells that retain their fibroblast configuration.

[a] **Theca interna** cells are endocrine cells distinguished by scattered lipid droplets, tubular sER, and mitochondria with tubular cristae. These features resemble other steroid-secreting cells (testes, suprarenal cortex). *Thecal endocrine cells secrete estrogen.*

[b] The **theca externa** cells are protective, supportive connective tissue cells.

[4] The *follicular epitheliocytes* secrete a fluid **liquor follicularis**, which accumulates and separates the cells in places. The *ovocyte*, however, retains an eccentric connection to the peripheral *follicular epithelium* at a site named the **cumulus oöphorus**. Accumulating **liquor follicularis** balloons the growing follicle to such a degree that it protrudes on the surface of the ovary.

(4) *Ovulation* occurs when the **ovum**, plus adhering follicular epitheliocytes, is flushed out of the follicle into the abdominal *ostium* of the *uterine tube.*

(a) Escaping follicular fluid contains blood from ruptured vessels of the vascularized **theca interna**. Seeping blood from torn capillaries clots within the empty follicle, forming a recognizable **corpus hemorrhagicum**. The clot is removed, eventually, by connective tissue phagocytes.

(b) The collapsed follicle differentiates into a **corpus luteum** (yellow body) with two distinctive cell types: remaining *follicular epitheliocytes* and *corpus luteum endocrine cells*. The latter, distinguished by cytoplasmic lipid droplets, secrete the steroid hormone *progesterone* for the 14 days following ovulation.

(5) Failure of fertilization results in cessation of progesterone production, causing the corpus luteum to regress as the **corpus luteum cyclicum** (of menstruation). Invading connective tissue transforms it to white scar tissue, the **corpus albicans**, which disappears with time.

(6) Successful fertilization initiates enlargement of the corpus luteum into a **corpus luteum graviditatis** (of pregnancy), which persists for the first two trimesters and then undergoes regression as the **corpus luteum regressum**. Involution occurs rapidly after parturition, but a much larger **corpus albicans** may take years to disappear. Its persistence permits determination of the number of pregnancies.

(7) *Atretic follicles* (formed as scar tissue) result from involution of primary, secondary, or tertiary follicles. Starting with the 16-week fetus until birth, more than 2 million ovogonia from and rapidly succumb to *atresia*. At birth, some 400,000 quiescent primary ovocytes await puberty for *FSH* stimulation, while follicular atresia

continues. If the average female commences ovulation at age 10 and ceases ovulation at age 50, then some 500 primary ovocytes reach maturation. What happens to the others?

(a) Follicular *atresia* occurs before most follicles ever begin maturation.

(b) Many follicles initiate maturation and then succumb to *atresia*.

(c) Other follicles undergo atresia late into advanced stages of maturation. These may be identified by a residual refractile zona pellucida and thicker thecal walls.

b. The *medulla* of the ovary (central vascular zone) is recognized by large numbers of blood vessels. Some connective tissue cells filling the areas between blood vessels are the *interstitial endocrine cells*, which resemble corpus luteum cells. The exact hormone and activity in humans has not been clearly defined. These cells may migrate into the stroma from the hypertrophied theca interna of regressing follicles. Smaller vessels and capillary plexuses arborize throughout the medulla and cortex from medullary ovarian vessels.

B. *Uterine tube* (formerly: Fallopian tube, oviduct)

1. The *uterine tube*, extending from the ovary to the **uterus**, conducts the ovum into the uterine cavity. Dimensions of the uterine tube are 15 cm in length and 1 cm in diameter. *Three regions* are characterized:

a. the **ampulla**, distal one third of the tube, is where *fertilization* commonly occurs. This flared trumpet-shaped end consists of

(1) an **infundibulum**, the flared end fringed with **fimbriae**. Large **plicae** (folds) are branched and quite complicated. The plicae run parallel to the longitudinal axis of the uterine tube.

(2) an *abdominal ostium*, the tube opening into the abdominal peritoneal cavity.

b. the *isthmus*, middle one third, extending from the ampulla to the uterus, has smaller and less complicated plicae. Closer to the uterus, the tunica muscularis thickens and the number of ciliated epithelial cells decreases.

c. The **pars uterina**, the proximal third of the tube, has a smaller lumen and much smaller plicae, particularly the portion within the uterine wall.

2. *Layers* of the *uterine tube*

a. The **tunica mucosa** is folded into longitudinal branched **plicae** (folds). So complex are these plicae in the distal third that the lumen appears as a maze. Little wonder then, that a fertilized ovum may be entrapped, resulting in a tubal pregnancy.

(1) The simple columnar epithelium consists of
(a) *ciliated epitheliocytes*, which are most populous around the fimbriae and gradually decrease in number toward the uterus.

[1] Ciliary activity not only creates the necessary strong currents that drive the ovum toward the uterine cavity, but also imposes an major obstacle for spermatozoa. Surely, one reason for the massive numbers of sperm is to overcome the enormous losses occurring in the female reproductive tract.

[2] *Ciliogenesis* depends on estrogen. Thus, in premenopausal women, there are a substantial number of active cilia. In postmenopausal women, the number and height of ciliated cells is diminished. Estrogen therapy provided to postmenopausal women results in proliferation of ciliated cells (Verhage et al, 1979).

(b) *microvillous epitheliocytes*, which are nonciliated cells distinguished by *microvilli* covering the luminal surface of the cells. Secretory granules (containing a nourishing protein polysaccharide) occupy the apical cytoplasm. The secretion may nourish the ovum on its journey and coat the ovum plasmalemma with substances to facilitate sperm penetration.

(2) **Lamina propria mucosae** is loose connective tissue housing a variety of cells and fibers (predominantly reticular). The rich vasculature, resembling erectile tissue, engorges with blood to extend the fimbriae to the ovary. Contractions of the tunica muscularis bring the "erect" fimbriae over the ovulatory site, to capture of the ovum. Ciliary activity directs the ovum into the *ostium* of the uterine tube.

(3) A **lamina muscularis mucosae** cannot be distinguished.

b. A **tunica muscularis** consists of bundles of smooth myocytes arranged in an inner **stratum circulare** and an outer **stratum longitudinale**. The indistinct boundary between the two strata results from intermingling of the two strata. The tunica muscularis increases in thickness as the uterus is approached. Its rhythmic contractions extend the *ostium* to the ovulatory site and *transport* the **ovum** through the uterine tube.

c. A **tunica serosa** supported on a **tela subserosa** completes the layers of the tube.

3. *Fertilization:* Ejaculated spermatozoa must travel a hostile route through the vagina, uterus, and uterine tube to its distal third, the **ampulla**. Here they may lie in disorganized array for up to 3 or 4

days. If they do not fertilize the ovum, they die. If a discharged ovum enters, the entourage of spermatozoa align in perfect formation, head first, and "swim" furiously and purposefully toward the arriving ovum. Normally only one spermatozoön penetrates the ovum, to stimulate the sudden appearance of a *fertilization membrane* which prevents other sperm from entering. The fertilized ovum moves to the uterus by muscular contractions and ciliary activity.

C. Uterus (Norris et al, 1973)

1. *General:* The uterus is a single structure, formed by the union of the medial parts of the uterine tubes. In lower animals (eg, mouse) the uterus is bifid, with each uterine tube continuous with half a uterus.

a. *Shape:* The human uterus resembles an inverted "pear," in which the uterine tubes open into the uterine cavity at its upper widest part, the *body of the uterus.* The narrower lower portion, the *neck of the uterus,* projects into the **vagina.**

b. *Dimensions:* In adult *nulliparous* women (no viable infant born) the uterus measures: length, 7.6 cm; width, 5 cm; thickness, 2.5 cm. In *multiparous* women (two or more pregnancies that resulted in viable offspring), it is larger.

2. The *uterine wall* consists of three major tunics. From the outside in they are **tunica serosa [perimetrium], tunica muscularis [myometrium],** and the **tunica mucosa [endometrium].**

a. **Tunica serosa,** also **perimetrium,** covers some outer surfaces of the uterus; others are sheathed with tunica adventitia. The underlying tela subserosa, a connective tissue layer, covers one stratum of the myometrium.

b. **Tunica muscularis,** also **myometrium,** has several strata of smooth myocyte bundles, providing the most complex muscular structure of the body. Under normal conditions, smooth myocytes measure about 50 μm in length. During pregnancy, these may hypertrophy up to 500 μm in length. In addition to the hypertrophied myocytes, residual embryonic connective tissue cells may differentiate into new smooth myocytes to increase the total mass. The *smooth myocyte* layers, from outside in are

(1) stratum subserosum: a thin layer oriented longitudinally.

(2) stratum supravasculosum: a longitudinal layer covering a circular layer. (It should be recalled that usage of the terms longitudinal and circular refer to the coursing of bundles of myocytes in loose or tight spirals.)

(3) stratum vasculosum: a layer with many large vessels that present the appearance of a spongiosum. Fibers spiral obliquely over circular spirals.

(4) **stratum submucosum**: layers spiral in a longitudinal path, but circular and oblique are also found.

c. **Tunica mucosa [endometrium]**, the spongy layer containing glands, blood vessels, and tissues involved in menstruation.

(1) **Epithelium** is *simple columnar* consisting of

(a) tall *ciliated cells* that predominate in the very young, but are rare following menstruation and pregnancies,

(b) tall *microvillous cells* (nonciliated) that are covered with microvilli. Electron-dense secretory granules occupy the apical portion of the cell, glycogen deposits aggregate below a basal polarized nucleus, and rER is distributed evenly throughout the cell.

(2) The **lamina propria mucosae [stroma endometrialis]** is populated by reticular fibers in a loose connective tissue arrangement.

(a) Coiled unbranched glands undergo cyclic changes during menstruation. Tortuous *spiral arteries* in the lamina propria mucosae encircle the glands.

(b) Wandering leucocytes phagocytize foreign substances.

(3) *Structural components* of the **uterus**

(a) The *body* is the major portion of the uterus engaged in menstruation. Its tunica mucosa [endometrium] is subdivided into

[1] **stratum basale endometrii**, the lower one third of the tunica mucosa, supports the *basal arteries* which give rise to the *spiral arteries.*

[2] **stratum functionale endometrii**, the upper two thirds of the tunica mucosa, is further divisible into an upper **stratum compactum endometrii** and a lower **stratum spongiosum endometrii**. At menstruation, most of the **stratum functionale** is discharged with the *menses.*

(b) The **cervix uteri** (lower segment) consists of a **portio prevaginalis** and a **portio vaginalis**.

[1] The **portio prevaginalis** leads to the inner cervical canal. The **tunica mucosa [endometrium]**, with fewer glands than the tunica mucosa of the body, is less involved in menstruation. The ciliated cells and mucous exocrine cells of the simple columnar epithelium are not shed in the menstrum. The arteries are not involved, consequently there is no bleeding from this zone. The **tunica mucosa** (in the cervical canal) requires a thinner lamina propria mucosae and a very dense **tunica muscularis [myometrium]**. The superficial simple columnar epithelium is corregated into longitudinal folds, the **plicae palmatae**. The superficial columnar epithelium continues into short-

necked *cervical glands* where tall *mucous exocrine cells* secrete the mucus that plugs the cervical canal during pregnancy.

[2] The **portio vaginalis:** At the *external os* (opening) of the cervical canal leading into the vagina, the epithelium changes abruptly from simple columnar to the stratified squamous variety continuous with that lining the vagina.

[a] *Glycogen* in the surface cells of the stratified squamous epithelium washes out in routine histologic preparations.

[b] Small *lymphatic nodules* appear in the lamina propria mucosae.

[c] The *Pap technique* scrapes some of the superficial cells, smears, and stains them to detect early cellular changes. This (now routine) technique has proven successful and invaluable in controlling early onset of cervical cancer.

(4) *Menstruation* (Fig. 19-3) (Noyes, 1973)

(a) *Menstrual phase* is recognized by the first sign of bleeding, which is considered day 1. Between day 1 and day 4, the stratum functionale is shed, leaving the stratum basale at a thickness of 0.5 mm to 3 mm. Constricted *spiraled arteries* produce an ischemia that characterizes the stratum functionale. However, blood continues to circulate in the stratum basale. After several hours, the constricted arteries open for some time, causing damaged surface vessels to erupt and blood to stream into the mucosal stroma. (Normally menstrual blood does not clot.) The blood-drenched stratum functionale separates, tearing glands and vessels. The blood loss by day 4 is approximately 35 ml.

(b) The *postmenstrual phase* is a quiescent period between day 4 and day 5, in which some spotting may occur. There is no epithelium, and the tunica mucosa consists of a 0.5-mm-thick "raw" stratum basalis.

(c) The *follicular phase* (proliferative), day 5 through day 14, is marked by stimulation of follicular development by *FSH*. The tunica mucosa may thicken from 1 to 4 mm.

[1] The bases of uterine glands grow in height and proliferate (by mitoses) new cells for the growing glands and for the superficial epithelium.

[2] Around the 8th day, the glands begin secreting a thin aqueous fluid rich in carbohydrates.

[3] About the 10th day, glycogen accumulates in the apical cytoplasm of the tall columnar cells.

(d) The *luteal phase* (progesterone phase, secretory

phase), day 14 to day 26, is marked by further thickening of the tunica mucosa up to 6 mm in height.

[1] On or about day 14 the ovum is discharged from the ovary (ovulation), and the **corpus luteum** begins to secrete *progesterone*, which contributes to the preparation of the uterine mucosa to receive a blastocyst.

[2] Major changes occur in the stratum functionale are marked by

[a] *glycogen* from the apical regions of tall glandular columnar cells is shed into highly sacculated glands distended with fluid, mucus, and glycogen.

[b] *edema* of the stroma.

[c] *lengthening* of arteries with increased complexity of spiraling.

[3] *Decidual reaction* is characterized by stromal cells of the tunica mucosa becoming larger while they accumulate glycogen and lipid.

[a] *Intrauterine implantation* stimulates stromal cells to differentiate into large pale *decidual cells*. Initially confined to the zone around the implanted blastocyst, the reaction soon spreads throughout the entire tunica mucosa endometrium. The presence of chorionic villi in pathological tissues is useful in verifying an intrauterine pregnancy.

[b] *Ectopic implantation* also initiates *decidualization*. However, the absence of chorionic villi in decidualized uterine tissue requires one to rule out an ectopic pregnancy in the proper clinical setting.

[c] *Other stimuli:* The normal menstrual cycle, trauma, electrical stimulation, or intraluminal injection of oil also stimulate the decidual reaction, but chorionic villi may not develop.

(e) The *ischemic phase* may occur from day 26 to 28, when the arteries begin to constrict intermittently. This phenomenon occurs at the junction between the stratum basale and the stratum functionale, with concomitant intermittent blanching of the stratum functionale. Leucocytes in the vessels migrate into the stroma, as the stratum functionale enters the menstrual phase, to start another cycle.

(5) *Hormonal factors involved in menstruation*

(a) The **hypophysis** secretes *FSH* to initiate the follicular phase. *FSH* stimulates development of a new follicle. In two weeks that follicle matures and ovulation occurs.

(b) The **theca interna** *endocrine cells* secrete *estrogen*, which stimulated proliferation of the tunica mucosa (endometrium).

Estrogen also stimulates the hypophysis to secrete *LH*, which in turn initiates ovulation and induces formation of the **corpus luteum.**

(c) The **corpus luteum** secretes *progesterone*, which acts on the uterine tunica mucosa to initiate the luteal phase. Secretory activity commences in the uterine glands. *Progesterone* also "informs" the hypophysis to cease production of *FSH*.

(d) When *FSH* is diminished no other follicles can develop. Without follicles = *no estrogen.*

(e) No estrogen = *no LH* = *no progesterone.*

(f) No progesterone = menstruation begins and *FSH* restarts the cycle.

D. *Vagina*

1. *Surrounding layers*

a. The **tunica mucosa** is lined by noncornified stratified squamous epithelium that thickens toward the external opening, the *introitus*. In tissue sections three features are readily discerned:

(1) *Glycogen* in the superficial cells. Estrogen increases the quantity of glycogen. Released glycogen is acted upon by indigenous bacteria to produce an acid fluid that coats the vagina. The high acidity environment provides another major obstacle to spermatozoa.

(2) *Lymphatic nodules* in the lamina propria mucosae release lymphocytes that penetrate the epithelium and intermingle with desquamated superficial squamous cells.

(3) *Venous plexuses*, in the lamina propria mucosae, function as erectile tissue to dilate the vaginal lumen in preparation for coitus.

b. The **tunica muscularis**

(1) has an inner **fasiculus circularis** (rather than a true stratum) of smooth myocytes (fasiculus = bundle) and an outer **stratum longitudinale** of nonstriated (smooth) myocytes.

(2) forms a sphincter of striated skeletal myocytes around the *introitus*.

c. A **tunica adventitia** of connective tissue surrounds the muscular layers.

2. A *hymen*, obstructing the introitus in virgins, is a thin fold of cribriform mucosa covered by stratified squamous epithelium.

E. The *external genitalia* (the **vulva**) surround the separate openings of the urethra and vagina.

1. Two lip-like lateral longitudinal folds meet in the midline, but can be readily separated to provide access to the urethra or vagina.

a. The **labia majus pudendi**, the outer larger lips, are skin folds containing large amounts of adipose tissue and a thin layer of nonstriated muscle. The external surface is covered with short hairs and keratinized stratified squamous epithelium. The inner surface is glabrous and relatively smooth. Sebaceous glands and sudoriferous glands populate both surfaces.

b. The **labia minus pudendi**, beneath the labia majus, are totally glabrous. These lips possess lightly cornified stratified squamous epithelium and a connective tissue core resplendent with elastic fibers, sebaceous glands, and blood vessels.

2. Both labia converge over the urethral orifice to protect the **clitoris** (the structural equivalent of the penis).

a. Structurally and functionally, it resembles the corpora caverosa of the penis in possessing a pair of cylindrical bodies of erectile tissue, the **corpora cavernosa clitoridis.**

b. The distal free end is capped by the **glans clitoridis**, also composed of erectile tissue of the **corpora spongiosum.** Very sensitive stratified squamous epithelium covers the glans.

c. The **clitoris** differs from the penis in that the urethra does not travel in it. However, *minor vestibular glands* similar to the penile urethral glands open onto the clitoris.

3. The *major vestibular glands* (of Bartholin), on the lateral walls of the **vulva**, open onto the inner surface of the **labia minus**. About a centimeter in diameter during active sexual life, they regress after age 30 and begin the process of involution. The glandular tissue, which secreted a lubricating mucus, gradually ceases functions.

III. The *female breast* (Cowie, 1974)

A. *General:* The breasts are modified sweat glands derived from ectodermal cells. Each breast is composed of 10 to 25 individual, radially arranged *mammary glands* which may be visualized as inverted trees. Smaller branches represent small ducts leading to a single large *lactiferous duct* (the tree trunk). Therefore, 10 to 25 large *lactiferous ducts* converge upon the *nipple* and open to the exterior as *papillary ostia* (milk pores).

B. *Mammary glands:* Each of the mammary glands is surrounded by a **stratum fibrosum** of dense connective tissue, which in turn is surrounded by a **stratum adiposum** of adipose connective tissue. The latter imparts the contours of the breasts, which reach maximal development at age 20.

1. In the *nonlactating* breast, glands consist of ducts and their

branches. There are no terminal secretory **alveoli** in the nonlactating breast.

2. During *pregnancy*, **alveoli** develop fully, so that each mammary gland could be compared to a tree in full bloom with branches (ducts) obscured by leaves (alveoli).

3. From the **alveoli**, ducts may be traced as follows:

a. **alveolus** to *lactiferous alveolar duct*. In the nonlactating breast, alveolar cells form a solid cord of potential secretory cells. The alveolar duct possesses an epithelium of low cuboidal cells.

b. *intralobular lactiferous ducts*, the next larger order, have cuboidal epithelium. Many alveolar ducts lead into it.

c. *interlobular lactiferous ducts*, possessing cuboidal to low columnar epithelium, are fed by the previous ducts. (These are analogous to the main branches of a tree.)

d. *lobar lactiferous duct*, a single duct, is the largest duct terminating in the nipple. The *lobar* ducts have a local dilatation, the *lactiferous sinus*, under the areola. They are lined by columnar epithelium.

4. A fat-free loose connective tissue surrounds the basement membranes of the alveoli and ducts. During pregnancy and lactation, distensibility of ducts is faciliated by this loose connective tissue. The *interlobular* connective tissue is quite dense and forms *interlobular septae*.

C. Areola: The areola is a circular area of pigmented skin from which the nipple arises. Unusually long papillae of connective tissue carry capillaries almost to the epithelial surface, causing the areola to appear pink in fair-skinned individuals and in the immature.

1. During puberty and pregnancy, melanocytes increase their activity and darken both the areola and the nipple.

2. At the periphery of the areola are small *areolar glands* (formerly: glands of Montgomery), somewhat similar in structure to sweat glands and mammary glands. Also present are sweat glands and sebaceous glands in a ring at the outer margin of the areola.

D. *Nipple:* The nipple projects from the areola and receives the lactiferous ducts. Sebaceous glands populate the summit and lateral surfaces of the nipple where usually there are no hairs. Longitudinal and circularly arranged smooth myocytes are found in the connective tissue stroma. Contraction of the circular muscles causes nipple elongation, whereas contraction of the longitudinal muscles shortens the nipple and may even retract it below the level of the areola.

E. The *lactating mammary gland* (Vorherr, 1978)

1. During pregnancy, the mammary gland alveoli proliferate and grow under the influence of estrogen and progesterone.

2. Alveolar milk cells, **exocrinocytus lactus** (*lactocytes*), begin to secrete via stimulus of *prolactin*, but the secretion remains in the alveoli and in the lactiferous ducts.

3. During the preparatory periods, the pars intermedia of the hypophysis secretes *MSH*, causing pigmentation of the areola and nipple.

4. A new baby, suckling on the nipple, sets up a series of neuronal stimuli causing release of *oxytocin* from the neurohypophysis. Oxytocin causes contraction of smooth myocytes and *myoepithelial cells*, causing *ejection* of milk.

5. *Myoepithelial cells* (Fig. 19-4) of ectodermal origin, between the basement membrane and glandular cells, contract like smooth myocytes to force milk out of the alveoli.

6. The *lactocytes* (gland cells) (Fig. 19-4) are columnar cells with a well-developed apical golgi complex and rER at the base and sides of the nuclei.

Figure 19-4 The lactocyte and related myoepithelial cells.

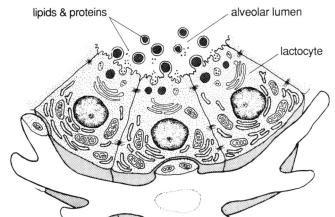

    a. Membrane-bound protein molecules are released from the luminal surface via exocytosis.

    b. Lipid droplets formed within the cytoplasm migrate to the surface, push the plasmalemma up, and are cast off enclosed in a portion of the plasmalemma.

    7. *Milk* consists of lipid droplets, casein, lactose (a sugar), salts, calcium, and cellular fragments. Frequently, lymphocytes from the lamina propria are found in the duct lumen.

    8. *Colostrum,* the first milk, is secreted by a mother shortly after birth. Besides fluid, there are many fat-filled antibody-containing leucocytes in this colostrum, to provide the neonate with a degree of temporary immunity. The special laxative properties of colostrum are beneficial in establishing regular colonic evacuation.

Questions

DIRECTIONS: For each numbered item, select the one heading most closely associated with it. Each lettered heading may be selected once, more than once, or not at all.

Questions 1 – 4
A. Tunica vaginalis
B. Tunica albuginea
C. Mediastinum testis
D. Testicular septulae

    1. Divide the testis into compartments
    2. Peritoneal tunica serosa
    3. At the concave hilum of the testis
    4. Capsule of the testis

Questions 5-8
A. Spermatocytogenesis
B. Spermiogenesis
C. Meiosis
D. Spermatogenesis

5. The overall process
6. Spermatogonia undergo mitosis
7. Spermatids are formed
8. Spermatids mature into spermatozoa

Questions 9-12
A. Sustentacular cells (Sertoli)
B. Interstitial endocrine cells (Leydig)
C. Ciliated columnar cells
D. Nonciliated columnar cells

9. Efferent ductules
10. Prominent crystalloids
11. Blood-testis barrier
12. Involved in fluid absorption

Questions 13-16
A. The most muscular tube
B. Tall branched microvilli (stereocilia)
C. Honeycombed pouches
D. Composite of 50 glands

13. Seminal vesicle
14. Prostate
15. Ductus epididymis
16. Ductus deferens

Questions 17-20
A. Prostate
B. Seminal vesicle
C. Epididymis
D. Bulbourethral glands

17. Produces flavin, identified by its fluorescence
18. Produces substance with the characteristic odor of semen
19. Produces secretion identified by its opalescence
20. Produces fibrinolysin

Questions 21–24
A. Theca externa
B. Theca interna
C. Zona pellucida
D. Superficial epithelium

21. Contributed to by the ovum
22. Contributed to by follicular epitheliocytes
23. Derived from stromal cells
24. Secretes estrogen

Questions 25–28
A. Corpus albicans
B. Corpus luteum cyclicum
C. Corpus luteum graviditatis
D. Corpus hemorrhagicum

25. Persists for two trimesters of pregnancy
26. May take years to disappear
27. Forms after failure of fertilization
28. Appears immediately after ovulation

Questions 29–32
A. Thicker closer to the uterus
B. Lack a complete serosa
C. Possesses vasculature like erectile tissue
D. Thinner closer to the uterus

29. Uterine tube ciliated cells
30. Uterine tube lamina propria mucosae
31. Uterine tube tunica muscularis
32. Uterine tube fimbriae

Questions 33–36
A. Tela serosa [perimetrium]
B. Lamina propria mucosae
C. Tunica muscularis [myometrium]
D. Tunica mucosa [endometrium]

33. Stratum vasculosum
34. Stratum functionale
35. Stratum spongiosum
36. Stratum submucosum

Questions 37–40
A. Menstrual phase
B. Follicular phase
C. Luteal phase
D. Ischemic phase

37. Blood-drenched stratum functional separates
38. Bases of glands grow and proliferate new epithelium
39. Glycogen accumulates in sacculated glands
40. Arteries constrict intermittently

Questions 41–45
A. Lamina propria veins
B. Clitoris
C. Release glycogen to increase acidity
D. Major vestibular glands (Bartholin)
E. Corpus spongiosum

41. Open onto the inner surface of the labia minus
42. Superficial cells of the vaginal epithelium
43. Function as erectile tissue of the vagina
44. Structural equivalent of the penis
45. Glans clitoridis

Questions 46–50
A. Myoepithelial cells
B. Lactocytes
C. Sebaceous gland cells
D. Smooth myocytes
E. Melanocytes

46. Secrete protein and lipids
47. Respond to MSH
48. At the outer margin of the areola
49. Between the basement membrane and the parenchymal cell
50. Populate the surface of the nipple

Explanatory Answers

1. D. The testicular septulae, composed of dense connective tissue, radiate out from the mediastium to the convex surface to meet the

tunica albuginea (albuginea = white, for white collagen fibers). Some 250 compartments house the testicular lobules.

2. A. A sac of peritoneum tunica serosa descends through the inguinal canal to form the tunica vaginalis around the dense fibrous tunica vaginalis. This sac may be involved in development of a hernia if the prolongation from the peritoneum remains patent.

3. C. The mediastinum testis is the thickened connective tissue in the hilum of the testis. Housed in this tissue are the straight tubules, the rete testis, and a portion of the efferent ductules.

4. B. The capsule of the testis is the dense fibrous tunica albuginea. When accumulating fluid and maturing spermatozoa fill the testicular lobules, and the pressure cannot stretch the tunica albuginea any further, the first components of the seminal fluid begin to move out under passive pressure.

5. D. The overall process of formation of spermatozoa is spermatogenesis. This process is similar to ovogenesis in the female, whereby a haploid ovum is the final product. The subdivisions are in sequence: spermatocytogenesis, meiosis, and spermiogenesis.

6. A. Spermatocytogenesis is the process whereby ovogonia divide by mitosis to produce more ovogonia, some of which become spermatocytes.

7. C. In meiosis, there are two successive maturation divisions to reduce the diploid chromosome number (46 in humans) to the haploid (23 in humans).

8. B. Spermatogenesis consists of a series of maturation changes whereby spermatids mature into spermatozoa.

9. C. About 12 efferent ductules exit the testis from the rete testis to form the vascular cones. These ductules are lined by pseudostratified columnar epithelium in which the ciliated columnar cells move the maturing spermatozoa through the vascular cones and eventually into the epididymis.

10. B. The interstitial endocrine cells of the testis (Leydig cells) are characterized by cytoplasmic structures reflecting their ability to synthesize the steroid hormone testosterone. A prominent feature is the presence of crystalloids (of Reinke). The precise nature of these crystals is unknown, but they help to distinguish these cells from other steroid-secreting cells.

11. A. The tight junctions close to the base of the sustentacular cells divide the width of the seminiferous tubules into a basal one third and a luminal two thirds. Cells in the upper two thirds are haploid and produce androgen-binding proteins (ABP), which would be detrimental if allowed to enter the vascular system. Thus, an effective blood–testis barrier is provided.

12. D. Nonciliated cells in the efferent tubules are involved in absorption of fluid. The microvillous surface coated with a glycocalyx is reminiscent of the intestinal absorptive cells. In the apical region there are definite morphological indications of the absorptive process, namely, apical pits, apical vesicles, and vacuoles.

13. C. The seminal vesicles are elongated pouches with one exiting duct, which empties into the ampulla of the ductus deferens. The tunica mucosa forms primary secondary and tertiary pouches that confer a honeycomb appearance to the interior of the pouch.

14. D. The prostate is a composite of about 50 glands that are arranged in three layers. Those in the tunica mucosa are the smallest, the next larger size (necessitating longer ducts to reach the prostatic urethra) are those residing in the tela submucosa. The largest glands are the most peripheral. These latter glands are usually the site of onset of prostatic carcinoma.

15. B. The ductus epididymis was believed to contain cilia. When studies determined that these cilia were not motile they were designated "stereocilia." The introduction of electron microscopy revealed that these were not cilia at all, but very tall branched microvilli.

16. A. Relative to the diameter of the lumen, the tunica muscularis makes the ductus deferens the most muscular tube in the body.

17. B. The seminal vesicles produce a yellow lipochrome pigment, flavin, identified by its fluorescence. This is an important medicolegal component of seminal fluid.

18. A. The prostate discharges a secretion containing the polyamine phosphate of spermine. This is the only component of semen that has a characteristic odor. All the other components are odorless.

19. A. The prostate secretion may be identified by its opalescence. This thin milky emulsion contains fine lipid droplets and proteins.

20. A. The prostate produces a number of proteolytic enzymes that are important in identifying semen. One of the most important is fibrinolysin, which assists in the liquefaction of semen.

21. C. The zona pellucida (Latin: *pella*, skin) is an acidophilic refractile carbohydrate-rich material that surrounds the maturing FSH-stimulated follicle. It is built up by secretions produced by the ovum and the follicular epitheliocytes.

22. C. Follicular epitheliocytes contribute to the formation of the zona pellucida. Long microvilli of the ovum are anchored into it, as are shorter microvilli of the follicular epitheliocytes.

23. B. The stromal cells give rise to the thecal cells. The layer closest to the follicular epitheliocytes differentiates into the theca interna, which are the endocrine cells producing estrogen during follicular development and progesterone after ovulation.

24. B. The theca interna cells produce estrogen (cf 23).

25. C. A normal corpus luteum is transformed into a very large corpus luteum graviditatis (of pregnancy), which persists for the first two trimesters.

26. A. The corpus albicans may form after any corpus luteum undergoes involution. The smaller they are the sooner they disappear. The very large corpus luteum graviditatis, however, is so large that it may take years to disappear.

27. B. If fertilization fails to occur, then progesterone production ceases and the corpus luteum regresses as the corpus luteum cyclicum (of menstruation). Eventually it too involutes and becomes a corpus albicans, which will disappear before the corpus luteum graviditatis.

28. D. Immediately after ovulation, the follicle, emptied of its ovum and corona radiata follicular epitheliocytes, fills with follicular fluid and seeping blood from torn capillaries of the vascularized theca interna cells. The clotted blood in this corpus hemorrhagicum is removed by connective tissue phagocytes.

29. D. The uterine tube ciliated cells are very populous around the fimbriae, but thin out as the uterus is approached.

30. C. The uterine tube lamina propria mucosae possesses erectile-like vasculature that causes the fimbriae to become erect at ovulation to clasp the ovary. Contractions of the tunica muscularis bring the infudibulum and attached fimbriae over the ovary to capture the released ovum.

31. A. The uterine tube tunica muscularis acquires additional smooth myocyte bundles as the uterus is approached.

32. B. The fimbriae fringing the infundibulum are for the most part surrounded by ciliated cells. A serosa along the outer surface of the fimbriae is not unusual.

33. C. The stratum vasculosum is a layer of the tunica muscularis of the uterus. This is the layer that gives it the spongy look. Layers of smooth myocytes are woven between blood vessels.

34. D. At menstruation most of the stratum functionale of the tunica mucosa [endometrium] is discharged with the menses.

35. D. The stratum functionale, making up two thirds of the tunica mucosa, is divisible into a stratum spongiosum and a stratum compactum.

36. C. The stratum submucosum is the layer of smooth myocytes immediately surrounding the tunica mucosa. It is the most internal layer of the tunica muscularis [myometrium].

37. A. The menstrual phase is characterized by constricted spiral arteries, which open after several hours, causing surface vessels to tear and stratum functionale to become blood soaked. Most of the func-tionale fragments into the menses.

38. B. During the follicular phase, proliferation of glandular remnants in the stratum basale commence growth. The developing cells spread over the denuded tunica mucosa and form new epithelium.

39. C. The luteal phase is marked by continued growth of the tunica mucosa. Following ovulation, the corpus luteum secretes progesterone.

40. D. The ischemic phase follows unsuccessful fertilization and withdrawal of hormones. The spiraled arteries begin agonal intermittent constrictions, which produce concomitant intermittent blanching of the stratum functionale. Then the arteries constrict for a day or so, depriving the stratum functionale of nutrition and oxygen. In effect the tissue dies. When the arteries open up, the rush of blood (menstrual phase) is sufficient to burst capillaries and weakened vessels in the stratum functionale.

41. D. The major vestibular glands, the size of a pea during active sexual life, discharge their lubricating mucus onto the inner surface of the labia minus.

42. C. The superficial cells of the vaginal noncornified (moist) stratified squamous epithelium build up glycogen under hormonal stimulus. When released, bacterial activity produces an acidic fluid that coats the epithelium.

43. A. The venous plexuses residing in the vaginal lamina propria mucosae act as erectile tissue, to dilate the vaginal lumen during intercourse.

44. B. The structural equivalent of the penis is the miniature clitoris. A major difference is that the clitoris lacks a urethra.

45. E. The distal free end of the clitoris is capped by the glans clitoridis, which is corpus spongiosum tissue covered by a very sensitive stratified squamous epithelium.

46. B. The lactocyte produces proteins and lipids as components of milk.

47. E. Epithelial melanocytes of the areola and nipple respond to MSH to darken these areas. Prior to puberty, capillaries in the long dermal papillae make these areas pink. With the onset of menstruation, the continued impact of MSH darkens the areola.

48. C. At the peripheral margin of the areola, both sweat glands and sebaceous glands form a ring.

49. A. Oxytocin-stimulated myoepithelial cells contract and squeeze milk out of the alveoli. Oxytocin, stored in the neurohypophysis, is released by neuronal stimuli.

50. C. The summit and lateral surfaces of the nipple, where there are usually no hairs, are populated by sebaceous glands.

20 The Eye and the Ear

I. The *eye* is the photoreceptor organ that communicates with the brain via the second cranial nerve, the *optic nerve* (Fine and Yanoff, 1972).

A. *Development:* The optic nerves and eyes develop as hollow outgrowths of the brain walls and thus are considered extensions of the brain. (Moore, 1988).

1. In early embryogenesis, two lateral *optic bulbs* protrude from the lateral walls of the brain via hollow *optic stalks*. As the optic bulb of neural ectoderm grows through the intervening mesoderm to contact the superficial ectoderm, the phenomenon of *induction* occurs. Appropriate signals, probably chemical in nature, evoke two simultaneous reactions (Fig. 20-1).

a. The optic bulb invaginates to form a double-walled cup. The inferior surface of the cup and part of the hollow optic stalk are indented to form the *choroidal fissure.*

b. At the point of contact, the surface ectoderm forms a thickened disc, the *lens placode*, which sinks into the underlying mesenchyme and pinches off as a hollow vesicle. The ovoid vesicle inserts into the open end of the cup to establish permanent residence as the **lens**.

2. The outer thin layer of the *optic cup* differentiates to a monolayer of *pigmented epithelium*, which is surrounded by the highly vascularized *choroid layer* (derived from mesenchyme).

3. The invaginated inner layer of the optic cup transforms into three definitive structural regions:

a. a thicker multicellular region lining the major portion of the cup forms the *visual receptor area* of the **retina**.

b. a distal area lacking photoreceptor cells at the outer circumference of the cup develops into the

420

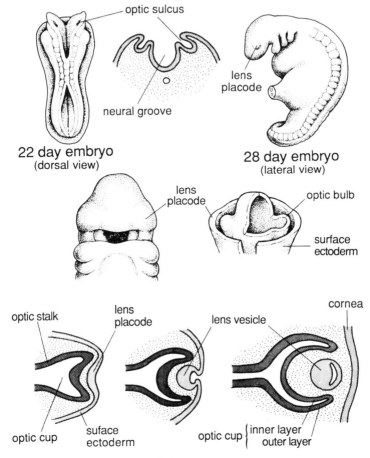

Figure 20-1 Development of the eye.

    (1) *ciliary body,* a muscular mass that controls the thickness of the lens during focusing,

    (2) iris, a muscular velum covering the **lens.**

    (3) *pupil,* a central aperture in the iris, which dilates or constricts to allow more or less light into the eye.

    c. Ora serrata: The junction between the *retina* and *cilliary body* lacks photoreceptor cells and is marked by a sawtooth border, the **ora serrata.**

4. The entire developing eye is surrounded by mesenchymal cells, which penetrate every available space, even between the iris and the outer surface ectoderm.

a. Cornea: In front of the iris, the ectoderm and underlying mesenchyme become the transparent **cornea**. Transparency permits light to enter without significant abberations.

b. *Conjunctiva:* At the periphery of the iris, the ectoderm and connective tissue under it are opaque and form the *conjunctiva* over the exposed surface of the eye wall, which is reflected under the eyelid.

c. Sclera. The portion of the *eyeball* behind the conjunctival reflection is covered only by dense connective tissue. This mesenchymal tissue, forming the fibrous tunic of the eye, condenses as regular connective tissue, the **sclera**.

B. *Fibrous tunic* of the *bulb* is the outermost coat of the bulb, consisting of the **cornea** and the **sclera** (Fig. 20-2).

1. Cornea (Jakus, 1956): The transparent **cornea** is the first important structure required for good vision. Its position renders it vulnerable to a variety of injuries, particularly exposure to various wavelengths of the spectrum and atmospheric conditions. Histologists

Figure 20-2 Meridional section of the eye.

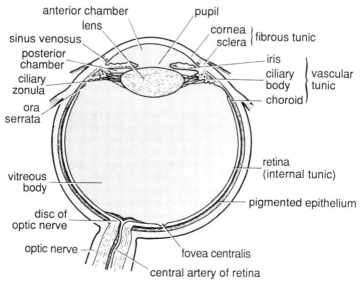

exert extreme caution when using osmium tetroxide as a TEM fixative, for its vapors will cornify the surface epithelium of the cornea. Loss of corneal transparency results in blindness. Corneal transplants to replace opaque corneas are fairly routine procedures. A *section* through the **cornea** reveals five definable layers (from outside in):

    a. *anterior epithelium*, derived from the superficial ectoderm of the embryo. Nonkeratinized stratified squamous cells of about five or six cell layers attach to one another by typical desmosomes.

    b. *anterior limiting lamina* (formerly: Bowman's membrane) is derived from embryonic mesenchyme. Light microscopy resolves a homogeneous layer about 7 to 12 μm thick, whereas electron microscopy clearly reveals an irregular network of very fine reticular fiber bundles.

    c. **substantia propria**, comprising about 90% of the 1-mm thick cornea, is composed of alternating lamellae (layers) of collagen fibers. Within one lamella, component fibrils lie parallel to one another while, in the next adjoining layer, parallel fibrils are situated at right angles to the previous layer. Compressed fibroblasts are scattered randomly throughout the substantia propria.

    d. *posterior limiting membrane* (formerly: Descemet's membrane) appears homogeneous and highly refractile via light microscopy. Histological and histochemical techniques indicate the presence of elastic fibers, from the positive staining for *elastin*. Electron microscopy, however, shows an atypical form of collagen and no elastic fibers. Masses of granules spaced at 107 nm, in a 3-D network, are bridged by fine fibrils to form a precise hexagonal pattern.

    e. *posterior epithelium* of the **cornea** (corneal endothelium), derived from mesenchyme surrounding the embryonic optic bulb, forms a single layer of low cuboidal cells lining the interior surface of the cornea.

    2. Sclera: The sclera is the dense coat of fiber bundles forming the opaque portion of the outer coat. Three definable layers blend at their interfaces:

    a. *episcleral lamina* (outermost): loose fibroelastic tissue; the tendon fibers of the ocular muscles penetrate through this layer.

    b. **substantia propria**, the middle layer, comprises the major portion of the sclera. Collagen fiber bundles, closely woven with some elastic fiber networks, form a strong framework. The collagen fibers of the ocular muscle tendons anchor into these fibers.

    c. **lamina fusca** of the **sclera** forms the pigmented inner layer adjacent to the choroid. Its connective tissue stroma, interspersed with *melanocytes*, forms a transition between the choroid coat and the sclera. The melanin pigment in *melanocytes* imparts a brownish color to this portion of the sclera. An increased number of elastic fibers (over that of the substantia propria) characterizes this layer.

C. The *vascular tunic* of the eye (**uvea**), consists of the choroid, ciliary body, and the iris (Fig. 20-2).

    1. *Choroid:* four layers, from outside to inside:

       a. *suprachoroid lamina*, similar in structure to the inner layer (lamina fusca) of the sclera. A potential space, the *perichoroidal space,* between this layer and the sclera is bridged by numerous connective tissue fibers. The loose stroma of collagen and elastic fibers forms a bed for a variety of free and fixed connective tissue cells, plus *choroidal melanocytes.*

       b. *vascular lamina*, vaguely divisible into an outer layer of large vessles and an inner layer of smaller vessels. The veins are arranged in whorls, which unite into single emissary *vortex veins.* Two superior and two inferior vortex veins exit directly through the sclera.

       c. *choroidocapillary lamina* consists of very-large-diameter capillaries that form a unique *uniplanar network.* The interstitial spaces beween the capillaries are filled with delicate loose connective tissue fibers and cells.

       d. *basal complex* (formerly: the lamina vitrea or Bruch's glassy membrane) is the basement membrane of the *pigment epithelium* of the retina. Three portions are recognized:

         (1) stratum elasticum, with a condensation of elastic fibers penetrating the choroidocapillary layer,

         (2) stratum fibrosum, the fibrous layer of pigmented epithelium, which adheres to the

         (3) lamina basalis or basement membrane.

    2. *Ciliary body:* This is the thickened, triangular anterior portion of the middle coat, which is localized at the junction of the choroid and the iris. All layers of the choroid except the choroidocapillary lamina are represented in the ciliary body and, in addition, epithelial layers from the retina continue over it. From outside in, the following layers are noted:

       a. stratum musculare of smooth myocytes forms the *ciliary muscle.*

         (1) Three directional bundles are formed:

            (a) *meridional* (formerly: Brucke's fibers) located at the outer surface of the ciliary body under the sclera,

            (b) *radial* (formerly: Iwanow's fibers)

            (c) *circular* (formerly: Müller's fibers). These are the innermost fibers, which appear between the ages of 2 and 3.

(2) *Contraction* of all muscles simultaneously draws the ciliary body and choroid forward, thus relieving tension on the suspensory ligaments of the lens. As a result the lens increases curvature, permitting one to focus on nearby objects.

(3) *Relaxation* of all muscles allows the ciliary body to return to its normal position, thus the ligaments decrease curvature for distance vision.

(4) Coordinated fine activity of muscular contractions (some more than others, etc) accommodates for objects situated between infinity and maximal close-ups.

b. stratum vasculosum. This inner vascular layer of the ciliary body is continuous with the vascular lamina of the choroid. The vessels are predominately capillaries and venules of varying diameters.

c. pars ciliaris retinae (pigmented layer) consists of two layers of cells:

(1) *pigmented cells* of simple columnar epithelium resting on the basal lamina (above). This layer, together with the stratum vasculosum at the root of the iris, is thrown into about 70 radially arranged small irregular folds. These are the *ciliary processes*, which give the ciliary body in this area the appearance of glands.

(2) *nonpigmented cells* of simple cuboidal (or columnar) epithelium. These cells are united at the apices by tight junctions which function as the *blood-aqueous barrier* (cf below).

3. Iris continues forward from the ciliary body as the final extension of the tunica vasculosum (middle coat).

a. As it penetrates the space between the cornea and the lens (actually lies on the anterior surface of the lens) two chambers are created whereby aqueous fluid in the posterior chamber flows freely to the anterior chamber through the *pupil*:

(1) *anterior chamber:* the space between the cornea and the anterior surface of the iris.

(2) *posterior chamber:* the space between the posterior surface of the iris and the anterior surface of the lens and the *zonule* (the grouping of ligaments suspending the lens from the ciliary body).

b. The periphery of the iris is appropriately named the *ciliary margin* for its union with the ciliary body. The central margin at the pupil is the pupillary margin.

c. *Surfaces*

(1) *anterior surface:* covered by simple squamous epithelium, continuous with the epithelium lining the inner surface of the cornea. This surface is rippled by several concentric folds and several crypts.

(2) *posterior surface:* covered by the *pigmented cells* of the

iris, which is continuous with the dual-layered pigmented stratum of the ciliary body. Both layers of heavily pigmented cells rest on a typical basement membrane. Pigmentation by the melanin granules obscures all cell morphology.

(3) Between these two surfaces are two internal layers:

(a) **stroma** of the iris lies immediately under the anterior surface epithelium and its basement membrane. This tissue is composed of a cellular connective tissue with more cells than fibers. *Melanocytes* scattered in the stroma deposit pigment granules that determine iris color. Various iris colors are accounted for by a gradual increase in pigment granules as follows:

[1] − *pigment* = blue
[2] +   = gray
[3] ++   = green
[4] +++   = light brown
[5] ++++   = brown
[6] +++++ = dark brown

(b) *vascular stratum* underlies the stroma, with radially arranged, thick-walled vessels that accommodate changes of the iris. The vessels are embedded in loose connective tissue.

d. **Stratum musculare** is composed of smooth myocytes derived from ectodermal pigment epithelium. The cell arrangement permits the **iris** to dilate or constrict the pupil.

(1) *Sphincter muscles* are arranged as a doughnut ring at the *pupillary margin*. Contraction of these myocytes (and relaxation of dilator myocytes) in bright sunlight closes the pupil to restrict entering light.

(2) *Dilator muscles* are arranged radially like the spokes of a bicycle wheel. Contraction of these myocytes (and relaxation of sphincter myocytes) at dusk or in the dark dilates (opens) the pupil to permit more light to enter.

D. The *internal [sensory] tunic* of the bulb, the **retina** (Fig. 20-2): The **retina**, derived from the inner layer of the double walled optic cup, extends from the posterior entrance point of the optic nerve to the anterior ora serrata (Rodieck, 1973).

1. The *optic nerve*
a. *Disc* of the *optic nerve*, a depression located at the entrance site of the optic nerve, is a blind spot lacking the necessary photoreceptors that make vision possible. It is the point of convergence of all nerve fibers relaying visual messages to the brain.

  b. Lamina cribrosa is a small cribriform portion of the sclera, directly behind the disc of the retina through which *fibers* of the *optic nerve* emerge and return to the brain.

  c. *Optic nerve formation:* As the nerve fibers emerge, they acquire a myelin sheath (the jelly roll). The numerous myelinated fibers contribute substantially to the general increase in total diameter of the nerve. The coverings of the brain (dura mater, arachnoid mater, and pia mater) also envelop the optic nerve because it is an extension of the brain wall.

  d. *Vessels:* The *central artery* and *vein* of the retina help to distinguish the optic nerve (histologically) from any other nerve.

  2. Fovea centralis is another depression located about 2.5 mm to the temporal side of the *disc.* In contrast to the "blind" disc, this is the site of most acute vision. Yellow pigment in and surrounding the fovea forms the **macula lutea,** the yellow spot. In histological sections of the retina, several layers are recognized. These are due primarily to the position of various photoreceptor cells, bipolar relay cells, and various supporting cells.

  3. *Four basic layers* must be penetrated by light waves before impinging upon the pigment epithelium of the choroid. Each of these layers is divided into sublayers. Figure 20-3 depicts 10 sublayers of the major four layers, which are *A, inner mantle layer; B, outer mantle layer; C, ependymal layer;* and *D, pigmented layer* (of the choroid).

  a. *Glial supporting cells* (formerly: Muller's supporting fibers) are represented in Figure 20-3 by the elongated cell with the largest amount of cytoplasm. Although only two glial cells are represented in Figure 20-3, it should be realized that many glial cells contribute to the structural integrity of the retinal stroma. Branches support any parenchymal cell in the vicinity. The ovoid nucleus resides in the *outer mantle layer,* contributing to the overall appearance of the *inner nuclear layer* of *bipolar cells.*

  (1) The outer terminations of the glial cells form the *external limiting membrane* of *glial cells.*

  (2) The inner terminations of the same glial cells form the *internal limiting membrane* of *glial cells.*

  b. The *pigmented layer* of the *choroid:* Consider that light penetrated through all layers to reach the *pigmented epithelium.* The free surfaces of these extend microvilli-like processes into the layer of *rods* and *cones* to interdigitate with the elongated outer elements of the rods and cones.

  (1) The pigmented cells and the tips of the rods and cones

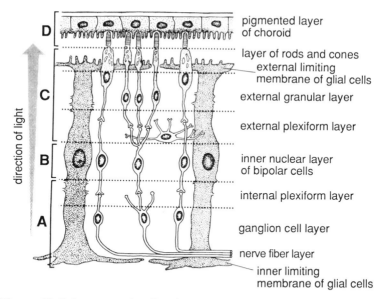

direction of light

D — pigmented layer of choroid

layer of rods and cones
external limiting membrane of glial cells

C — external granular layer

external plexiform layer

B — inner nuclear layer of bipolar cells

internal plexiform layer

A — ganglion cell layer

nerve fiber layer
inner limiting membrane of glial cells

Figure 20-3 Layers and cells of the retina (cf text).

do not fuse, but can be separated artifactually in most histological preparations. Clinically, this situation becomes reality in the condition known as *detached retina*.

(2) Within the pigment cells, large oval granules concentrate around the nucleus.

(a) *Increasing* the intensity of light causes migration of pigment granules into the microvilli, to prevent diffusion of light between photoreceptors.

(b) *Decreasing* the light intensity causes the pigment granules to retreat into the cell body.

c. *Photoreceptors:* Light wavelengths are received by two types of photoreceptors, the slender *rods* and the plump *cones*.

(1) The *external granular layer* is formed by the nuclei of the rods and cones.

(a) Both rods and cones consist of the following parts:

[1] *external segments* that interdigitate with the pigment cell microvillous processes. These segments are joined to the internal segments by a few cilia situated to one side. TEM resolves a series of *laminated discs*, which are the photoreceptor end organs. *Rod discs*

are continuously replenished in the following manner: new protein synthesized in the internal segment is transferred to the external segment where new discs are built by invaginations of the cell membranes. The oldest discs are, therefore, found at the extremities of the external segments where they continually shed into the pigmented epithelium. *Cone discs* are not replaced nor are they generally discarded as occurs in the rods.

[2] *internal segments* containing aggregations of mitochondria.

[3] *nuclear portions* that make up the *external granular layer.*

[4] *nerve cell processes* that synapse with the bipolar cells.

(b) *Rods:* In the diagram, three rods represent several rods synapsing with one bipolar cell, thus summating low light intensities. The rods faciliate vision in darkened situations, but cannot discriminate colors. The *external segment* contains the photoreceptor substance *rhodopsin* or *visual purple.*

(c) *Cones:* The cones establish a one-to-one relationship with the ganglion cells and are responsible for vision in high light intensity to mediate color. Such a situation may be appreciated when noting that the **fovea centralis**, the area of greatest visual acuity, possesses only cones. The *external segment* contains the photoreceptor substance *iodopsin.*

(2) The *inner nuclear layer* of *bipolar cells* houses the nuclei of bipolar cells, which synapse with the rods and cones, and the nuclei of the glial cells.

E. *Spaces of the eye*

1. The *anterior* and *posterior spaces* have been defined above (cf *iris*).

2. The *space* posterior to the lens and zonule is filled with a transparent gel-like substance, the *vitreous body.* This is a connective tissue similar to that of the embryo and can be termed embryonic connective tissue. In the developing eye, the *hyaloid artery*, emanating from the center of the optic nerve, passes through the center of the *vitreous body.* With advancing development, the hyaloid artery atrophies, leaving a *hyaloid* canal surrounded by condensed embryonic connective tissue resembling a membrane. This canal is filled with aqueous fluid.

3. *Sinus venosus* of the *sclera* (canal of Schlemm) is a ring-like vein situated in the sclera at the corneal junction. It encircles the

cornea at the root of the anterior surface of the iris. This sinus possesses a highly irregular endothelial-lined lumen, receiving scleral tributaries that drain the anterior chamber.

 a. *Aqueous fluid*, most probably produced by blood vessels in the connective tissue of the ciliary body, flows into the posterior chamber and subsequently into the anterior chamber.

 b. *Aqueous fluid* from the anterior chamber is drained by afferent channels leading to the circular **sinus venosus**, which communicates with the venous system. Normally *no blood is found in these channels*. This system of spaces provides a means of continual drainage of the intraocular aqueous fluids.

 c. *Aqueous fluids* provide nutrition, exchange metabolites, and maintain a constant intraocular pressure to stabilize the tissues of the eye. Inadequate drainage causes the intraocular pressure to increase to such an extent that serious eye damage may occur, resulting in *glaucoma*.

 d. *Blood–aqueous barrier:* The slightly alkaline fluid resembling cerebrospinal fluid, in addition to the functions outlined above, also nourishes the lens, which lacks a blood supply.

  (1) The difference between this fluid and blood plasma is that the aqueous fluid has

   (a) a lower content of proteins, urea, and glucose.

   (b) a higher content of ascorbate, pyruvate, and lactate.

  (2) To maintain this fluid which is different from plasma, the *blood–aqueous barrier* comes into play. Plasma components can get through ciliary epithelium and stroma, but are finally blocked by tight junctions between the apices of the nonpigmented cells of the ciliary epithelium. This in fact is the morphological blood–aqueous barrier.

 F. The **lens** is an encapsulated, transparent, biconvex body with elastic properties.

 1. The *capsule* is a homogeneous carbohydrate-rich substance coating the entire lens. Under the capsule, on the anterior surface, is a simple cuboidal epithelium that becomes columnar in shape at the equator of the lens and fibrillar posteriorly in the bulk of the lens.

 2. *Aging:* Though highly elastic in youth, the lens gradually begins to harden, and at about age 40, the patient complains of difficulty in focusing. At this time it may be necessary to prescribe bifocals or even trifocals.

 3. *Cataract:* Loss of transparency of the lens or its capsule results in a cataract, which must be removed surgically. The patient is prescribed thickened cataract glasses in place of the removed lens or lenses. Advances in ophthalmology have made possible the insertion of plastic implants in place of a removed lens.

4. The *ciliary zonule* suspends the lens in its permanent position. Ligaments radiate from the region of the ciliary body to the anterior rim of the lens equator and to the posterior sheets of ligaments. The space between the sheets is spanned by similar filaments, but is primarily an access route for newly formed aqueous humour to flow into the posterior chamber.

G. *Accessory organs of the eye*

1. *Eyelids*, examined grossly, are noted to be composed of skin on the external surface and a mucous membrane on the internal ocular surface, covered by a transparent nonkeratinized stratified squamous epithelium.

a. Between these two surfaces, histological examination reveals in sequence:

(1) *loose connective tissue* under the skin, relatively free of adipocytes, but striated skeletal myocytes of the orbicularis oculi muscle may be encountered.

(2) *tarsal plate:* dense regular connective tissue forms the *tarsal plate* (collagen fibers with some elastic fibers), which extends to the free margin of the lid. The opposite margin of the tarsal plate provides an excellent insertion point for striated skeletal myocytes of the *superior palpebral muscle*, whch elevates the lid.

(a) *Tarsal glands* (formerly: Meibomian glands), distributed within the tarsal plate, secrete a lipid-like lubricant that prevents the free margins of opposing eyelids from sticking together. Eversion of the eyelid and examination through the transparent mucous membrane reveals a row of individual glands with long perpendicular ducts opening on the free margin of the lid. The long central ducts, lined by simple cuboidal epithelium, are surrounded by numerous alveoli opening into them.

(b) **Cilia** or *eyelashes* characterize the free margins of each eyelid. The cilia lack arrector pili muscles. *Sebaceous glands* (formerly: glands of Zeis) are associated with each cilium. Between follicles of the cilia are the spiraled *ciliary glands* (sweat glands, formerly called glands of Moll).

(3) *loose connective tissue* under the mucous membrane is also relatively free of adipocytes and may have isolated myocytes of the orbicularis oculi muscle.

2. *Conjunctiva:* Internally, the eyelid is lined with an epithelium two cells thick, the *palpebral conjunctiva*, which is reflected upon the sclera as the *bulbar conjunctiva* to the margins of the cornea.

3. The *lacrimal glands*, at the superior temporal margin of the bony orbits, secrete lubricating aqueous *tears*. The parenchymal *lacrimocytes* are more columnar, but bear striking similarities to the serous cells of the parotid. Between the *lacrimocytes* and the basement membrane reside numerous *myopithelial cells* that apparently contract to "squeeze" tears out of the glands into the excretory ducts. The supporting loose connective tissue stroma is characterized by lymphatic tissue in the adult.

II. The *Ear* is a complex organ of hearing divided into three structural compartments, the *external ear*, the *middle ear*, and the *inner ear* (Fig. 20-4) (Flock and Wersall, 1986).

A. The *external ear* is composed of the *auricle, external acoustic meatus*, and *tympanic membrane*.

1. The *auricle* is the cup-like structure on the side of the head, designed to catch sound waves. A thin curved plate of elastic cartilage is surrounded by a layer of thin skin possessing poorly developed hairs, sudoriferous glands, and sebaceous glands. Thin fibers of vestigial striated skeletal myocytes may be found beneath the skin. Occa-

Figure 20-4 Relationships between the external ear, middle ear, and internal ear.

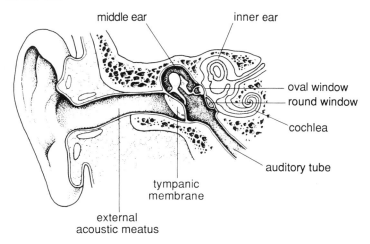

sionally, some individuals with a well-developed musculature display a voluntary ability to contract these muscles, causing the ears to move.

2. The *external acoustic meatus* is the roughly oval, rigid, skin-lined canal that funnels sound to the *tympanic membrane* (Perry, 1957).

a. *Skin dermis* attaches directly to elastic cartilage of the outer one-third of the meatus and to bone in the internal two-thirds of the canal, because there is no subcutaneous connective tissue.

b. *Hairs:* Large protective hairs guard the outer walls of the meatus. Deep within the meatus, smaller hairs protrude only from the glands.

c. *Glands:* Most conspicuous in the skin of the canal are large coiled sweat glands, the *ceruminous glands*, which can open directly onto the skin surface or into the excretory ducts of the *sebaceous glands*. Secretions of both glands combine to form *cerumin*, a brownish waxy substance that protects the canal and the tympanic membrane.

3. The *tympanic membrane* (Greek: *tympanon*, drum), measuring about 1cm in diameter and 0.1 mm thick, separates the external acoustic meatus from the middle ear, and thus possesses an external surface and an internal surface. This thin, semitransparent disc has a central indentation caused by the bony **malleus** (an ossicle of the middle ear) attached to its internal surface. The membrane is formed of two epithelial layers, sandwiching a flattened **lamina propria** of connective tissue:

a. a thin **stratum cutaneum**, continuous with the epidermis of the external auditory meatus, covers the external surface.

b. a thin **stratum mucosum** on the internal surface covered with epithelial cells that vary between squamous to cuboidal. This middle ear **stratum mucosum**, derived from the first pharyngeal pouch, adheres to the **malleus**, one of the three auditory ossicles.

c. A thin fibrous **lamina propria**, between the stratum cutaneuem and the stratum mucosum, consists of two parts:

(1) a lax **pars flaccida**, located superiorly, forms only a minor part.

(2) a taut **pars tensa**, forming the rest, consists of two strata, an outer **stratum radiale** and an inner **stratum circulare**.

B. *Middle ear:* The *tympanic cavity* receives atmospheric air through the *auditory tube* to equilibrate pressure on both sides of the tympanic membrane.

1. To appreciate the structure of the middle ear, perform this simple exercise with a thin attache case. Stand the case on end and open it. The open side facing you represents the opened *right* tympanic cavity of a subject who is facing you.

    a. The inside of the *left* lid represents the bony lateral wall bearing the tympanic membrane. The outer rim of the tympanic membrane attaches firmly to a ring of fibrocartilage.

    b. The inside of the *right* lid represents the bony medial wall of the *right* tympanic cavity.

    c. The posterior hinged end represents that portion of the *temporal bone* containing the *mastoid air cells.*

    d. The anterior wall, floor, and roof of the tympanic cavity is formed when the attache case is closed.

2. The *medial wall* is marked by a large circular prominence, the *promontory*, elevated by the underlying *vestibule cavity* of the *bony labyrinth* (*inner ear*).

    a. Posterior to this *promontory*, two tiny membrane-covered windows seal off the internal ear, an *oval window* in the upper left quadrant and a *round window* at the middle level.

    b. Three *auditory ossicles* form a miniature chain of articulating bones that mediate the transference of sound waves from the tympanic membrane to the oval window. The ossicles are:

    (1) the *stapes* (stirrup shaped), which attaches its oval footrest portion to the oval window of the medial wall.

    (2) the *malleus* (hammer shaped), which attaches to the tympanic membrane.

    (3) the **incus** (anvil shaped), which articulates between the malleus and the stapes.

    c. Contractions of two small striated skeletal muscles, the **tensor tympani** and a smaller **stapedius**, dampen the oscillations of the ossicles to protect the inner ear from injury following loud noises or high frequencies.

    (1) Tensor tympani: *origin*, anterior wall; *insertion*, handle of the malleus; *innervation*, trigeminal (V) nerve; *action*, tense tympanic membrane.

    (2) Stapedius (smallest human striated skeletal muscle): *origin*, posterior wall; *insertion*, head of stapes; *innervation*, facial (VII) nerve; *action*, pulls backwards on the stapes to tilt the base and increase the tension of fluid in the internal ear.

    d. A **stratum mucosum**, covering the tympanic membrane and other structures in the middle ear, consists of a **lamina propria** binding

epithelium to underlying structures. Simple squamous epithelium covers most areas and ciliated cuboidal or pseudostratified ciliated columnar appears near the opening of the auditory tube.

(1) *Normal:* A few goblet cells elaborate a thin humidifying fluid which cilia wave into the *auditory tube.* Normally no other secretory cell types or glands are found.

(2) *Pathological:* Blockage of the auditory tube by prolonged colds reduces pressure in the tympanic cavity, causing an increase in the number of goblet cells and development of mucous glands in the thin layer lamina propria. Accumulation of secretion results in *secretory otitis media,* which impairs hearing. If chronic, the condition could form scar tissue and permanent hearing impairment.

3. The *auditory tube* consists of a *bony portion* contiguous with the bony walls of the middle ear and a *cartilaginous portion* in the remainder.

    a. The posterior wall of the cartilaginous portion is shaped like a "C" in cross section, while the anterior wall is a wrinkled *fibrous membrane* closing off the "C." The fibrous membrane usually collapses into the cartilaginous "C" to keep the tube closed, except when swallowing or chewing.

    b. A lining of cilated epithelium commences as cuboidal near the tympanic cavity and increases in thickness to pseudostratified columnar (continuous with the epithelium of the nasopharynx). *Goblet cells* and mucous *tubal glands* occur.

    c. While serving admirably to funnel atmospheric air from the nasopharynx into the tympanic cavity, the *auditory tube* also is an unfortunate access for pathogens invading the middle ear.

C. The *internal ear* consists of a continuous series of fluid-filled ducts and saccules, the *membranous labyrinth* (Fig. 20-5), suspended in a *bony labyrinth.*

1. *Basic structure:* The *membranous labyrinth* is a closed system of labyrinthine *ducts* and *saccules* communicating via a fluid *endolymph.* Two portions are identified:

    a. a portion associated with *balance:*

    (1) The *semicircular ducts,* composed of three arched tubules coursing through the semicircular canals: *superior, lateral,* and *posterior ducts.* Each commences in the *utricle* as a dilated *ampulla* and terminates as a thin tubule: (a) the *lateral duct* terminates directly in the utricle; (b) the superior and posterior ducts unite to form a single channel, the *crus commune,* which terminates in the *utricle.*

    (2) The *utricle,* a dilated membranous sac, possesses two

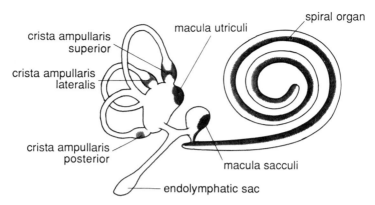

Figure 20-5 The membranous labyrinth.

surfaces: a larger convex surface facing the semicircular ducts and a smaller concave surface joined via a small *utriculosaccular duct* to the *saccule*, a smaller, more spherical sac.

    b. a portion associated with *hearing* (containing the *spiral organ*, formerly the organ of Corti) is joined to the saccule via a small **ductus reuniens**.

    2. The *bony labyrinth* consists of a series of bony canals in the petrous portion of the temporal bone. Two united cavities form the bony labyrinth:

    a. the *vestibule*, an oddly shaped oval cavity housing the *utricle* and the *saccule*,

    b. the **cochlea**, a spiral canal anteromedial to the vestibule, consisting of two and three-quarter turns around a central pillar of bone, the **modiolus**. The apex of the cochlea is directed somewhat inferiorly in an anterolateral direction.

    3. *Microscopic structure*

    a. The *utricle, saccule, semicircular ducts,* and the *ampullae* are lined with simple squamous or low cuboidal epithelium, except for narrow elevated zones and ridges of these components, which are covered with specialized sensory cells.

    (1) The **macula utriculi** and the **macula sacculi** are narrow elevated zones bearing sensory cells in the utricle and saccule respectively.

    (2) The **crista ampullaris** is the elevated narrow transverse ridge bearing sensory cells in the ampullae of each of the semicircular canals.

(3) Two types of cells distinguish the elevated zones, *supporting cells* and *sensory epithelial hair cells.*

(a) *Supporting cells* are tall columnar types with nuclei polarized toward the basement membrane. A cuticular plate is prominent near the free surface. These cells, at the edge of the *macula*, grade down to the squamous epithelium common to the rest of the tubes or sacs.

(b) *Sensory hair cells*, occupying the upper three quarters of the *maculae* are distinguished by TEM into two types, *piriform epitheliocytes* and *columnar epitheliocytes.* Head movements in one of several planes move the endolymph within the semicircular canals, stimulating the hair cells to convey impulses to the *vestibular nerve.*

[1] *Piriform epitheliocytes* are pear-shaped cells enveloped by the cup-shaped end of the sensory nerve. The luminal surface is covered by rather unusual microvilli and a single cilium embedded in a gelatinous *membrane* of **statoconia** (formerly: otoconia). The **statoconia** are small crystalline bodies of calcium carbonate and protein suspended in the gelatinous matrix.

[2] *Columnar epitheliocytes* have slightly different microvilli and single cilium on the luminal surface. This cell differs from the piriform epitheliocyte by the several nerve synaptic terminals contacting the basal and lateral surfaces. The terminals are differentiated as *afferent* or *efferent.*

b. The *endolymphatic sac* (Fig. 20-5): One small duct from the *utricle* and one small duct from the *saccule* unite to form the *endolymphatic duct.* The duct terminates in a dilated *endolymphatic sac* lined by two cell types:

(1) electron-dense columnar cells with relatively smooth luminal surfaces,

(2) less dense columnar cells with long microvilli on the luminal surfaces *absorb* endolymph, cellular debris, and foreign materials and transport them intracellularly to underlying capillaries of a rich vascular network surrounding the endolymphatic sac.

c. The *cochlear duct* is a spiraled evagination of the saccule containing the *spiral organ* (formerly: organ of Corti).

(1) *Longitudinal section* (Fig. 20-6): Pulled out of the bony cochlea like an escargot, and unrolled, the cochlear duct forms a long straight tube filled with endolymph. This is the **scala media** (Fig. 20-7).

(a) A separate tube (with no communication to the mem-

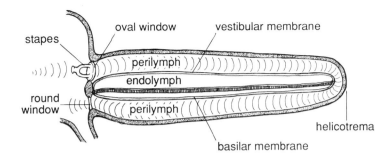

Figure 20-6 The cochlear duct (filled with endolymph) is unwound to reveal relationships with the perilymph-filled tubes: scala vestibuli (upper) and scala tympani (lower).

braneous labyrinth), filled with *perilymph*, surrounds the longitudinal axis of the cochlear duct. Its component continuous divisions are an upper tube and a lower tube.

[1] The upper portion of the tube, the **scala vestibuli** (Fig. 20-7), begins at the *oval window* (facing the cavity of the middle ear) where it contacts the base of the **stapes**.

Figure 20-7 Schematic representation through one segment of a turn of the cochlear duct.

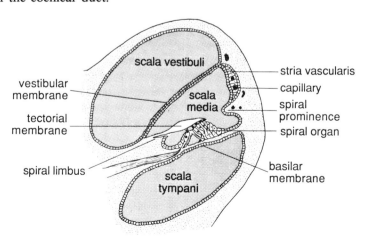

[2] The **helicotrema**, a continuation, is the constricted part that bends around the tip of the cochlear duct.

[3] The lower portion of the tube, the **scala tympani** (Fig. 20-7), extends to the round window where it terminates against the *round window* of the middle ear.

(2) A *cross section* (Fig. 20-7) through the complex shows the **scala vestibuli** above and the **scala tympani** below the **scala media**. Each scala is lined by simple squamous epithelium.

(a) The *vestibular membrane* forms from the union of the epithelium of the scala vestibuli and the scala media (formerly: Reissner's membrane) is formed. Blood vessels are lacking in this membrane.

(b) The *basilar membrane* forms from the union of the epithelium of the **scala tympani** and the base of the *spiral organ.*

(c) The **scala media**, compressed into a pie-shaped section by the surrounding *perilymphatic space*, has the following features:

[1] A **stria vascularis** forming the outer wall is lined by an unusual stratified epithelium composed of three cell types named according to location: *basal cells, intermediate cells,* and *marginal cells.*

[a] The unusual nature of this epithelium stems from the presence of capillaries coursing between the cells parallel to the surface. Only a thin basement membrane contributed by the epithelial and endothelial cells separates the two cell types.

[b] The **stria vascularis** is the major source of *endolymph.* (Recall: cells that absorb endolymph occur in the *endolymphatic sac.*)

[2] Inferiorly is the *spiral prominence*, an elevation of vascularized periosteum where the **stria vascularis** terminates. Gradually its covering of cuboidal cells elongate as the *outer supporting cells* (formerly: cells of Claudius) and *outer limiting cells* (formerly: cells of Henson) of the spiral organ. These cells rest on the connective tissue of the *basilar membrane.*

(3) The *spiral organ* is the specialized system of cells maintained in appropriate positions by the supporting cells. Special names are given to portions and regions of cells, but attention is focused on two types of *sensory epithelial hair cells* and the mechanism of stimulation (Hudspeth, 1983).

(a) *Internal sensory epithelial hair cells (piriform)* are arranged in a single row running the length of the **scala media**.

[1] These resemble the *piriform epitheliocytes* of the *utricle*, but lack the single cilium in adults.

[2] *Efferent* as well as *afferent nerve endings* terminate at the base and sides of the cells.

[3] Long unusual **microvilli** (hairs) populate the luminal surface of these cells.

[4] Mitochondria and sER are found just under the dense apical cytoplasm and at the base of the cell under a spherical nucleus.

(b) *External sensory epithelial hair cells (columnar)* are more highly specialized for hearing than the internal hair cells.

[1] Nerve terminals resemble those of the internal hair cells.

[2] The unusual microvilli (hairs) stud the luminal surface of the cell and also lack the single cilium.

[3] Rough ER, interspersed with dense lipid droplets, occupies the apical portion of the cell.

[4] Mitochondria, related to sER vesicles, aggregate at the base of the cell and along the lateral walls.

(c) *Spiral limbus*, a tissue primarily periosteal in origin, bulges into the **scala media** from the *internal wall* (pie point) between the points of the modiolus origin of the vestibular and basilar membranes. It forms an edge protruding toward the spiral organ, covering an *inner tunnel*. The specialized cells on the surface of the spiral limbus secrete the *tectorial membrane* which overlies the hairs of the *hair cells* of the spiral organ. Evidence indicates that these hairs are embedded into the membrane.

4. *Endolymph* and *perilymph* (Guild, 1927)

a. *Endolymph* fills all components of the *membranous labyrinth*, including the **scala media** with the thick fluid *endolymph*.

(1) While the **stria vascularis** produces endolymph, evidence indicates that the lining cells of the membranous labyrinth contribute to the production of endolymph.

(2) Similarly, while cells of the *endolymphatic sac* absorb endolymph, EM evidence indicates that the lining cells of the membranous labyrinth also absorb endolymph.

b. *Perilymph* surrounds the entire membranous labyrinth to provide a spongy support for the epithelial lining.

(1) The **scala vestibuli** and **scala tympani** are also filled with perilymph.

(2) Perilymph is a reticulum composed of highly attenuated processes of primitive reticular cells embedded in a viscous extracellular matrix. Capillary beds in the perilymph provide metabolic requirements of the membranous labyrinthine epithelium.

5. *Hearing*

a. Sound waves are trapped by the *external ear* and funneled into the *external acoustic meatus.*

b. Sound waves vibrating the *tympanic membrane* are dampened through the chain of auditory ossicles to the *oval window.*

c. Vibrations of the *oval window* change the pressure in the perilymph of the **scala vestibuli.**

d. Pressure changes in perilymph are reflected on the *round window* to release the pressure. This occurs is one of two ways:

(1) *directly:* by passing through scala vestibuli, the heliocotrema, and the scala tympani to reach the oval window.

(2) *indirectly:* by passing from the scala vestibuli *across* the *vestibular membrane* through the endolymph of the scala media to *displace* the *tectorial membrane,* thence to the *basilar membrane* to access the perilymph of the **scala tympani** for transmission to the round window.

e. Stimulation of the sensory hair cells transmits the sensory impulse to appropriate receptors in ganglion cells of the *cochlear nerve.*

f. Differences in sound frequencies are accounted for by the position of the site of displacement of the basilar membrane.

(1) *High frequencies* are transmitted by hair cells of the spiral organ closest to the *oval window.*

(2) *Low frequencies* are transmitted by hair cells of the spiral organ closest to the *round window.*

(3) *Intermediate frequencies,* from high to low, are transmitted by hair cells located in the spiral organ between the sites where high and low frequencies are received.

Questions

DIRECTIONS: For each of the items in this section, one or more of the numbered options is correct. Select

    A if only *1, 2, and 3* are correct
    B if only *1 and 3* are correct
    C if only *2 and 4* are correct
    D if only *4* is correct
    E if *all* are correct

---

1. Components of the fibrous tunic of the eye are
   1. cornea
   2. lens
   3. sclera
   4. choroid

2. The morphological blood–aqueous barrier of the eye is the
   1. anterior chamber
   2. posterior chamber
   3. sinus venosus of sclera (canal of Schlemm)
   4. tight junctions between ciliary nonpigmented cells

3. Rods and cones consist of
   1. internal segments, containing mitochondria
   2. nuclear portions in the external granular layer
   3. cell processes that synapse with bipolar cells
   4. external segments containing laminated discs

4. Pertaining to the rods and cones, which statements are correct?
   1. Rods cannot discriminate color
   2. Cones discriminate color in the high light intensity
   3. Each cone synapses with one bipolar cell
   4. Several rods synapse with one bipolar cell

5. Histological examination of the eyelids reveals
   1. sebaceous glands
   2. sweat glands
   3. tarsal glands
   4. lacrimal glands

6. The thin tympanic membrane is derived from
   1. ectoderm
   2. mesoderm
   3. endoderm
   4. ectoderm and mesoderm

7. Which structures of the middle ear are covered by epithelium?
   1. Simple squamous
   2. Pseudostratified ciliated cuboidal
   3. Pseudostratified ciliated columnar
   4. Simple columnar with microvilli

8. The auditory tube possesses a
   1. "C"-shaped cartilaginous tube
   2. fibrous membrane
   3. bony portion
   4. ciliated epithelium

9. The narrow elevated zones of the utricle, saccule, and ampullae are distinguished by which of the following cell types?
   1. Supporting
   2. Piriform
   3. Columnar
   4. Modiolus

10. Endolymph may be produced by
    1. spiral organ
    2. most of the lining cells of the membranous labyrinth
    3. light-dense columnar clls of the endolymphatic sac
    4. stria vascularis

Explanatory Answers

1. B. 1 and 3 are correct. These are not neural derivatives, but mesenchymal. The lens is an ectodermal derivative. The choroid is part of the vascular tunic (uvea) of the eye.

2. D. 4 is correct. The anterior chamber is the space between the cornea and anterior surface of the iris. It communicates with the posterior chamber, which is the space between the posterior surface of the iris and anterior surface of the lens. The sinus venosus drains the anterior chamber. The fluid is maintained in its purity by the tight junctions of the nonpigmented cells, which prevent blood-borne plasma components from gaining entrance to the chamber fluid.

3. E. All are correct. The rods are the slender photoreceptors, and the cones are the more plump photoreceptors.

4. E. All are correct. Several rods, by synapsing with one bipolar ganglion cell, summate low light intensities, thus facilitating vision in darkened situations. The cones, especially in the fovea centralis (where there are only cones), provide for great visual acuity and thus mediate color vision.

5. A. 1, 2, and 3 are correct. The major gland of the eyelid is one of several aligned tarsal glands that secrete a lipid-like lubricant which prevents the free margins of the opposing eyelids from sticking together. Sebaceous glands (Zeiss glands) are associated with each cilium (eyelash). Between follicles of the cilia are the ciliary glands, which are sweat glands (Moll glands). The lacrimal glands, with parotid-like serous-type cells, are located at the superior margin of the bony orbits and not in the eyelid.

6. A. 1, 2, and 3 are correct. The ectoderm of the skin gives rise to the stratum corneum. The endoderm of the first pharyngeal pouch gives rise to the stratum mucosum (facing the middle ear). The mesoderm gives rise to the lamina propria between the stratum corneum and stratum mucosum.

7. A. 1, 2, and 3 are correct. The majority of the middle ear is covered by simple squamous epithelium that is bound to underlying structures by a lamina propria. Closer to the auditory tube, the epithelium becomes pseudostratifed ciliated cuboidal and then columnar. There is no simple absorptive (microvillous) columnar epithelium. In fact, scattered goblet cells are present to humidify the middle ear. The ciliated cells wave the fluid into the auditory tube.

8. E. All are correct. The fibrous membrane is a wrinkled sheet that is usually collapsed into the "C"-shaped cartilaginous tube to close off the tube, except when swallowing or chewing. The ciliated epithelium, cuboidal in the first part and pseudostratified near the nasopharynx, possesses goblet cells and mucous tubal glands.

9. A. 1, 2 and 3 are correct. The supporting cells are tall columnar cells with nuclei polarized toward the basement membrane. The piriform epitheliocytes (pear-shaped cells) are covered by long unusual microvilli and one cilium embedded in the gelatinous membrane of statoconia. The columnar epitheliocytes, with slightly different microvilli and one cilium, are in contact with afferent and efferent nerve terminals on their basal and lateral surfaces. The modiolus is the pilar of bone around which the cochlea makes its two and three-quarter turns.

10. C. 2 and 4 are correct. The stria vascularis is the only known epithelium that has capillaries coursing through it. This unusual relationship facilitates the production of endolymph. Evidence also indicates that most of the lining cells of the membranous labyrinth can produce endolymph. The spiral organ (of Corti) possesses the specialized cells of hearing and does not produce endolymph. The lining cells of the endolymphatic sac possess specialized columnar cells that are involved in absorption. Capillaries surrounding the sac receive the absorbed endolymph.

Bibliography

Abramowitz, M. 1985. *Microscope Basics and Beyond*. Olympus Corporation, Lake Success, NY.

Abramowitz, M. 1987. *Contrast Methods in Microscopy. Transmitted Light*. Olympus Corporation, Lake Success, NY.

Allison, A.C. and P. Davies 1974. Mechanisms of exocytosis and endocytosis. Symp. Soc. Exp. Biol. *28:*419.

Amenta, P.S. 1961. Fusion of nucleoli in cells cultured from the heart of *Triturus viridescens*. Anat. Rec. *139:*155.

Amenta, P.S. 1962. The effects of ultraviolet microbeam irradiation on the eosinophil granular leukocytes of *Triturus viridescens*. Anat. Rec. *142:*81.

Amenta, P.S. 1967. Lymphotaxis induced by ultraviolet microbeam irradiation of fibroblasts cultured from mouse embryos. Anat. Rec. *159:*199.

Amenta, P.S. 1987. Elias-Pauly's *Histology and Human Microanatomy*, 5th edition, John Wiley & Sons/Piccin, New York/Padova.

Amenta, P.S., I. Gersh, and E. Gersh 1973. Persistence of individuality of chromosomes during interphase. In: *Submicroscopic Cytochemistry*, Vol. I, Edited by I. Gersh, Academic Press, New York.

Anderson, P.H. et al 1984. The clinical anatomy of the cardiac conduction system. In: *Recent Advances in Cardiology*, Vol. 9, Edited by D.J. Rowland, Churchill-Livingstone, New York.

Ariens-Kappers, J. and J. Schade (eds) 1965. Structure and function of the epiphysis cerebri. In: *Progress in Brain Research*, Vol. 10, Elsevier, Amsterdam.

Arstila, A.U. 1967. Electron microscopic studies on the structure and histochemistry of the pineal gland of the rat. Neuroendocrinology (Suppl.) *2:*1.

446

Axelrod, J. and T. Reisine 1984. Stress hormones: their interaction and regulation. Science *224*:452.

Bach, J. and M. Papiernik 1981. Cellular and molecular signals in T-cell differentiation. In: *Ciba Foundation Symposium*, Edited by R. Porter and J. Whelan, Pittman, London.

Bainton, D. and M. Farquhar 1966. Origin of granules in the polymorphonuclear leukocytes. Two types derived from opposite faces of the Golgi complex. J. Cell Biol. *26*:277.

Bainton, D. and M. Farquhar 1970. Segregation and packaging of granule enzymes in eosinophilic leukocytes. J. Cell Biol. *45*:54.

Bainton, D., J. Ullyot, and M. Farquhar 1971. The developmet of neutrophilic polymorphonuclear leukocytes in human basement membranes. Origin and contents of azurophilic and specific granules. J. Exp. Med. *134*:907.

Barajas, L. and H. Latta 1967. Structure of the juxtaglomerular apparatus. Circ. Res. *20-1*:15.

Barer, R. 1955. Phase contrast, interference contrast and polarizing microscopy. In: *Analytical Cytology*, 3, Edited by R. Mellors, McGraw-Hill, New York.

Becker, R.P. and P.P.H. DeBruyn 1976. The transmural passage of blood cells into myeloid sinuses and entry of platelets into the sinusoidal circulation; a scanning electron microscopic investigation. Am. J. Anat. *145*:183.

Beeson, P.B. and D.A. Bass 1977. The *Eosinophil*, W.B. Saunders, Philadelphia.

Beeuwkes, R. 1980. The vascular organization of the kidney. Am. Rev. Physiol. *42*:531.

Bennett, M.L.V. et al 1981. Gap junctions and development. Trends Neurosci. *4*:159.

Bergland, R. and R. Page 1979. Pituitary-brain vascular relations: a new paradigm. Science *204*:18.

Bessis, M. 1966. Life cycle of the erythrocyte. Sandoz Monographs, Sandoz Ltd, Basle.

Bevan, M.J. and P.J. Fink 1978. The influence of thymus H-2 antigens on the specificity of maturing killer and helper cells. Immunol. Rev. *42*:3.

Billingham, R. and W. Silvers 1968. Dermal-epidermal interactions and epidermal specificity. In: *Epithelial-Mesenchymal Interac-*

tions, Edited by R. Fleischmayor and R. Billingham, Williams & Wilkins, Baltimore.

Blue, J. and L. Weiss 1981. Vascular pathways in non-sinusal red pulp: an electron microscopic study of cat spleen. Amer. J. Anat. *161:*135.

Blumenstein, R. and P.S. Amenta 1981. An interferometric analysis of nucleoli in cultured mesothelial cells. Anat. Rec. *201:*13.

Bolander, M.E. et al 1988. Osteonectin cDNA sequence reveals potential binding regions for calcium and hydroxyapatite, and shows homologies with both a basement membrane protein (SPARC) and a serine protein inhibitor (ovomucoid). Proc. Natl. Acad. Sci. *85:*2919.

Bolzer, E. 1962. Smooth muscle. In: *Muscle As A Tissue*, Edited by K. Rodahl and S.M. Horvath, McGraw-Hill, New York.

Bonner, T. and M. Brownstein 1984. Vasopressin, tissue specific defects and the Brattleboro rat. Nature *310:*17.

Bourne, G.H. 1972. *The Biochemistry and Physiology of Bone*, 2nd Edition, Vol. I–IV, Academic Press, New York.

Boyden, E.A. 1971. Development of the human lung. In: *Brennemann's Practice of Pediatrics*, Vol. 4, Harper & Row, New York.

Branton, D. et al 1975. Freeze-etching nomenclature. Science *190:*54.

Bray, D. and D. Gilbert 1981. Cytoskeletal elements in neurons. Annu. Rev. Neurosci. *4:*505.

Brenner, B. and F. Rector 1976. *The Kidney*, Vol. I, W.B. Saunders, Philadelphia.

Brightman, M.W. 1977. Morphology of blood-brain interfaces. Eye Res. (Suppl) 1.

Brinkley, B.R. 1965. The fine structure of the nucleolus in mitotic divisions of Chinese hamster cells in vitro. J. Cell. Biol. *27:*411.

Burnside, B. 1975. The form and arrangement of microtubules: an historical, primarily morphological review. Ann. N.Y. Acad. Sci. *253:*14.

Bussolati, G. and G. Pearse 1967. Immunofluorescent localization of calcitonin in the C-cells of pig and dog thyroid. J. Endocrinol. *37:*205.

Campbell, F.R. 1968. Nuclear elimination from the normoblast of fetal guinea pig liver as studied with electron microscopy and serial section techniques. Anat. Rec. *160:*539.

Carmichael, S. 1983. *The Adrenal Medulla*, Vol. 3, Eden Press, Quebec.

Cauna, N. and K. Hinderer 1969. Fine structure of blood vessels of the human nasal respiratory mucosa. Ann. Otolaryngol. *78*:865.

Chakrabarti, B. and J.W. Park 1980. Glycosaminoglycans: structure and interaction. CRC Crit. Rev. Biochem. *8*:225.

Charonis, A. et al 1985. Binding of laminin to type IV collagen. A morphological study. J. Cell Biol. *100*:1848.

Chen, L. and L. Weiss 1973. The role of the sinus wall in the passage of erythrocytes through the spleen. Blood *41*:529.

Chen, L. 1978. Microcirculation of the spleen: an open or closed circulation? Science *201*:157.

Christiansen, A.K. 1975. Leydig cells. In: *Handbook of Physiology: Endocrinology*, Vol. 5, Sec. 7, *Male Reproductive System*. American Physiological Society, Washington, D.C.

Clark, A. and K. MacLennan 1986. The many facets of thymic involution. Immunol. Today *100*:1848.

Clemente, C.D. 1985. *Gray's Anatomy of the Human Body*, 30th American Edition. Lea & Febiger, Philadelphia.

Cohen, C.M. 1983. The molecular organization of the red cell membrane skeleton. Semin. Hematol. *20*:141.

Cohen, J. and W.H. Harris 1958. The three dimensional anatomy of the Haversian systems. J. Bone Joint Surg. [Br.] 40-A:419.

Cooke, P. 1976. A filamentous cytoskeleton in vertebrate smooth muscle fibers. J. Cell Biol. *68*:539.

Cooper, R.R. et al 1966. Morphology of the osteon. An electron microscopic study. J. Bone Joint Surg. [Am.] *48*:1239.

Cooperstein, S. and D. Watkins 1981. *The Pancreatic Islets*. Academic Press, New York.

Cowie, A.T. 1974. Overview of the mammary gland. J. Invest. Dermatol. *63*:2.

Davies, H.G. 1958. The determination of mass and concentration by microscopic interpherometry. In: *General Cytochemical Methods*, Edited by J. Danielli, Vol. I:57. Academic Press, New York.

Davis, R. and A.C. Enders 1961. Light and electron microscopic studies on the parathyroid gland. In: *The Parathyroids*, Edited by

R.O. Greep and R. Talmadge, Charles C. Thomas, Springfield, IL.

Davson, H. 1967. *Physiology of the Cerebrospinal Fluid*, Little, Brown & Co., Boston.

Dawson, I. 1977. The endocrine cells of the gastrointestinal tract and neoplasms which arise from them. Curr. Concepts Pathol. *63*:222.

deBold, A.J. and T.G. Flynn 1983. Cardionatrin I, a novel heart peptide with potent diurectic and naturetic properties. Life Sci. *33*:297.

DeBruyn, P.P.H. 1944. Locomotion of blood cells in tissue culture. Anat. Rec. *89*:43.

DeBruyn, P.P.H. 1981. Structural substrates of bone marrow formation. Semin. Hematol. *18*:179.

DeDuve, C. 1963. Lysosomes. Sci. Am. *208*:5.

DeLuca, H.F. et al 1981. *Osteoporosis: Advances in Pathogenesis and Treatment*. University Park Press, Baltimore.

Dennis, M.J. 1981. Development of the neuromuscular junction: inductive interactions between cells. Annu. Rev. Neurosci. *4*:43.

DePace, D.M. 1982. Evidence for a blood ganglion barrier in the superior cervical ganglion of the rat. Anat. Rec. *204*:357.

DeSousa, M. et al 1969. The lymphoid tissues in mice with congenital aplasia of the thymus. Clin. Exp. Immunol. *4*:637.

Devlin, T. 1986. *Textbook of Biochemistry*, 2nd Edition. John Wiley & Sons, New York.

Dewey, M.P. and L. Barr 1962. Intercellular connection between smooth muscle cells: the nexus. Science *137*:670.

Dierickx, K. and F. Vandesande 1977. Immunocytochemical localization of the vasopressinergic and oxytocinergic neurons in the human hypothalamus. Cell Tissue Res. *184*:203.

Dvorak, A.M. 1978. Morphology of basophilic leukocytes. In: *Immediate Hypersensitivity, Modern Concepts of Developmental Immunology Series*, Edited by M.K. Bach, Marcel Dekker, New York.

Dym, M. 1973. The fine structure of the monkey (*Macaca*) Sertoli cell and its role in maintaining the blood-testis barrier. Anat. Rec. *175*:639.

Ebashi, S. 1974. Regulatory mechanism of muscle contraction with special reference to the Ca-troponin-tropomyosin system. Essays Biochem. *10*:1.

Ekholm, R. and L. Erickson 1968. Ultrastructure of the parafollicular cells of the rat. J. Ultrastruct. Res. *23*:378.

Elgsaeter, A. et al 1986. The molecular basis of erythrocyte shape. Science *234*:1217.

Erlandsen, S. and D. Chase 1972. Paneth cell function, phagocytosis and intracellular digestion of microorganisms. J. Ultrastruct. Res. *41*:296.

Erlandsen, S. 1980. Types of pancreatic islet cells and their immuno-cytochemical identification. Int. Acad. Pathol. *91*:77.

Farquhar, M.G. 1961. Fine structure and function in capillaries of the anterior pituitary gland. Angiology *12*:270.

Farquhar, M.G. 1975. The primary glomerular filtration barrier-basement membrane or epithelial slits? Kidney Int. *8*:197.

Farquhar, M.G. and G.E. Palade 1981. The golgi apparatus (complex) — 1954–1981 — from artifact to center stage. J. Cell Biol. (Suppl.) *91*:77.

Fawcett, D.W. 1961. Cilia and flagella. In: *The Cell, Biochemistry, Physiology, Morphology*, Vol. II:217, Edited by J. Brachet and E. Mirsky, Academic Press, New York.

Fawcett, D.W. 1975. The mammalian spermatozoon. Dev. Biol. *44*:394.

Fawcett, D.W. 1976. The male reproductive system. In: *Reproduction and Human Welfare: A Challenge to Research*, Edited by R.O. Greep, M.A. Koblinsky, and F.S. Jaffe, p. 165. MIT Press, Cambridge, MA.

Fernandez-Moran, H. et al 1964. A macromolecular repeating unit of mitochondrial structure and function. J. Cell Biol. *22*:71.

Fine, B.S. and M. Yanoff 1972. *Ocular Histology*, Harper & Row, New York.

Finian, J.B. 1977. The development of ideas on membrane structure. Subcell. Biochem. *1*:363.

Fink, B.R. 1975. *The Human Larynx. A Functional Study.* Raven Books, New York.

Fishmann, D.A. and E.D. Hay 1962. Origin of osteoclasts from mononuclear leucocytes in regenerating new limbs. Anat. Rec. *143*:329.

Fitzpatrick, T. et al 1979. Biology of the melanin pigmentary system. In: *Dermatology in General Medicine*, 2nd Edition, Edited by T. Fitzpatrick et al, McGraw-Hill, New York.

Flock, A. and J. Wersall 1986. Cellular mechanisms of hearing. *Nobel Symposium 63. Hearing Research*, Elsevier, Amsterdam.

Forsmann, W.G. et al 1983. The right auricle is an endocrine organ. Anat. Embryol. *168*:307.

Frank, R.M. 1979. Tooth enamel: current state of the art. J. Dent. Res. *58B*:684.

Franzini-Armstrong, C. 1986. The sarcoplasmic reticulum and transverse tubules. In: *Myology*, Vol. I, Edited by A.G. Engel and B. Banker, McGraw-Hill, New York.

Franzini-Armstrong, C. et al 1981. Striated muscle: contractile and control mechanisms. J. Cell Biol. *88*:166.

Fujimoto, S. and R.G. Murray. 1970. Fine structure of degeneration and regeneration in denervated rabbitt vallate taste buds. Anat. Rec. *168*:393

Fujita, H. and T. Murakani 1974. Scanning electron microscopy on the distribution of the minute vessels of the dog, rat and rhesus monkey. Arch. Histol. Jpn. *36*:181.

Gapp, D.A. 1986. The gastrointestinal endocrine system. In: *Fundamentals of Comparative Vertebrate Endocrinology*, Edited by I. Chester-Jones et al, Plenum, New York.

Gardner, L. (Ed.) 1975. Development of the normal fetal and neonatal adrenal. In: *Endrocrine and Genetic Diseases of Childhood and Adolescence*, 2nd Edition, W.B. Saunders, Philadelphia.

Gauthier, G.F. 1986. Skeletal muscle fiber types. In: *Myology*, Vol. I, Edited by A.G. Engel and B.Q. Banker, McGraw-Hill, New York.

Gerace, L. 1986. Nuclear lamina and organization of the nuclear envelope. Int. Rev. Cytol. [Suppl.] *4*:72.

Geren, B.B. 1956. Structural studies on the formation of the myelin sheath in peripheral nerve fibers. In: *Cellular Mechanisms in Differentiation and Growth*. Princeton University Press, Princeton.

Ghosh, S. 1976. The nucleolar structure. Int. Rev. Cytol. *44*:1.

Ginsburg, H. and L. Sachs 1963. Formation of pure suspensions of mast cells in tissue culture by differentiation of lymphoid cells from the mouse thymus. J. Natl. Cancer Inst. *31:*1.

Glees, P. 1955. *Neuroglia: Morphology and Function*, Charles C. Thomas, Springfield, IL.

Golden, D.W. and M.J. Cline 1974. Regulation of granulopoiesis. N. Engl. J. Med. *231:*1388.

Goldstein, A.D. 1984. *Thymic Hormones and Lymphokines*. Plenum Press, New York.

Goldstein, A.M. et al 1982. New observations on the microarchitecture of the corpora cavernosa in man and their possible relationship to the mechanism of erection. Urology *20:*259.

Gould, V.E., R. Moll, I. Moll, I. Lee and W. Frank. 1985. Neuroendocrine (Merkel) cells of the skin: Hyperplasias, dysplasias and neoplasms. Lab Invest. *53:*334.

Gray, E.G. 1959. Axo-somatic and axo-dendritic synapses of the cerebral cortex: an electron microscopic study. J. Anat. *231:*1388.

Gray, P. 1973. *The Encyclopedia of Microscopy and Microtechnique*, Van Nostrand Reinhold, New York.

Greaves, M.F., J.J. Owen, and M.C. Raff 1974. *T and B Lymphocytes. Origins, Properties and Roles in Immune Responses.* Excerpta Medica, New York.

Groom, A.C. et al 1971. Physical characteristics of red cells collected from the spleen. Can. J. Physiol. Pharmacol. *49:*1092.

Groom, A.C. and S.H. Song 1962. Effects of norepinephrine on washout of red cells from the spleen. Am. J. Physiol. *221:*255.

Guild, S.R. 1927. Circulation of the endolymph. Am. J. Anat. *39:*57.

Hadley, M.E. et al 1981. Biological actions of melanocyte stimulating hormone. In: *Peptides of the Pars Intermedia.* Ciba Symposium 81, Pitman Medical, London.

Hall, B.K. 1983. *Cartilage*, Vol. I. Academic Press, New York.

Hamaj, M. and T. Harrison 1984. Blood vessels and lymphatics of the adrenal gland. In: *Blood Vessels and Lymphatics in Organ Systems,* Edited by D. Abramson and P. Dobrin, Academic Press, New York.

Hamashima, Y. 1982. *The Use of the Olympus Fluorescence Microscope.* Olympus Optical Co., Tokyo.

Hamilton, D.W. 1975. Structure and function of the epithelium lining the ductuli efferentes, ductus epididymis, and ductus deferens in the rat. In: *Handbook of Physiology, Endocrinology*, Vol. 5, Sec. 7, *Male Reproductive System*, Edited by R.O. Greep. American Physiological Society, Washington, D.C.

Hancox, N.M. 1972. *The Biology of Bone*, Cambridge University Press, Cambridge.

Harmsen, A.G. et al 1985. The role of macrophages in particle translocation from lungs to lymph nodes. Science *230:*1277.

Harris, J.W. and R.W. Kellermeyer 1970. *The Red Cell.* Harvard University Press, Boston.

Hay, E.D. 1981. *Cell Biology of Extracellular Matrix.* Plenum Press, New York.

Hayat, M.A. 1972. *Basic Electron Microscopic Techniques.* Van Nostrand Reinhold, New York.

Hayat, M.A. 1978. *Introduction to Biological Scanning Electron Microscopy.* University Park Press, Baltimore.

Hearle, J., J. Sparrow, and P. Cross 1972. *The Use of the Scanning Electron Microscope.* Pergamon Press, Baltimore.

Heuser, J. 1976. Morphology of synaptic vesicle discharge and reformation, neuromuscular junction. In: *Motor Innervation of Muscle*, Edited by S. Thesleff, Academic Press, New York.

Heuser, J. et al 1979. Synaptic vesicle exocytosis by quick freeze and correlated with quantal transmitter release. J. Cell Biol. *81:*275.

Heuser, J. and T. Reese 1973. Evidence for recycling of synaptic vesicle membrane during transmitter release at the frog neuromuscular junction. J. Cell Biol. *57:*315.

Hewitt, A.T., H.K. Kleinman, J.P. Pennypacker, and G.R. Martin. 1980. Identification of an adhesive factor for chondrocytes. Proc. Natl. Acad. Sci (USA) *77:*748.

Hirsch, J.G. 1965. Phagocytosis. Annu. Rev. Microbiol. *19:*339.

Holtrop, M.E. 1972. The ultrastructure of osteoclasts during stimulation and inhibition of bone resorption. IV Int. Congr. Endocrinol. Washington, D.C.

Hudspeth, A.J. 1983. The hair cells of the inner ear. Sci. Am. *248:*54.

Huggins, C. and B.H. Blocksom 1936. Changes in outlying bone marrow accompanying a local increase of temperature within physiological limits. J. Anat. *64:*253.

Hurley, H. and W. Shelly 1960. *The Human Apocrine Sweat Gland in Health and Disease.* Charles C. Thomas, Springfield, IL.

Huxley, H.E. 1960. Muscle cells. In: *The Cell: Biochemistry, Physiology, Morphology,* Vol. 4, Edited by J. Brachet and A.E. Mirsky. Academic Press, New York.

Huxley, H.E. 1971. The structural basis of muscular contraction. Proc. R. Soc. Lond. [Biol.] *178:*131.

Huxley, H.E. and G. Zubray 1961. Preferential staining of nucleic acid containing structures for electron microscopy. J. Biophys. Biochem. Cytol. *11:*273.

Inoue, S. 1981. Cell division and the mitotic cycle. J. Cell Biol. (Suppl.) *93:*131s.

Ito, S. 1965. The surface coat of enteric microvilli. J. Cell Biol. *27:*475.

Ito, T. and S. Shibasaki 1968. Electron microscopic study on the hepatic sinusoidal wall and the fat storing cells in the human normal liver. Arch. Histol. Jpn. *29:*137.

Jacobson, M. 1978. *Developmental Neurobiology.* 2nd Edition. Plenum Press, New York.

Jaffe, D. et al 1971. Coronary arteries in newborn children. Acta Paediatr. Scand. [Suppl.] *219:*1.

Jakus, M.A. 1956. Studies on the cornea. II The fine structure of Descemet's membrane. J. Biophys. Biochem. Cytol. (Suppl.) *2:*243.

Jamieson, J.D. and G.E. Palade 1964. Specific granules in atrial muscle cells. J. Cell Biol. *100:*1647.

Johannison, E. 1968. The fetal cortex in the human. Its ultrastructure at different stages of development and in different functional stages. Acta Endocrinol. 58:[Suppl.] *130:*7.

Kanwar, Y.S. and M.G. Farquhar 1979. Presence of heparan sulfate in the glomerular basement membrane. Proc. Natl. Acad. Sci. *76:*1303.

Keller, T.C. et al 1985. Role of myosin in terminal web contraction in isolated intestinal brush borders. J. Cell Biol. *100:*1647.

Kelley, D. and M. Cahill 1972. Filamentous and matrix components of skeletal muscle Z-discs. Anat. Rec. *172:*623.

Kendall, M.D. 1981. *The Thymus Gland.* Academic Press, London.

Kessel, R.G. 1968. Annulate lamellae. J. Ultrastruct. Res. (Suppl.) *10:*1.

Kitamura, Y.K. et al 1981. Spleen colony-forming cells as common precursors for tissue mast cells and granulocytes. Nature *291:*159.

Kinsely, M.H. 1936. Spleen studies. I. Microscopic observations of the circulatory system of living unstimulated mammalian spleen. Anat. Rec. 65:23.

Kolmer, W. 1927. Handbuch des Microskopischen Anatomie des Menschen, p. 154, (ed) V. Mollendorf, Springer, Berlin.

Kornberg, R. 1977. Structure of chromatin. Annu. Rev. Biochem. 46:931.

Kriz, W. et al 1980. Comparative and functional aspects of thin loop ultrastructure. In: Functional Ultrastructure of the Kidney, Edited by A. Maunsbach et al, Academic Press, London.

Kuettner, K.E. et al 1986. Articular Cartilage Biochemistry, Raven Press, New York.

Ladman, A.J. and A. J. Mitchell 1955. The typographical relations and histological characteristics of tubuloacinar glands of the Eustachian tube in mice. Anat. Rec. 121:167.

Lazarides, E. 1980. Intermediate filaments as mechanical integrators of cellular space. Nature 283:249.

LeBlond, C.P. 1981. Life history of cells in renewing systems. Am. J. Anat. 160:113.

Lehninger, A.L. 1964. The Mitochondrion. W.B. Benjamin, New York.

Lennarz, W.J. 1980. The Biochemistry of Glycoproteins and Proteoglycans. Plenum Press, New York.

Lerner, A.B. and J. McGuire 1981. Effects of alpha and beta melanocyte stimulating hormones on skin colour in man. Nature 189:176.

Levi-Montalcini, R. 1964. Events in the developing nervous system. In: Progress In Brain Research, Vol. 4, Edited by D. Purpura and J. Shade, Elsevier, Amsterdam.

Lindberg, O. 1970. Brown Adipose Tissue. Elsevier, New York.

Lindhal, U. and M. Hook 1978. Glycosaminoglycans and their binding to biological macromolecules. Annu. Rev. Biochem. 47:385.

Ludwig, H, and A. Metzger 1976. The Human Female Reproductive Tract: A Scanning Electron Microscopic Atlas. Springer-Verlag, Berlin/Heidelberg/New York.

Luther, S. and J. Squire 1978. Three dimensional structure of the vertebrate muscle M-region. J. Mol. Biol. 125:313.

Madri, J. et al 1980. Ultrastructural localization of fibronectin and laminin in the basement membranes of the murine kidney. J. Cell Biol. *86*:682.

Mark, M.P. et al 1987. A comparative immunocytochemical study on the subcellular distributions of 44kDa bone phosphoprotein and bone carboxyglutamic acid. J. Bone Min. Res. *2*:337.

Marshall, S.F. and W.F. Becker. 1949. Thyroglossal cysts and sinuses. Ann. Surg. *129*:642.

Martin, G. R. et al 1985. The genetically distinct collagens. TIBS *10*:285.

Martin, G.R. and R. Timpl 1987. Laminin and other basement membrane components. Annu. Rev. Cell Biol. *3*:57.

Mascarro, J. and R. Yates 1970. Microscopic observations on abdominal sympathetic paraganglia. Tex. Rep. Biol. Med. *28*:59.

Mason, D. and D. Chisholm 1975. *Salivary Glands in Health and Disease.* W.B. Saunders, London.

Massaro, G.D. 1988. Non-ciliated bronchiolar epithelial (Clara) cells. In: *Lung Cell Biology*, Edited by G.D. Massaro. Marcel Dekker, New York.

Maul, G.G. 1971. Structure and formation of pores in fenestrated capillaries. J. Ultrastruct. Res. *36*:768.

Maximow, Alexander 1930. *Textbook of Histology*, First Edition, Edited by W. Bloom, W.B. Saunders, Philadelphia.

Maynard, E.A. et al 1957. Electron microscopy of the vascular bed of the rat cerebral cortex. Am. J. Anat. *100*:409.

Mazia, D. 1964. The cell cycle. Sci. Am. *230*:54.

McCuskey, R. and P. McCuskey 1977. In vivo microscopy of the spleen. Bibl. Anat. *16*:121.

McCuskey, R. and P. McCuskey 1985. In vivo and electron microscopic studies of the splenic microvasculature in mice. Experientia *41*:179.

McNeal, J.E. 1973. The prostate and prostatic urethra, a morphologic synthesis. J. Urol. *197*:1008.

McNeil, P.A. and M.W. Berns. 1981. Chromosome behavior after laser microirradiation of a single kinetochore in mitotic PtK2 cells. J. Cell. Biol. *88*(3):543.

McNutt, N.S. and D.W. Fawcett 1974. Myocardial ultrastructure. In: *Mammalian Myocardium.* John Wiley & Sons, New York.

Merklin, R. 1973. Growth and distribution of human fetal brown fat. Anat. Rec.*178*:637.

Metz, J. et al 1984. Immunohistochemical localization of cardiodilatin in myoendocrine cells of cardiac atria. Anat. Embryol. (Berl) *170*:123.

Miller, E.J. and S. Gay. 1987. The collagens: an overview and update. *Methods in Enzymology 144*:1.

Miller, J.F. 1962. Effect of neonatal thymectomy on the immunological responsiveness of the mouse. Proc. R. Soc. Lond. [Biol.] *156*:415.

Minns, R.J. and F.S. Stevens 1977. The collagen fibril organization in human articular cartilage. J. Anat. *123*:437.

Mitchel, J. and A. Abbott 1971. Antigens in immunity. XVI. A light and electron microscopic study of antigen localization in the rat spleen. Immunology *21*:207.

Montagna, W. and P. Parakkal 1974. *The Structure and Function of Skin*, 3rd Edition. Academic Press, New York.

Montagna, W. and R. Dodson 1969. Hair growth. Adv. Biol. Skin *9*:585.

Montagna, W. and W. Lobitz 1964. *The Epidermis.* Academic Press, New York.

Montagna, W. et al 1970. The dermis. Adv. Biol. Skin *10*:1–302.

Moore, K.L. 1988. *The Developing Human. Clinically Oriented Embryology*, 4th Edition. W.B. Saunders, Philadelphia.

Mooseker, M.S. 1985. Organization, chemistry, and assembly of the cytoskeletal apparatus of the intestinal brush border. Annu. Rev. Cell Biol. *1*:209.

Morel, F. et al 1971. Quantitation of human red blood cell fixation by glutaraldehyde. J. Cell Biol. *48*:91.

Mota, P.M. 1984. *Ultrastructure of Endocrine Cells and Tissues*, Martinus Nijhoff, Boston.

Muir, A.R. 1975. Electron microscopic study of the embryology of the intercalated disc in the heart of the rabbit. J. Biophys. Biochem. Cytol. *3*:193.

Munger, B.L. and S.I. Roth 1963. The cytology of the normal parathyroid glands of man and Virginia deer: a light and electron microscopic study with morphologic evidence of secretory activity. J. Cell Biol. *16:*397.

Munn, E. 1975. *Structure of Mitochondria.* Academic Press, New York.

Murphy, P. 1976. *The Neutrophil.* Plenum Press, New York.

Murray, R. 1969. Cell types in rabbit taste buds. In: *Olfaction and Taste,* Vol. 3, Edited by C. Paffman. Rockefeller University Press, New York.

Murray, R. 1986. The mammalian taste bud type III cell: a critical analysis. J. Ultrastruct. Mol. Struct. Res. *95:*175.

Neville, A. and M. O'Hare 1982. *The Human Adrenal Cortex.* Springer-Verlag, Berlin.

Nichols, B.A. et al 1971. Differentiation of monocytes: origin, nature and fate of their azurophil granules. J. Cell Bol. *50:*498.

Nickerson, P. and A. Brownie 1975. Effect of hypophysectomy on the volume and ultrastructure of the zona glomerulosa in the rat adrenal. Endocrinol Exp. *9:*187.

Nishimoto, S.K. and P.A. Price 1980. Secretion of the vitamin K-dependent protein of bone by rat osteosarcoma cells. J. Biol. Chem. *255:*6579.

Norris, H.J. et al (eds.) 1973. *The Uterus.* Williams & Wilkins, Baltimore.

Novikoff, A. and J.M. Allen 1973. Symposium on "Peroxisomes." J. Histochem. Cytochem. *21:*941.

Novikoff, P.M. et al 1971. Golgi apparatus, GERL, and lysosomes of neurons in rat dorsal ganglia. J. Cell Biol. *50:*859.

Noyes, R.W. 1973. Normal phases of the endometrium. In: *The Uterus,* Edited by H.J. Norris et al, Williams & Wilkins, Baltimore.

Oldberg, A. et al 1986. Cloning and sequence analysis of rat bone sialoprotein (osteopontine) cDNA reveals an Arg-Gly-Asp cell binding sequence. Proc. Natl. Acad. Sci. *83:*8819.

Olmstead, J.B. and G.B. Borisy 1973. Microtubules. Annu. Rev. Biochem. *42:*507.

Osmond, D.G. 1975. Formation and maturation of bone marrow lymphocytes. J. Reticuloendothel. Soc. *17:*99.

Palade, G.E. 1952. The fixation of tissues for electron microscopy. J. Exp. Med. *95:*285.

Palade, G.E. 1955. A small particulate component of the cytoplasm. J. Biophys. Biochem. Cytol. *1:*59.

Palade, G.E. and K.E. Porter 1954. Studies on the endoplasmic reticulum. I. Its identification in cells in situ. J. Exp. Med. *100:*641.

Palay, S.L. et al 1968. The axon hillock and the initial segment. J. Cell Biol. *38:*193.

Palmer, J.M. and D.O. Hall 1972. The mitochondrial membrane system. Prog. Mol. Biol. *24:*125.

Parrott, D. and M. DeSousa 1971. Thymus dependent and thymus-independent populations: origin, migratory patterns and lifespan. Clin. Exp. Immunol. *8:*663.

Parrott, D., M. DeSousa, and J. East 1966. Thymus-dependent areas in the lymphoid organs of neonatally thymectomized mice. J. Exp. Med. *123:*191.

Pearse, A.G. 1974. The endocrine cells of the G.I. tract: origins, morphology and functional relationships in health and disease. Clin. Gastroenterol. *3:*491.

Pearse, A.G., J.M. Polak, and S.R. Bloom 1977. The newer gut hormones, cellular sources, physiology, pathology and clinical aspects. Gastroenterology *72:*746.

Pellitier, G. et al 1978. Identification of human pituitary cell types by immunoelectron microscopy. J. Clin. Endocrinol. *46:*534.

Pennington, D.G. 1979. Cellular biology of megakaryocytes. Blood Cells *5:*5.

Perry, E.T. 1957. *The Human Ear Canal.* Charles C. Thomas, Springfield, IL.

Perry, R.P. 1964. Role of the nucleolus in ribonucleic acid metabolism and other cellular processes. Natl. Cancer Inst. Monog. *18:*325.

Peters, A. 1966. The node of Ranvier in the central nervous system. Q. J. Exp. Physiol. *51:*229.

Peters, A. et al 1976. *The Fine Structure of the Nervous System,* 2nd edition. W.B. Saunders, Philadelphia.

Peters, H. and K.P. McNatty 1980. *The Ovary.* University of California Press, Berkeley.

Phifer, R. and S. Spicer 1973. Immunohistochemical and histologic demonstration of thyrotropic cells of the human adenohypophysis. J. Clin. Endocrinol. *36:*1210.

Phifer, R. et al 1970. Specific demonstration of human hypophyseal cells which produce adrenocorticotrophic hormone. J. Clin. Endocrinol. *31*:347.

Platt, W.R. 1969. *Colar Atlas and Textbook of Hematology.* Lippincott, Philadelphia.

Pollard, T.D. 1981. Cytoplasmic contractile proteins. J. Cell Biol. (Suppl.) *93*:156s.

Porter, K.R. 1953. Observations on a submicroscopic basophilic component of the cytoplasm. J. Exp. Med. *97*:725.

Porter, K.R. and J.B. Tucker 1981. The ground substance of the living cell. Sci. Am. *244*:40.

Porter, K.R. et al 1983. The cytoplasmic matrix. Mod. Cell Biol. *2*:259.

Powers, J.B. et al 1979. Olfactory and vomeronasal system participation in male hamster's attraction to female vaginal secretions. Physiol. Behav. *22*:77.

Pratt, S.A., M.H. Smith, A.J. Ladman, and T.N. Fintey 1971. The ultrastructure of alveolar macrophages from human cigarette smokers and nonsmokers. Lab Invetig. *24*:331.

Quevedo, W.C. Jr. 1972. Epidermal melanin units: melanocyte-keratinocyte interactions. Am. Zool. *12*:35.

Rambourg, A. 1966. Presence of a cell coat rich in carbohydrates at the surface of cells in the rat. Anat. Rec. *154*:41.

Rambourg, A. and D. Segretain 1980. Three-dimensional electron microscopy of mitrochondria and endoplasmic reticulum in the red muscle fiber of the rat diaphragm. Anat. Rec. *197*:33.

Rambourg, A., Y. Clermont, A. Mirraud 1974. Three dimensional structure of the osmium impregnated Golgi apparatus as seen in the high voltage microscope. Amer. J. Anat. *140*:27.

Rapport, A.M. 1958. The structural and functional unit in the human liver (liver acinus). Anat. Rec. *130*:673.

Ramsey, W.A. 1972. Locomotion of human polymorphonuclear leukocytes. Exp. Cell Res. *72*:489.

Reiter, R.J. 1980. The pineal and its hormones in the control of reproduction in mammals. Endocr. Rev. *1*:109.

Revel, J.P. and D.W. Hamilton 1969. The double nature of the intermediate dense line in peripheral nerve myelin. Anat. Rec. *163*:7.

Reynolds, E.S. 1963. The use of lead citrate at high pH as electron-opaque stain in electron microscopy. J. Cell Biol. *17:*208.

Rhodin, J.A.G. 1967. The ultrastructure of mammalian arterioles and precapillary sphincters. J. Ultrastruct. Res. *18:*181.

Rhodin, J.A.G. 1968. Ultrastructure of mammalian venous capillaries, venules and small collecting venules. J. Ultrastruct. Res. *25:*452.

Richards, J.S. 1980. Maturation of ovarian follicles; actions and interactions of pituitary and ovarian hormones on follicular cell differentiation. Physiol. Rev. *60:*51.

Rifkin, R.A. and P.A. Marks 1975. The regulation of erythropoiesis. Blood Cells *1:*417.

Rodieck, R.W. 1973. *The Vertebrate Retina.* W.H. Freeman, San Francisco.

Rooney, S.A. 1985. The surfactant system and lung phospholipid biochemistry. Am. Rev. Respir. Dis. *131:*439.

Roseman, S. 1975. Sugars of the cell membrane. In: *Cell Membranes: Biochemistry, Cell Biology and Pathology*, Edited by G. Weisman, Hospital Practice, New York.

Roth, S.I. 1962. Pathology of the parathyroids in hyperparathyroidism with a discussion of recent advances in the anatomy and pathology of the parathyroid glands. Arch. Pathol. *73:*492.

Roth, S.I. 1971. Anatomy of the parathyroid glands. In: *Endocrinology*, Vol. 2, Edited by L.J. DeGroot, Grune and Stratton, New York.

Ryan, U. et al 1975. Fenestrated endothelium of the adrenal gland: freeze-fracture studies. Tissue Cell *7:*181.

Sabatini, D. et al 1983. Biogenesis of epithelial cell polarity. Mod. Cell Biol. *2:*419.

Sarles, H. 1977. The exocrine pancreas. Int. Rev. Physiol. *12:*173.

Sato, K. 1983. The physiology and pharmacology of the eccrine sweat gland. In: *Biochemistry and Physiology of the Skin*, Edited by L. Goldsmith, Oxford University Press, New York.

Scharrer, B. 1969. Neurohumors and neurohormones: definitions and terminology. J. Neurovisc. Rel. (Suppl.) *9:*1.

Scharrer, E. and B. Scharrer 1954. Neurosekretion. In: *Handbuch der Mikroskopischen Anatomie des Menschen*, Vol. 6, Part 5, Edited by von Mollinkoff/Bargmann. Springer-Verlag, Berlin.

Schlegel, R.A. et al 1987. *Molecular Regulation of Nuclear Events in Mitosis and Meiosis.* Academic Press, New York.

Schoenberg, C.F. and D.M. Needham 1976. A study of the mechanism of contraction in vertebrate smooth muscle. Biol. Rev. *51*:53.

Schwartz, S.M. and E.P. Benditt 1972. Studies on the aortic intima. I. Structure and permeability of rat thoracic aortic intima. J. Pathol. *66*:241.

Seljelid, R. et al 1970. The early phase of endocytosis in the rat thyroid follicle cell. Lab. Invest. *23*:595.

Sheehan, D.C. and B.B. Hrapchak 1973. *Theory and Practice of Histochemistry.* C.V. Mosby, St. Louis.

Shelanski, M.L. and R.K. Liem 1979. Neurofilaments. J. Neurosci. *33*:5.

Shepard, T.H. 1975. Development of the thyroid gland. *In: Childhood and Adolescence.* 2nd Ed, Edited by L.I. Gardner, p. 220. W.B. Saunders Co., Philadelphia.

Shroeder, T.E. 1975. Dynamics of the contractile ring. In: *Molecule and Cell Movement,* Edited by S. Inoue and R.E. Stephens, Raven Press, New York.

Sicher, H. 1971. Orban's *Oral Histology and Embryology,* 6th Edition. C.V. Mosby, St. Louis.

Silverstein, S. et al 1977. Endocytosis. Am. Rev. Biochem. *46*:669.

Simionescu, N. and M. Simionsecu. 1981. The dynamic hydrophilic system of capillary endothelium. In: *A Benzon Symposium on "Water Transport in Epithelia,"* Edited by H. Ussig et al. Copenhagen: Munsgaad, p. 228.

Simionescu, N. 1981. Transcytosis and traffic of membranes in the endothelial cell. In: *Cell Biology* 1980–81, Edited by H. Schweiger. Springer-Verlag, p. 657. Heidelberg.

Simionescu, N. et al 1978. Open junctions in the endothelium of postcapillary venules of the diaphragm. J. Cell Biol. *79*:27.

Singer, S.J. and G.L. Nicholson 1972. The fluid-mosaic model of the structure of the cell membranes. Science *175*:720.

Sohval, A.R. et al 1971. Ultrastructure of crystalloids in spermatogonia and Sertoli cells of normal human testis. J. Ultrastruct. Res. *34*:83.

Somlyo, A.P. and A.V. Somlyo 1970. Vascular smooth muscle. I.

Normal structure, pathology, and biophysics. Pharmacol. Rev. *22:*249.

Somlyo, A.P. et al 1976. Vertebrate smooth muscle; ultrastructure and function. In: *Cell Motility*, Edited by R. Goldman et al, Cold Spring Harbor Laboratories, Cold Spring Harbor, NY.

Sorokin, S. 1968. Reconstruction of centriole formation and ciliogenesis in mammalian lungs. J. Cell Sci. *3:*207.

Sorokin, S. and R. Hoyt 1988. Neuroepithelial bodies and solitary small granule cells. In: *Lung Cell Biology*, Edited by D. Massaro, Marcel Dekker, New York.

Steinert, P.M. et al 1985. The molecular biology of intermediate filaments. Cell *42:*411.

Stoeckel, M.E. et al 1981. Fine structure and cytochemistry of the mammalian pars intermedia. In: *Peptides of the Pars Intermedia.* Ciba Symposium 81, Pitman-Medical, London.

Strauss, J. et al 1976. The sebaceous glands: twenty five years of progress. J. Invest. Dermatol. *67:*90.

Susi, F. 1969. Anchoring fibrils in the attachment of epithelium to connective tissue in oral mucous membrane. J. Dent. Res. *48:*144.

Tanaka, Y. and J. Goodman 1972. *Electron Microscopy of Human Blood Cells.* Harper and Row, New York.

Taurog, A. 1978. Thyroid hormone synthesis and release. In: *The Thyroid. A Fundamental and Clinical Test*, Edited by S. Werner and S. Ingbar, Harper and Row, New York.

Taylor, S. (Ed.) 1968. Calcitonin: Proceedings of the Symposium on Thyrocalcitonin and the C Cells. Heinemann Educational Books, Ltd. London.

Tavassoli, M. 1976. Marrow adipose cells—histochemical identification of labile and stable components. Arch. Pathol. Lab. Med. *100:*16.

Tavassoli, M. 1980. Megakaryocyte-platelet axis and the process of platelet formation and release. Blood *55:*537.

Tavassoli, M. and J.M. Yoffey 1983. *Bone Marrow Structure and Function.* Alan R. Liss, New York.

Termine, J.D. et al 1981. Mineral and collagen-binding proteins of fetal calf bone. J. Biol. Chem. *256:*10403.

Terranova, V.P., D.H. Rohrbach, and G.R. Martin. 1980. Role of laminin in the attachment of PAM 212 (epithelial) cells to basement membrane collagen. *22*:719.

Till, J.E. and E.A. McCullough 1980. Hemopoietic stem cell differentiation. Biochim. Biophys. Acta *605:*43.

Timpl, R. and M. Dzlamek 1986. Structure, development and molecular pathology of the basement membrane. Int. Rev. Exp. Pathol. *29*:1.

Tixier-Vidal, A. and M. Farquhar 1975. *The Anterior Pituitary.* Academic Press, New York.

Trelstad, R.I. 1974. Human aorta collagens: evidence for three different species. Biochem. Biophys. Res. Commun. *57:*717.

Troyer, H. 1980. *Principles and Techniques of Histochemistry.* Little, Brown and Company, Boston.

Truex, R.C. and M.Q. Smythe 1965. Recent observations on the human cardiac conduction system with special considerations of the atrioventricular node and bundle. In: International Symposium on *Electrophysiology of the heart,* Edited by B. Taccardi and G. Marchetti. Pergamon Press, New York.

Uzman, B. Geren 1964. The spiral configuration of myelin lamellae. J. Ultrastruct. Res. *11:*208.

Vander Rhee, H.J. et al 1979. Differentiation of monocytes into macrophages, epithelioid cells and multinucleated giant cells. Cell Tissue Res. *197:*355.

van Furth, R. 1982. Current view on the mononuclear phagocyte system. Immunobiology *161:*178.

Verhage, H.G. et al 1979. Cyclic changes in ciliation, secretion and cell height of the oviductal epithelium in women. Am. J. Anat. *154(4):*505.

Vorherr, H. 1978. Human lactation and breast feeding. In: *Lactation,* Vol. IV, Edited by B.L. Larson, Academic Press, New York.

Waksmann, B.H. et al 1962. Role of the thymus in immune reactions in rats. III. Changes in the lymphoid organs of thymectomized rats. J. Exp. Med. *116:*187.

Wang, N. 1974. The regional difference of pleural mesothelial cells in rabbits. Am. Rev. Respir. Dis. *110:*623.

Warner, F.D. and P. Satir 1974. The structural basis of ciliary bend formation. Radial spoke positional changes accompanying microtubule slide. J. Cell Biol. *63:*35.

Watson, J.D. (Ed.) 1982. Organization of the cytoplasm. Cold Spring Harbor Symp. Quant. Biol. *46*.

Weiss, L. 1974. A scanning electron microscopic study of the spleen. Blood *43*:665.

Weiss, L. 1976. The hemopoietic microenvironment of the bone marrow: an ultrastructural study of the stroma in rats. Anat. Rec. *186*:161.

Weiss, L., U. Geduldig, and W. Weidanz 1986. Mechanisms of splenic control of murine malaria. Reticular cell activation and the development of a blood-spleen barrier. Am. J. Anat. *176*:251.

Werner , S.C. and S.H. Ingbar (eds.) 1978. *The Thyroid.* 4th Edition. Harper and Row, N.Y.

Weston, J.A. 1963. A radioautographic analysis of the migration and localization of trunk neural crest cells in the chick. Dev. Biol. *6*:279.

White, J.G. and C.C. Clawson 1980. Overview article: biostructure of blood platelets. Ultrastruct. Pathol. *1*:333.

Winklemann, R.K. 1977. The Merkel cell system and a comparison between it and the neurosecretory or APUD cell system. J. Invest. Dermatol. *69*:41.

Winklemann, R.K. et al 1961. Cutaneous vascular patterns in studies with injection preparations and alkaline phosphatase reactions. Adv. Biol. Skin *2*:1.

Winkelmann, R.K. 1977. The Merkel cell system and a comparison between it and the neurosecretory or APUD cell system. J. Invest. Derm. *69*:41

Winkler, H. and E. Westhead 1980. The molecular organization of adrenal chromaffin granules. Neuroscience *6*:1803.

Wintrobe, M.M. 1962. *Clinical Hematology*, 5th Edition. Lea & Febiger, Philadelphia.

Wischnitzer, S. 1970. *Introduction To Electron Microscopy.* 2nd Edition. Pergamon Press, New York.

Wislocki, G.B. 1938. The vascular supply of the hypophysis cerebri of the rhesus monkey and man. Proc. Assoc. Res. Nerv. Ment. Dis. *17*:48.

Wolff, K. and G. Stingl 1983. The Langerhan's cell. J. Invest. Dermatol. *80*:17S.

Wolosowick, J. and K.R. Porter 1979. Microtubular lattice of the cytoplasmic ground substance: artifact or reality? J. Cell Biol. *82*:114.

Wolstenholme, G. and J. Knight 1970. *Taste and Smell in Vertebrates.* J. & A. Churchill, London.

Wolstenholme, G. and J. Knight 1971. *The Pineal Gland.* Ciba Foundation Symposium, Churchill, London.

Wurtman, R.J. 1966. Effects of light and visual stimuli on endocrine function. In: *Neuroendocrinology*, Edited by W. Ganong and L. Martini, Academic Press, New York.

Yamada, Y.M. et al 1985. Recent advances in research on fibronectin and other cell attachment proteins. J. Cell Biochem. *28*:79.

Yoshida, T. and K. Kobayashi 1985. Lymphokines. In: *The Reticuloendothelial System*, Vol. 8, *Pharmacology*, Edited by J.H. Hadden and A. Szentivanyi, Plenum Press, New York.

Zaias, N. and H. Baden 1979. Nails. In: *Dermatology in General Medicine*, Edited by T.B. Fitzpatrick et al, McGraw-Hill, New York.

Suggested Reading

Fawcett, D.W. 1986. Bloom and Fawcett *A Textbook of Histology*, 11th edition. W.B. Saunders Co., Philadelphia.

Fawcett, D.W. 1986. *The Cell*, 2nd edition. W.B. Saunders, Philadelphia.

Hammersen, F. 1985. Sobbotta *Histology Color Atlas of Microscopic Anatomy*, 3rd edition. Urban & Schwarzenberg, Baltimore/Munich.

Kelly, D.E., R.L. Wood, and A.C. Enders 1984. Bailey's *Textbook of Microscopic Anatomy*, 18th edition. Williams & Wilkins, Baltimore.

Kessel, R.G. and R.H. Kardon 1979. *Tissues and Organs: A Text-Atlas of Scanning Electron Microscopy.* W.H. Freeman, San Francisco.

Lillie, R.D. 1972. H.J. Conn's *Biological Stains*, 8th edition. Williams & Wilkins Co, Baltimore.

Monesi, V. 1984. *Istologia.* seconda edizione, Piccin Nuova Libraria, Padova.

Moran, D.T. and J.C. Rowley 1988. *Visual Histology*, Lea & Febiger, Philadelphia.

Orci, A.P. 1975. *Freeze-Etch Histology.* Springer-Verlag. New York/Heidelberg.

Paul, J. 1973. *Cell and Tissue Culture*, 4th edition. Churchill Livingstone, Edinburgh.

Porter, K.R. and M.A. Bonneville 1973. *Fine Structure of Cells and Tissues*, 4th edition. Lea & Febiger, Philadelphia.

Rhodin, A.G. 1975. *An Atlas of Histology*, Oxford University Press, New York/London.

Weiss, L. 1988. *Cell and Tissue Biology, A Textbook of Histology*, 6th edition. Urban & Schwartzenberg, Baltimore/Munich.

Index